Oncogene and Cancer: Advanced Topics

Edited by **Eden Dennis**

FOSTER
A C A D E M I C S

New Jersey

Published by Foster Academics,
61 Van Reypen Street,
Jersey City, NJ 07306, USA
www.fosteracademics.com

Oncogene and Cancer: Advanced Topics
Edited by Eden Dennis

International Standard Book Number: 978-1-63242-303-0 (Hardback)

Contents

Preface

The main aim of this book is to educate learners and enhance their research focus by presenting diverse topics covering this vast field. This is an advanced book which compiles significant studies by distinguished experts in the area of analysis. This book addresses successive solutions to the challenges arising in the area of application, along with it; the book provides scope for future developments.

This book offers the course of cancer development, beginning from normal cells to cancerous form and the genomic instability, also cancer treatment as well as its prevention in the form of the invention of a vaccine is covered. Certain diseases are also elucidated, like leukaemia, glioma, breast cancer, and cervical cancer. Comprehending cancer through its molecular mechanism is required to decrease the cancer incidence. Complications like metastasis and drug resistance and the procedure of treating cancer more efficiently are vividly illuminated in this book along with some research results that could be employed to treat the cancer patients in the not too distant future. This book includes sections namely, non coding RNA & micro RNA in tumorigenesis and oncogenes for transcription factors.

It was a great honour to edit this book, though there were challenges, as it involved a lot of communication and networking between me and the editorial team. However, the end result was this all-inclusive book covering diverse themes in the field.

Finally, it is important to acknowledge the efforts of the contributors for their excellent chapters, through which a wide variety of issues have been addressed. I would also like to thank my colleagues for their valuable feedback during the making of this book.

Editor

Non Coding RNA and Micro RNA in Tumorigenesis

Non-Coding RNAs and Cancer

Gianpiero Di Leva and Michela Garofalo

Additional information is available at the end of the chapter

1. Introduction

The question of which regions of the human genome constitute its functional elements—those expressed as genes or serving as regulatory elements—has long been a central topic in biology. In the 1970s and 1980s, early cloning-based methods revealed the presence of more than 7000 genes in human genome [1], and large-scale analyses of expressed sequence tags (ESTs) in the 1990s suggested that the estimated number of human genes range from 35,000 to 100,000 [2]. The completion of the human genome project narrowed the focus considerably by highlighting the surprisingly small number of protein-coding genes, which is now conventionally cited as less than 25,000 [3]. While the number of protein-coding genes (20,000–25,000) has maintained broad consensus, recent studies of the human transcriptome have revealed an astounding number of non-coding RNAs (ncRNAs) [4-6]. In fact, the increased sensitivity of genome tiling arrays provides an even more detailed view, revealing that the extent of non-coding sequence transcription is at least four times greater than coding sequence, and that the abundance of non-coding transcripts had been previously overlooked. The RNA world hypothesis proposes that early life was based on RNAs, which subsequently devolved the storage of information to more stable DNA, and catalytic functions to more versatile proteins. Consequently, despite crucial roles in the ancient processes of translation and splicing, RNA is assumed to have been largely relegated to an intermediate between gene and protein, encapsulated in the central dogma 'DNA makes RNA makes protein' [7]. However, the finding that most of the genome in complex organisms is transcribed and the discovery of new classes of regulatory non-coding RNAs (ncRNAs) challenges this assumption and suggests that RNAs have continued to evolve and expand alongside proteins and DNA.

ncRNAs are considered as RNA transcripts that do not encode for a protein. In the past decade, a great diversity of ncRNAs has been observed. Depending on the type of ncRNA, transcription can occur by any of the three RNA polymerases (RNA Pol I, RNA Pol II, or RNA Pol III). General conventions divide ncRNAs into two main categories: small ncRNAs less than 200 bp and long ncRNAs greater than 200 bps [8]. Within these two categories, there are also many individual classes of ncRNAs (Table1), although the degree of biological and experimental support for each class ranges substantially and should be evaluated individually. The relevance of ncRNAs in gene regulation has been rapidly unveiling during the last decade. However, the functional elements in the primary sequence of noncoding genes that determine their role as RNA molecules remain unknown. Protein-coding genes have a defined language with a set of grammatical rules: three nucleotides forms a codon that translates into a specific amino acid [9]. Aberrations in codons of a protein-coding gene can be interpreted in terms of the amino acids they encode. We can recognize a mutation in a codon and determine its contribution to a given disease. In contrast to the genetic code for protein synthesis, 'the ncRNA alphabet' – a specific set of RNA sequences or structural motifs important for ncRNA function – remains to be largely elucidated. However, it has become increasingly apparent that the ncRNAs are of crucial functional importance for normal development, physiology and disease [10]. The functional relevance of the ncRNAs is particularly evident for a class of small non-coding RNAs called microRNAs (miRNAs) [11-12]. In human diseases, particularly cancer, it has been shown that epigenetic and genetic defects in miRNAs and their processing machinery are a common hallmark of disease [13-16]. However, miRNAs are just the tip of the iceberg, and other ncRNAs such as small nucleolar RNAs (snoRNAs), PIWI-interacting RNAs (piRNAs), large intergenic non-coding RNAs (lincRNAs) and, overall, the heterogeneous group of long non-coding RNAs (lncRNAs), might also contribute to the development of many different human disorders. Here we discuss the most recent genetic studies on ncRNAs and their related proteins in the context of cancer and we will analyze the new regulatory elements of the noncoding language to interpret their contribution to the pathogenesis of cancer.

2. MicroRNAs

In 1993, Victor Ambros and colleagues discovered a gene, lin-4, that affected development in *Caenorhabditis elegans* and found that its product was a small nonprotein-coding RNA [31]. The number of known small RNAs in different organisms such as *Caenorhabditis elegans*, *Drosophila melanogaster*, plants, and mammals—including humans—has since expanded substantially, mainly as a result of the cloning and sequencing of size-fractionated RNAs. MiRNAs are single stranded RNAs (ssRNAs) of 19–25 nucleotides in length that are generated from endogenous hairpin transcripts [32]. They play an important role in the negative regulation of gene expression by base-pairing to partially complementary sites on the target messenger RNAs (mRNAs), usually in the 3′ untranslated region (UTR). Binding of a miRNA to the target mRNA typically leads to translational repression and exonucleolytic mRNA decay, although highly complementary targets can be cleaved endonucleolytically. A genomic analysis of miRNAs has revealed that more than 50% of mammalian miRNAs are located within the intronic regions of annotated protein-coding or non-protein-coding genes [33]. These miRNAs could therefore use their host gene transcripts as carriers, although it remains possible that some are actually transcribed separately from internal promoters. Other miRNAs, located in intergenic regions, apparently have their own transcriptional regulatory elements and thus constitute

Category	Name	Supporting data	Function	Role in cancer	Refs.
Housekeeping RNAs	Ribosomal RNAs (rRNA)	high	ribosome structure	no	17-18
	Transfer RNAs (tRNA)	high	protein translation	no	17-18
	Small nuclear RNAs (snRNA)	high	splicing	no	17-18
	Small nucleolar RNAs (snoRNA)	high	post-translational modification	yes	17-18
Short non coding RNAs (above 200nt in size)	MicroRNAs	high	translational repression	yes	20,21
	Tiny transcription initiation RNAs	high	may regulate gene expression	not known	18
	Repeat associated small interfering RNAs	high	gene regulation, transposon control and viral defence	not known	18
	Promoter-associated short RNAs	high	may regulate gene expression at chromatin level	not known	18, 22,24
	Termini associated short RNAs	high	may regulate gene expression at chromatin level	not known	18, 22,24
	Antisense termini associated short	high	may regulate gene expression at chromatin level	not known	17, 22,24
	Piwi-interacting RNAs	high	regulate transposon activity and chromatin state	yes	23
	Transcription start site antisense RNAs	moderate	may regulate transcription	not known	17
	Retrotraspon-derived RNAs	high	may regulate transcription	not known	24
	3'UTR-derived RNAs	moderate	may regulate transcription	not known	17
	Splice-site RNAs	poor	not known	not known	18
Long non coding RNAs (over 200nt in size)	Long or large intergenic ncRNAs	high	epigenetic regulation, protein complex subcellular compartments or localization	yes	25,26
	Transcribed ultraconserved regions	high	not known	yes	27
	Pseudogenes	high	competitive endogenous RNAs	yes	25, 28
	Enhancer RNAs	high	not known	yes	29
	Long intronic ncRNAs	moderate	not known	not known	17,18
	Repeat associated ncRNAs	high	not known	not known	23
	Antisense RNAs	high	gene expression	not known	28
	Promoter associated long RNAs	moderate	may regulate gene expression at chromatin level	not known	22, 30
	Long stress-induced non-coding transcripts	moderate	epigenetic regulation, protein complex subcellular compartments or localization	yes	17, 18

Table 1. Non coding RNA in human genome.

independent transcription units. Animal miRNAs are processed from longer primary transcripts (pri-miRNAs) that can contain multiple miRNAs [34,35]. Few pri-miRNA transcripts have been studied in detail, but in general miRNAs are regulated and transcribed similar to protein encoding genes by (Pol) II with the exception of the rapidly evolving RNA polymerase (Pol) III transcribed miRNA cluster [36]. MiRNA processing occurs in three essential steps (**Figure 1**). First, the nuclear endoribonuclease protein Drosha recognizes the miRNA hairpins in the primary transcript and cleaves each hairpin ~11 nt from its base [37-38]. It has been proposed that Drosha may recognize the pri-miRNA through the stem-loop structure and then cleave the stem at a fixed distance from the loop to liberate the pre-miRNA. How is the Drosha enzyme able to discriminate the pri-miRNA stem-loop structure from the other stem-loop cellular RNAs? Both cell culture experiments and in vitro Drosha cleavage assays have shown that proteins associated with Drosha confer specificity to this process. In fact, Drosha has been found to be part of a large, ~650-kDa protein complex known as the Microprocessor [39], where Drosha interacts with its cofactor DGCR8 (the DiGeorge syndrome critical region gene 8 protein) in the human and interacts with Pasha in *Drosophila melanogaster* [40]. The next step in miRNA biogenesis is recognition of the ~60 nt pre-miRNA by exportin-5 and export into the cytoplasm in a ran-guanine-GTP-dependent manner [41-43]. The Exp5/Ran-GTP complex has a high affinity for pre-miRNAs,

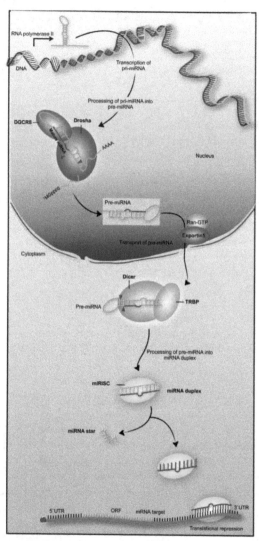

Figure 1. miRNA biogenesis and function. The primary miRNA (pri-miRNA) is transcribed by RNA pol II from its genomic location and cleaved by the microprocessor complex, which comprises Drosha and DGCR8. The resulting pre-miRNA is actively transported to the cytoplasm by exportin 5 (Expt.5), where the pre-miRNA undergoes further processing into the mature miRNA by Dicer and its co-factors, protein activator of interferon-induced protein kinase (PACT) and TAR RNA binding protein (TRBP). Normally, one strand of this duplex is degraded (miRNA star), whereas the other strand accumulates as a mature miRNA. From the miRNA-miRNA duplex, only the miRNA enters preferentially in the protein effector complex, formed by the RNA-induced silencing complex (RISC) and miRgonaute and binds with partial complementarity to the 3′ untranslated region (UTR) of target messenger RNAs (mRNAs) to mediate translational repression.

protecting them from the moment they are generated in the nucleus until they are ready for the next cleavage step in the cytoplasm, where GTP is hydrolyzed to guanosine diphosphate (GDP); at that point, the Exp5/Ran-GDP complex releases its cargo. Third, the endoribonuclease protein Dicer cleaves the pre-miRNA into ~22 nt duplexes and, with the help of cofactors such as TAR RNA binding protein (TRBP) and protein activator of the interferon-induced protein kinase (PACT), preferentially incorporates one of the duplex strands Into the RNA induced-silencing complex (RISC) [44-50]. The final product is a miRNA-miRNA duplex that needs to be unwound to act as a single-stranded guide in the RISC to recognize its target mRNAs. It was originally proposed that an ATP-dependent helicase (known as unwindase) separates the two small RNA strands, after which the resulting single-stranded guide is loaded into Ago proteins. However, it was later shown that *Drosophila* Ago2 [51], as well as human Ago2 [52], directly receive double-stranded small RNA from the RISC-loading complex. Ago2 then cleaves the passenger strand, thereby liberating the single-stranded guide to form mature Ago2-RISC. In mammals, miRNAs guide the RISC to complementary target sites in mRNAs, where endonucleolytically active Ago proteins cleave the RNA [53] (**Figure 1**). Finally, RISC can cleave [54-55] degrade [56-57] or suppress translation [58-59] of target mRNAs depending on the complementarity between miRNA and mRNA. Imperfect base pairing between small RNAs and their target mRNAs leads to repression of translation and/or deadenylation (removal of the polyA tail of the target), followed by destabilization of the target [60], whereas perfect base pairing usually leads to mRNA degradation.

3. MicroRNAs and cancer

Cancer is a multistep process in which normal cells experience genetic changes that progress them through a series of pre-malignant states (initiation) into invasive cancer (progression) that can spread throughout the body (metastasis). The dysregulation of genes involved in cell proliferation, differentiation and/or apoptosis is associated with cancer initiation and progression. Genes linked with cancer development are characterized as oncogenes and tumor suppressors. Recently, the definition of oncogenes and tumor suppressors has been expanded from the classical protein coding genes to include miRNAs [61-62]. MiRNAs have been found to regulate more than 60% of mRNAs and have roles in fundamental processes, such as development [63], differentiation [64], cell proliferation [65], apoptosis [66], and stress responses [67]. Over the past few years, many miRNAs have been implicated in various human cancers. The first evidence that miRNAs are involved in cancer comes from the finding that miR-15 and miR-16 are downregulated or deleted in most patients with chronic lymphocytic leukemia [68]. This discovery has projected miRNAs to the center stage of molecular oncology and, in the past few years, a myriad of genome-wide miRNA expression profiling analyses have shown a general dysregulation of miRNA expression in all tumors (**Table 2**) [69]. Surprisingly, the use of miRNA profiles is newly becoming highly preferred to the traditional mRNA signature for a variety of reasons. First, the remarkable stability of miRNAs, due to their short length, has allowed scientists to perform analyses also in samples considered to be technically challenging, such as formalin fixed specimens. High sensitive and refined miRNA detection technique provide high reliability in the use of miRNAs as a diagnostic tools. Finally, miRNA fingerprints have demonstrated the ability to identify the tissue of origin for cancer that have already spread in multiple metastatic sites, thereby reducing patient's psychological burden and overall procedure costs. To date, over 1000 miRNAs have been reported in humans (miRbase: 1527 at November 2011), and both loss and gain of miRNA functions contribute to cancer development through a range of different mechanisms that we will discuss in the following sections.

Cancer	Authors	Samples	Main findings	miRNA signature
Breast Cancer	Iorio et al. 2005	10 normal 76 tumors	First miRNA signature of breast cancer. 15 miRNAs predict the nature of the sample analyzed with 100% accuracy.	miR-21, -155 were up-regulated while miR-10b, -125b, -145 were down-regulated.
	Mattie et al. 2006	20 tumors	Unique sets of miRNAs are associated with ErbB2 and ER/PR status.	ErbB2 status (let-7f, let-7g, miR-107, -10b, -126, -154, -195) ER/PR status (miR-142-5p, -200a, -205, -25).
	Blenkiron et al. 2007	93 tumors	Striking differences in miRNA expression between breast tumor molecular subtypes (luminal A, luminal B, basal-like, HER2+ and normal breast-like).	-
	Sempere et al. 2007	> 100 pairs tumor-normal	In situ hybridization method to reveal the spatial distribution of miRNA expression in archived formalin-fixed breast tumors	20 miRNAs differentiate matched normal/tumor. miR-21 up-regulated in all tumor specimens, miR-145 and miR-451 were the only miRs high expressed in normal specimens and low expressed in tumor specimens. let-7a, miR-21,-141, -214 preferentially expressed in luminal cells, miR-145 and -205 in myoepithelial cells.
	Foekens et al. 2008	299 tumors	Identification of miRNAs associated with metastatic capability.	miR-7, -128a, -210, -516-3p associated with tumor aggressiveness in ER-positive patients with lymph node-negative disease. miR-210 associated with early relapse in ER-negative patients with lymph node-negative disease and with poor outcome.
	Volinia et al 2012	80 IDC 8 DCIS 6 normal	Identification of miRNA dysregulation during the transition from ductal carcinoma in situ to invasive ductal carcinoma	Let-7d, miR-210, and -221 down-regulated in DCIS and up-regulated in IDC. miR-210, -21, -106b⁶, -197, and let-7i associated with prognosis. Only miR-210involved in the invasive transition.
Lung Cancer	Yanaihara et al. 2006	104 pairs tumor-normal	miRNA expression profiles are diagnostic and prognostic markers of lung cancer.	43 miRNAs discriminate between normal ad tumors. let-7a-2, mir-155, -17-3p, -145, -21 were associated with adenocarcinoma patients survival.
	Raponi et al. 2009	10 normal 61 squamous	miRNAs may have greater clinical utility in predicting the prognosis of patients with squamous cell lung carcinomas than mRNA-based signatures.	15 miRNAs that were differentially expressed including miR-17/92 cluster, miR-155, let-7. miR-146b has the strongest prediction accuracy for stratifying prognostic groups.
	Landi et al. 2010	290 tumors 165AC-125S Q	miRNA expression profiles can distinguish adenocarcinoma (AC) from squamous carcinoma (SQ) and predict survival.	let-7g and miR-26 were the most down-regulated in SQ versus AC. miR-25, -34c-5p, -34a, -191 and let-7e strongly predicted SQ survival for the 107 male smokers with early-stage SQ tumors. miR-21 is overexpressed in AC and may be a marker of tumor progression in adenocarcinoma.
	Tan et al. 2011	34 pairs tumors-normal	miRNA expression profiles of squamous carcinoma vs normal tissues.	miR-210, -182, -486-5p, -30a, -140-3p discriminate between cancerous and normal lung tissues. miR-31 was associated with poor survival in squamous cell carcinoma.
	Lu et al. 2012	527 tumors	Identification of miRNA signatures that predict prognosis of stage I NSCLC.	Two miRNA signatures that are highly predictive of recurrence/relapse free survival were identified. The first contained 34 miRNAs derived from 357 stage I NSCLC patients independent of cancer subtype, whereas the second containing 27 miRNAs was adenocarcinoma specific.
	Guan et al. 2012	14 different dataset	A meta-analysis reviews 14 microRNA expression profiling studies that compared the microRNAs expression profiles in lung cancer tissues with those in normal lung tissues.	184 miRNAs discriminate lung cancer tissues from normal tissues; 61 miRNAs were reported in at least two studies. Up-regulated miRNA: miR-210 was reported in 9 studies and miR-21 in 7 studies. Down-regulated miRNA: miR-126 was reported in 10 studies and miR-30a in 8 studies.
Thyroid Cancer	Pallante et al. 2006	10 normals 30 tumors	Identification of the miRNA expression profile of papillary carcinomas.	A significant increase in miR-221, -222 and -181b was detected in papillary carcinomas in comparison with normal thyroid tissue.
	Visone et. al 2007	10 normals 76 tumors	Identification of the miRNA expression profile of anaplastic carcinomas from normal thyroid tissues.	A significant decrease in miR-30d, -125b, -26a, -30a-5p was detected in anaplastic carcinomas compared to normal thyroid tissue.
	Nikiforov a et al. 2008	60 normals 60 tumors	Identification of miRNA signature for the different thyroid tumors subtypes: Oncocytic, conventional follicular, papillary and medullary carcinomas.	miR-187, -221, -222, -146b, -155, -224, -197 were the most differentially overexpressed in thyroid tumors vs. hyperplastic nodules and combination of them classified the different subtypes.
	Yip et al. 2011	32 tumors	Identification of a specific signature in aggressive (17) compared with nonaggressive papillary carcinomas (15).	Upregulation of miR-146b, -221, -222, -155, -31 and downregulation of miR-1, -34b, -130b, -138 downregulation. miR-146 overexpression was associated with aggressive behavior in BRAF-positive tumors.
	Kitano et al 2011	47 tumors	miRNAs expression signature for samples representing difficult to diagnose histologic subtypes of thyroid neoplasm (21 benign, 26 malignant).	Out of 34 differentially expressed miRNA, miR-126 and miR-7 had high diagnostic accuracy and could be helpful in the classification of benign and malignant thyroid tumors.

a

Cancer	Authors	Samples	Main findings	miRNA signature
Colon Cancer	Schetter et al. 2008	84 pairs tumor-normal	miRNA expression profiles and clinical correlation for colon cancer.	37 miRNAs differentially expressed in tumors: high miR-21 was in adenomas and tumors with more advanced TNM staging. High miR-21 expression was also associated with poor survival and therapeutic outcome.
	Schepeler et al. 2008	10 normals 49 tumors	miRNA expression profiles of colon cancer with different microsatellite status and prognosis.	miR-145 showing the lowest expression in cancer relative to normal tissue. miR-142-3p, -212, -151, -144 were associated with tumor microsatellite status. High expression of miR-320 or -498 associated with good prognosis.
	Arndt et al. 2009	8 cell lines 4 normals 45 tumors	miRNA expression profiles for colon cancer.	37 miRNAs discriminate between colorectal cancer and normal tissues. 22 miRNAs were differentially expressed between normal and early stage cancer including increases in miR-21 and -224 and decreases in miR-133a and -145. A differential expression in miR-31, -7, -99b, -378*, -133a, -125a discriminates between early and late stage.
Prostate Cancer	Ambs et al. 2008	16 normals 60 tumors	First miRNA expression profiles for prostate cancer.	Up-regulated miRs: miR-32, -182, -31, -26a, -200c, -196a, -106b/25 cluster; down-regulated miRNAs included miR-520h, -494, -490, -1/133a cluster.
	Tong et al. 2009	40 pairs normal-tumor	miRNA expression profiles of paired microdissected malignant and non-involved areas from stage T2a/b, early relapse and non-relapse cancer patients.	miR-23b, -100, -145, -221, -222 were significantly downregulated in malignant tissues. Patients with post-surgery elevation of prostate-specific antigen (chemical relapse) displayed a distinct profile of 16 miRNAs, as compared with those with non-relapse disease.
	Schaefer et al. 2010	76 pairs normal-tumor	miRNA expression profiles for prostate cancer and clinical correlation.	miR-16, -31, -125b, -145, -149, -181b, -184, -205, -221, -222 were downregulated and miR-96, -182, -182, -183, -375 were upregulated. Expression of 5 miRNAs correlated with Gleason score or pathological tumor stage.
Liver Cancer	Murakami et al. 2006	25 pairs normal-tumor	miRNA expression profiles in hepatocellular carcinoma and non-tumorous tissues.	miR-18, precursor miR-18, -224, -199a*, -195, -199a, -200a, -125a differentially expressed between cancer and normal tissues; miR-92, -20, -18 and precursor miR-18 were significantly higher in poorly differentiated tumors. In contrast, miR-99a exhibited a positive correlation between expression levels and degree of tumor differentiation.
	Budhu et al. 2008	241 pairs normal-tumor	miRNA expression profiles in liver cancer predict metastasis.	A unique 20-miRNA metastasis signature was identified that could predict primary neoplastic tissues with venous metastases from metastasis-free solitary tumors. mir-219-1, -207, and -338 were most highly up-regulated, whereas mir-34a, -30c-1, -148a were most highly down-regulated in metastasis cases.
	Wang et al. 2008	4 normals 46 tumors	miRNA expression profiles in hepatocellular carcinoma and non-tumorous tissues.	miR-224 overexpression identified in all tumors and miR-200c, -200, -21, -224, -10b, -222 specific deregulation in benign or malignant tumors. miR-96 was overexpressed in HBV tumors, and miR-126* was down-regulated in alcohol-related hepatocellular carcinoma. Down-regulations of miR-107 and miR-375 were specifically associated with HNF1alpha and beta-catenin gene mutations, respectively.
	Ji et al. 2009	241 pairs normal-tumor	miRNA expression profiles in hepatocellular carcinoma and non-tumorous tissues and significant correlation to survival.	Reduced miR-26 in tumors and the expression of miR-26a and miR-26b in nontumor liver tissue was higher in women than in men. Low miR-26 is associated to a short overall survival but a better response to interferon therapy.
	Toffanin et al. 2011	89 tumors	miRNA expression profiles in hepatocellular carcinoma and non-tumorous tissues: identification of tumor subtypes and new oncomiRs.	3 main clusters of hepatocellular carcinoma: beta-catenin gene mutated tumors (36%), interferon-response–related genes (33%), and tumors with abnormal activation of IGF and mTOR-(PI)3K pathways (31%). A subset of tumors in last subclass (9%) overexpressed a family of miRNAs from chr19q13.42: miR-517a and miR-520c (from ch19q13.42) increased proliferation, migration, and invasion of HCC cells in vitro.

b

Cancer	Authors	Samples	Main findings	miRNA signature
Ovarian Cancer	Iorio et al. 2007	5 cell lines 15 normals 69 tumors	miRNA expression profiles of ovarian cancer vs normal and tumor subtype-specific miRNA signature.	29 miRNAs differentially expressed between normal and tumor with a classification rate of 89%. 4 up-modulated: miR-200a, -200b, -200c, -141; 25 down-modulated: miR-199a, -140, -145, -125b-1 among the most significant.
	Yang et al. 2008	10 normal cells 10 tumors	miRNA expression profiles of ovarian cancer vs normal ephitelial cells.	Up-regulation of miR-214, -199a*, -200a and down-regulation of miR-100; alterations of the first three miRNAs is associated with late-stage and high-grade ovarian tumors. miR-214 induces cell survival and cisplatin resistance by targeting the PTEN/Akt pathway.
	Wu et al. 2009	10 pairs normal-tumor	miRNA expression profiles of endometrioid ovarian cancer vs normal tissues.	17 up-regulated (miR-205, -449, -429) and 6 down-regulated (miR-204, -99b, -193b) miRNAs in endometrioid adenocarcinoma samples.
	Marchini et al. 2011	144 tumors	miRNA expression profiles of stage I ephitelial ovarian cancer assess the existence of a miRNA signature associated with overall and progression-free survival.	34 miRNAs were associated with survival. Between them miR-200c, -199a-3p, -199a-5p were highly associated with overall and progression-free survival.
	Devor et al. 2011	4 normal 23 tumors	miRNA signature in ovarian cancer vs normal and in serous (9) and endometrioid (14) subtypes	7 miRNAs was down-regulated and 13 miRNAs up-regulated in both adenocarcinomas. miR-133b the most repressed miRNA in both adenocarcinomas; miR-205 the most expressed miRNA. miR-135b, -200a, -200b, -200c, -141, -429 significantly overexpressed in both types of endometrial cancers.
Gastric Cancer	Luo et al. 2009	2 cell lines 3 normals 24 tumors	miRNA expression profiles of gastric cancer vs normal.	19 miRNAs down-regulated and 7 miRNAs up-regulated. miR-433 and miR-9 were remarkably down-regulated in the carcinoma samples.
	Ueda et al. 2010	160 pairs normal-tumor	miRNA expression profiles of gastric cancer vs normal and miRNA signature in histological subtypes	22 miRNAs upregulated and 13 downregulated in gastric cancer. Diffuse-type and intestinal-type subtypes were discriminated by miRNA expression. miR-125b, -199a, -100 were the most important microRNAs involved progression signature. Low let-7g and miR-433 and high expression of miR-214 were associated with unfavourable outcome in overall survival independent of clinical covariates, including depth of invasion, lymph-node metastasis, and stage.
	Brenner et al. 2011	45 tumors	miRNA expression profiles of primary tumor of patients with recurrent and non-recurrent gastric cancer.	miR-451, -199a-3p, -195 differentially expressed in gastric tumors from patients with good prognosis vs bad prognosis. High expression of each miR was associated with poorer prognosis for both recurrence and survival. miR-451 showed a positive predictive value for non-recurrence of 100%.
	Kim et al. 2011	34 normals 90 tumors	miRNA signature distinguishes gastric cancer from normal stomach epithelium from healthy volunteers, and a chemoreresistance miRNA signature that is correlated with time to progression after cisplatin/fluorouracil therapy	30 miRNAs inversely correlated with time to progression of disease after chemotherapy whereas 28 miRNAs positively correlated. Among the upregulated miRNAs associated with chemosensitivity: let-7g, miR-342, -16, -181, -1, -34 known to regulate apoptosis.
Esophageal Cancer	Guo et al. 2008	31 pairs normal-tumor	miRNA expression profiles of esophageal cancer vs normal tissues.	46 miRNAs differently expressed between the cancerous and adjacent normal tissues. A minimal set of 7 distinguishes malignant from normal esophageal tissues: miR-25, -424, -151 showed up-regulation and miR-100, -99a, -29c, -140* showed down-regulation. High miR-103/107 correlated with poor survival.
	Yang et al. 2009	32 pairs normal-tumor	miRNA expression profiles of esophageal cancer progression from Barret's low to high grade dysplasia to adenocarcinoma.	111 miRNAs differentiated the adenocarcinoma tissues with 100% accuracy. 11 miRNAs may be important in the progression from low-grade to high-grade dysplasia. let-7b/a/c/f, miR-345, -494, -193a were modulated in the progression from high-grade dysplasia to adenocarcinoma, and all of them were down-regulated in esophageal adenocarcinoma.
	Mathe et al. 2009	170 tumors	Identification of miRNAs involved in major histologic types of esophageal carcinoma and significant associations with prognosis.	In adenocarcinoma patients: high expression of miR-21, -223, -192, -194 and low miR-203 levels. In squamous carcinoma: high expression of miR-21 and low miR-375 levels. High miR-21 in normal tissue of squoamous carcinoma and low levels of miR-375 in cancerous tissue of adenocarcinoma patients with Barrett's were strongly associated with worse prognosis.
	Fassan et al. 2011	14 normals 23 dysplasias	miRNA expression profiles in Barrett's subtypes (7 low grade dysplasia, 5 high grade dysplasia, 11 Barrett's adenocarcinomas)	Up-regulation of miR-215, -560, -615-3p, -192, -326, -147 and down-regulation of miR-100. -23a, -605, -99a, -205, let-7c, -203.
	Feber et al. 2011	45 tumors	miRNA expression profiles provide prognostic utility in staging esophagus cancer patients and elucidate steps in the metastatic pathway and allow for development of targeted therapy.	Up-regulation of miR-143, -199a_3p, -199a_5p, -100, -99a predicted a worse survival. miR-99b, -199a_3p and _5p also associated with the presence of lymph node metastasis.

c

Table 2. miRNA profiling in cancer.

4. Oncogenic microRNAs

Although studies linking miRNA dysfunctions to human diseases are in their infancy, a great deal of data already exists, establishing an important role for miRNAs in the pathogenesis of cancer. Many miRNAs have been shown to function as oncogenes in the majority of cancers profiled to date (**Table 3**). *MiR-21* displays a strong evolutionary conservation across a wide range of vertebrate species in mammalian, avian and fish clades [70]. It has been demonstrated that a primary transcript containing *miR-21* (i.e., *pri-miR-21*) is independently transcribed from a conserved promoter that is located within the intron of the overlapping protein-coding gene *TMEM49* [71]. Several studies suggest that this miRNA is oncogenic [72-74] and that it may act as an antiapoptotic factor. For example, Chan et al. have found that miR-21 is commonly and markedly up-regulated in human glioblastoma and that inhibiting miR-21 expression leads to caspase activation and associated apoptotic cell death [72]. Moreover, Zhu and collaborators provided the first evidence that *miR-21* regulates invasion and metastasis, at least in part, by targeting metastasis-related tumor suppressor genes such as TPM1, programmed cell death 4 (PDCD4) and maspin [73]. Furthermore, examination of human breast tumor specimens revealed an inverse correlation of *miR-21* with PDCD4 and maspin [74]. The final proof of miR-21 oncogenic activity came from the Slack laboratory where the first conditional knock-in of miR-21 overexpressing mice was generated. The mice developed a severe pre-B-cell lymphoma but when miR-21 was reduced to endogenous levels, the mouse tumors completely disappeared, defining the concept of "oncomiR addition" [75].

Another important oncogenic miRNA is represented by *miR-155*. Several groups have shown that *miR-155* is highly expressed in pediatric Burkitt's lymphoma [76], Hodgkin's disease [77], primary mediastinal non-Hodgkin's lymphoma [77], chronic lymphocytic leukemia (CLL) [78], acute myelogenous leukemia (AML) [79], lung cancer [80], pancreatic cancer [81], and breast cancer [80]. Dr. Croce laboratory reported that *miR-155* transgenic mice develop acute lymphoblastic leukemia/high-grade lymphoma and that most of these leukemias start at approximately nine months, irrespective of the mouse strain, preceded by a polyclonal pre-B-cell proliferation [82].

Another example of "oncomiR" is represented by *miR-221&222* cluster that is highly upregulated in a variety of solid tumors, including thyroid cancer [83], hepatocarcinoma [84], estrogen receptor negative breast tumor [85], and melanoma [86]. Elevated *miR-221&222* expression has been causally linked to proliferation [85-87], apoptosis [88-89], and migration [89] of several cancer cell lines. We recently reported that the hepatocyte growth factor receptor (MET) oncogene, through c-Jun transcriptional activation, upregulates *miR-221&222* expression, which, in turn, by targeting *PTEN* and *TIMP3*, confers resistance to tumor necrosis factor–related apoptosis-inducing ligand (TRAIL) and enhances tumorigenicity of lung and liver cancer cells [89]. The results suggest that therapeutic intervention involving the use of miRNAs should not only sensitize tumor cells to drug-inducing apoptosis but also inhibit their survival, proliferation, and invasion [89].

The miR-106b-25 polycistron is composed of the highly conserved miR-106b, miR-93, and miR-25 that accumulate in different types of cancer, including gastric, prostate, and pancreatic neuroendocrine tumors, as well as neuroblastoma and multiple myeloma. Petrocca and collaborators [90] demonstrated that E2F1 regulates miR-106b, miR-93, and miR-25, inducing their accumulation in gastric tumors. Conversely, miR-106b and miR-93 control E2F1 expression, establishing a negative feedback loop that may be important in preventing E2F1 self-activation and apoptosis. On the other hand, miR-106b, miR-93, and

miRNA	*Target*	*Tumor*
	PTEN	cholangiocarcinoma
	TPM1	breast cancer
	PDCD4	breast cancer
miR-21	SPRY1	
	RECK, TIMP3	glioblastoma
	p63, JMY, TOPORS, TP53BP2, DAXX, HNRPK, TGFβRII	glioblastoma
	MARKS	prostate cancer
	ANP32A, SMARCA4	prostate cancer
	SOCS1	breast cancer
	CEBPB, PU.1 ,CUTL1, PICALM	AML
	BACH1, ZIC3	
	ETS1, MEIS1	human cord blood CD34+
	C-MAF	lymphocytes
	HGAL	diffuse large B-cell lymphoma
miR-155	JMJD1A	nasopharyngeal carcinoma
	WEE1	breast cancer
	TP53INP1	pancreatic cancer
	SMAD1, SMAD5, HIVEP2, CEBPB, RUNX2, MYO10	
	FOXO3A	breast cancer
	hMSH2, hMSH6, hMLH1	colon cancer
	SMAD5	diffuse large B-cell lymphoma
	p27(KIP1)	glioblastoma, prostate and thyroid carcinoma
	p57 (KIP2)	normal fibroblast
	PTEN, TIMP3	non small cell lung cancer and hepatocellular carcinoma
	FOXO3A	breast cancer
	KIT	Endotelial cells
miR-221/222	ESR1	breast cancer
	PUMA	glioblastoma
	TRSP1	breast cancer
	PTPμ	glioblastoma
	DICER	breast cancer
	APAF1	non small cell lung cancer
miR-106a~363	BIM, p21	gastric cancer
miR-106b~25	E2F1	prostate cancer
	PTEN	prostate cancer
	TSP-1, CTGF	colon
	E2F2, E2F3	prostate/Burkitt lymphoma/testis carcinoma/
	BIM PTEN	c-Myc induced lymphoma
	HIF1α	lung cancer
	PTPRO	cervix tumor cell line
miR-17-92	p63	myeloid cells
	BIM, PTEN, PRKAA1, PPP2R5e,	T-cell acute lymphoblastic leukaemia
	JAK1	endothelial cells
	HBP1	breast cancer
	p21(WAF1)	Ras induced senescent-fibroblasts
	TGFβII, SMAD4	glioblastoma
	MnSOD, GPX2, TRXR2	prostate
	HOXB1, HOXB3	pancreatic cancer
	HOXD10	breast cancer
miR-10a/10b	KLF4	esophageal cancer
	TIAM1	breast cancer
	NF1	Ewing's sarcoma

Table 3. *-oncomiRs*

miR-25 overexpression causes a decreased response of gastric cancer cells to TGFβ by downregulating p21 and Bim, the two most downstream effectors of TGFβ-dependent cell cycle arrest and apoptosis, respectively.

Another example of a miRNA locus with oncogenic properties is represented by the *miR-17-92* cluster, which consists of six miRNAs: miR-17-5p, -18, -19a, -19b, -20a, and -92-1. The miR-17-92 cluster is located in a region frequently amplified in several types of lymphoma and solid tumors [91-92]. It has been shown that mice deficient for miR-17-92 die shortly after birth with lung hypoplasia and a ventricular septal defect. This cluster is also essential for B cell development; its absence, in fact, leads to increased levels of the proapoptotic protein Bim and inhibits B cell development at the pro-B-to-pre-B transition [93]. All together these studies indicate that many miRNAs have oncogenic activity. Importantly, their knockdown through the use of antisense oligonucleotides, inhibits the development of cancer-associated phenotypes, laying the groundwork for the creation of miRNA-based therapies [94-96].

5. Tumor suppressor microRNAs

The first evidence that miRNAs are involved in cancer comes from the finding that miR-15 and miR-16 are downregulated or deleted in most patients with chronic lymphocytic leukemia (CLL) (**Table 4**) [68]. They are transcribed as a cluster (*miR-15a–miR-16-1*) that resides in the 13q14 chromosomal region. Deletions or point mutations in region 13q14 occur at high frequency in CLL, lymphoma, and several solid tumors [97]. Their expression is inversely correlated to *BCL2* expression in CLL [98]. The tumor suppressor function of *miR-15a/16-1* has also been addressed in vivo. In immunocompromised nude mice, ectopic expression of *miR-15a/16-1* was found to cause dramatic suppression of tumorigenicity of MEG-01 leukemic cells that exhibited a loss of endogenous expression of *miR-15a/16-1*. Furthermore, Klein et al. [99] generated transgenic mice with a deletion of the *miR-15a–miR-16-1* cluster, causing development of indolent B-cell-autonomous, clonal lymphoproliferative disorders, recapitulating the spectrum of CLL-associated phenotypes observed in humans. Recently, Bonci et al. reported that the *miR-15a–miR-16-1* cluster targets not only *BCL2* but also *CCND1* (encoding cyclin D1) and *WNT3A* mRNA, which promote several prostate tumorigenic features, including survival, proliferation, and invasion [100]. Together, these data suggest that *miR-15a/16-1* genes are natural antisense interactors of *BCL2* and probably other oncogenes and that they can be used to suppress tumor growth in therapeutic application for a variety of tumors [100].

In mammalians, the miR-34 family comprises three processed miRNAs that are encoded by two different genes: miR-34a is encoded by its own transcript, whereas miR-34b and miR-34c share a common primary transcript. The miR-34 family has been shown to form part of the p53 tumor-suppressor network: their expression is directly induced by p53 in response to DNA damage or oncogenic stress [101-102]. He et al. identified different miR-34 targets such as cyclin E2 (CCNE2), CDK4, and MET. Silencing these selected miR-34 targets through the use of small interfering RNAs (siRNAs) led to a substantial cell cycle arrest in G1.

Moreover, ectopic miR-34 delivery caused a decrease in levels of phosphorylated retinoblastoma gene product (Rb), consistent with lowered activity of both CDK4 and CCNE2 complexes [102]. BCL2 and MYCN were also identified as miR-34a targets and likely mediators of the tumor suppressor phenotypic effect in neuroblastoma [103]. It has been also reported that p53 activation suppressed the EMT-inducing transcription factor SNAIL via induction of the miR-34a/b/c genes. In fact, suppression of miR-34a/b/c by anti-miRs caused up-regulation of SNAIL and cells displayed EMT markers, enhanced migration and invasion [104].

MicroRNA-122 (miR-122) is a liver-specific microRNA and is frequently downregulated in liver cancer [105]. Xu et al. reported that restoration of miR-122 in hepatocellular carcinoma cells could render cells sensitive to chemotherapeutic agents adriamycin or vincristine through downregulating antiapoptotic gene Bcl-w and cell cycle related gene cyclin B1 [106]. Another group found that over-expression of miR-122 inhibits hepatocellular carcinoma cell growth and promotes the cell apoptosis by affecting Wnt/β-catenin signalling pathway [107]. Coulouarn et al. showed that miR-122 is specifically repressed in a subset of primary hepatocellular tumors that are characterized by poor prognosis [108]. They further reported that loss of miR-122 resulted in an increase of cell migration and invasion and that restoration of miR-122 reverses this phenotype [108]. The final understanding of the tumor suppressor role for mir-122 role in liver cancer came from a recent study where miR-122 knockout mice were studied. When miR-122 KO mice aged, hepatic inflammation ensued, preceding the progressive onset of fibrosis and, eventually, tumors resembling human liver cancer. These pathologic manifestations were associated with hyperactivity of oncogenic pathways and hepatic infiltration of inflammatory cells that produce pro-tumorigenic cytokines, including IL-6 and TNF [109].

miRNA	Target	Tumor
miR-15/16	BCL2	CLL
	COX-2	colon cancer
	CHEK1	follicolar lymphoma
	CEBPβ, CDC25a, CCNE1	fibroblast
	VEGF, VEGFR2, FGFR1	fibroblast
	FGF2, FGFR1	cancer associated fibroblast
	CCNE1	
	FGFR1, PI3KCa, MDM4, VEGFa	multiple myeloma
	WIP1	
	BMI-1	ovarian cancer
	CCND1, CCND2, CCNE1	lung cancer
	SIRT1	colon cancer
miR-34	BCL2, NOTCH, HMGA2	
	MYC	fibroblast
	AXL	lung cancer
	MET	ovarian cancer
	NANOG, SOX2, MYCN	embryonic fibroblast
	SNAIL	colon cancer

Table 4. Tumor suppressor *miRS*

6. MetastamiRs

Metastasis is the result of cancer cells detaching from a primary tumor, consequently adapting to distant tissues and organs, and forming a secondary tumor [110] and this ability of cancer cells to metastasize is a hallmark of malignant tumors [111-112]. To successfully metastasize, a tumor cell must complete a complex set of processes, including invasion, survival and arrest in the circulatory system, and colonization of foreign organs. Despite great advancements in knowledge of metastasis biology, the molecular mechanisms are still not completely understood. Several miRNAs have been shown to initiate invasion and metastasis by targeting multiple proteins that are major players in these cellular events, thus they have been denominated as metastamiRs (Table 5). It seems that these metastasis-associated miRNAs do not influence primary tumor either in development or initiation steps of tumorigenesis, but they regulate key steps in the metastatic program and processes, such as epithelial-mesenchymal transition (EMT), apoptosis, and angiogenesis. Ma et. al reported that miR-10b is highly expressed in metastatic breast cancer cells and positively regulates cell migration and invasion. Overexpression of miR-10b in otherwise non-metastatic breast tumors initiates robust invasion and metastasis [113]. The team led by Joan Massague found that miR-335, miR-126, and miR-206 are metastasis-suppressors in breast cancer [114]. MiR-126 and miR-206 restoration reduced overall tumor growth and proliferation, whereas miR-335 inhibits metastatic cell invasion through targeting of the progenitor cell transcription factor SOX4 and extracellular matrix component tenascin C [114]. Others miRNAs with prominent roles in breast cancer metastasis have been reported. It has been reported that miR-31 inhibited multiple steps of metastasis including invasion, anoikis, and colonization leading to almost complete reduction of lung metastasis [115]. Clinically, miR-31 levels were lower in breast cancer patients with metastasis. In addition, miR-9, which is up-regulated in breast cancer cells, directly targets CDH1, the E-cadherin-encoding messenger RNA, leading to increased cell motility and invasiveness [116].

Another important aspect of the metastatic dissemination is represented by the epithelial-to-mesenchymal transition (EMT) that allow neoplastic cells to abandon their primary site and survive in the new tissue. During EMT, an epithelial neoplastic cell looses cell adhesion by repressing E-cadherin expression and thereby the cell increases its motility. Numerous studies have shown that different microRNAs are modulated during EMT and one of the best-studied example is represented by the miR-200 family. These miRs are commonly lost in aggressive tumors such as lung, prostate, and pancreatic cancer. It has been shown that miR-200 family members directly target ZEB1 and ZEB2, transcription repressors of E-cadherin [117]. In fact, in the highly aggressive mouse lung cancer model where KRAS is constitutively activated and p53 function is perturbed, miR-200 ectopic expression prevented metastasis by repressing ZEB1 and ZEB2 and preventing E-cadherin down-regulation [117]. However, overexpression of the miR-200 family is associated with an increased risk of metastasis in breast cancer and this overexpression promotes metastatic colonization in mouse models, phenotypes that cannot be explained by E-cadherin expression alone [118]. By using proteomic profiling of the targets of mesenchymal-to-epithelial (MET)-inducing miR-200, the authors discovered that miR-200 globally targets secreted proteins in breast cancer cells. Between the 38 modulated target genes, Sec23a, which is involved in transporting protein cargo from the endoplasmic reticulum to the Golgi, shows a superior association with human metastatic breast cancer as compared to the currently recognized miR-200 targets ZEB1 and the EMT marker E-cadherin. EMT is first acquired in the onset of transmigration and then reversed in the new metastatic site. Korpal et al. have shown that the miR-200 status predicts predisposition of the cancer to successful metastasis [119].

miRNA	Target	Tumor
	HOXB1, HOXB3	pancreatic cancer
	HOXD10	breast cancer
miR-10a/10b	KLF4	esophageal cancer
	TIAM1	breast cancer
	NF1	Ewing's sarcoma
	PRDM1/BLIMP-1	lymphomas
miR-9	CDH1	breast cancer
	CAMTA	glioblastoma
miR-31	ITGA5, RDX, RHOA FZD3, M-RIP, MMP16	breast cancer
	SATB2	cancer associated fibroblast
	ZEB1, ZEB2	breast cancer
	ERRFI-1	bladder cancer
	ZEB1, CTNNB1	nasopharyngeal carcinoma
	BMI-1	pancreatic cancer
	PLCγ1	breast cancer
miR-200 family	FAP1	
	SUZ12	breast cancer
	FLT1/VEGFR1	lung cancer
	JAG1, MALM2, MALM3	
	FN1, LEPR, NTRK2, ARHGAP19	breast and endometrial cancer
	p38α	ovarian cancer

Table 5. *metastamiRS*

7. Other non-coding RNAs: Biology and implications in cancer

7.1. snoRNAs: From post-transcriptional modification to cancer

Small nucleolar RNAs (snoRNAs) have, for many years, been considered one of the best-characterized classes of non-coding RNAs (ncRNAs) [120-123] but despite the common assumption that snoRNAs only have cellular housekeeping functions, in the past few years, independent reports have converged in implicating snoRNAs in the control of cell fate and oncogenesis [124-130]. SnoRNAs are small RNAs of 60-300nt in lenght that specifically accumulate in the nucleolar compartment of the cell where are in charge of the 2'-O-ribose methylation and pseudouridylation of specific ribosomal RNA nucleotides, essential modification for the efficient and accurate production of the ribosome [120-122]. The snoRNAs carry out their function in the form of small nucleolar ribonucleoproteins (snoRNPs), each of which consists of a box C/D or box H/ACA guide RNA, and four associated C/D or H/ACA snoRNP proteins (**Figure 2**). In both cases, snoRNAs hybridize specifically to the complementary sequence in the rRNAs, and the associated protein complexes then carry out the appropriate modification on the nucleotide that is identified by the snoRNAs. Biogenesis of vertebrate snoRNPs is remarkable and highly variable: in fact snoRNA gene organization ranges from independently transcribed genes, endowed with their own promoter elements, to intronic coding units lacking an independent promoter. In both yeast and animals, processing of intron-encoded snoRNAs is largely splicing-dependent; in contrast, the production of plant snoRNAs from introns seems to rely on a splicing-independent process [131]. Moreover, in both contexts (intergenic or intronic), genes can be either single or part of clusters. In the latter case, the generation of individual snoRNAs involves the enzymatic processing of polycistronic precursor RNAs. Such a processing, at least in yeast, appears to involve the same combination of endo- and exoribonucleases required for the maturation of monocistronic pre-snoRNAs [132-134]. The first indication that snoRNAs might have important roles in human disease was provided by the genetic studies on Prader–Willi syndrome (PWS), an inherited human disorder characterized by a complex phenotype, including mental retardation, decreased muscle tone and failure to thrive at birth, short stature, hypogonadism, sleep apnea, behavioral problems and hyperphagia (an insatiable appetite) that can lead to severe obesity [135]. The disease is caused by the genomic loss of the imprinted chromosomic 15q11-q13 locus which is normally only active on the paternal allele. The only characterized and conserved genes within this 121-kb-long genomic interval are the numerous HBII-85 snoRNA gene copies, thus suggesting that loss of expression of these repeated small C/D RNA genes might play a role in conferring some (or even all) phenotypes of the human disease and PWS-like phenotypes in mice (neonatal lethality, growth retardation and hypotonia). In fact, it has been shown that a site-specific deletion of the entire murine MBII-85 gene cluster led to post-natal growth retardation with low postnatal lethality (<15%) only seen in some genetic backgrounds, but no obesity [136]. Although all the imprinted C/D RNAs that have been tested accumulate within the nucleolus, none of them appear to act as RNA guides to modify rRNAs or spliceosomal U-snRNAs; they are called 'orphan C/D RNAs'. So far, the MBII-52 gene clusters have attracted much attention, given that the neuronal-specific MBII-52 small RNA is predicted to interfere (A-to-I RNA editing and/or alternative RNA splicing) with the post-transcriptional regulation of the pre-mRNA that encodes the 5-HT$_{2C}$ (5-hydroxytryptamine 2C) receptor, playing a key role in regulating serotonergic signal transduction [137-138]. These observations raised the possibility that snoRNAs could have functions completely independent from their traditional activities and carry out other regulatory roles. The first insights into the potential roles of snoRNAs in cancer began with a study that identified C/D box snoRNA U50 and its host gene U50HG at the breakpoint in the t(3;6) (q21;q15) translocation in a diffuse large B cell lymphoma [139]. Moreover, snoRNAU50 gene has been found to undergo to a frequent copy number loss and a transcriptional downregulation in breast and prostate cancer samples [139,140]. In addition, a 2-bp deletion in U50 sequence also occurred both somatically and in germline, leading to increased incidence of homozygosity for the deletion in cancer cells [140].

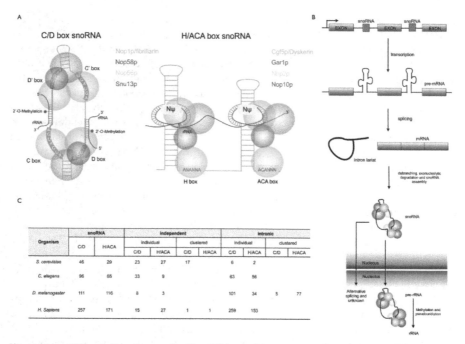

Figure 2. snoRNAs. A. Boxed sequences C and D (named from conserved, nuclease-resistant sequences that were originally identified in snoRNA U3) are hallmarks of the C/D box snoRNAs; boxed sequences H (Hinge region) and ACA are hallmarks of the H/ACA box snoRNAs. These conserved boxed sequences are important for the associations with protein components that are required to form the functional small nucleolar ribonucleoprotein (snoRNP) complexes and for accumulation in the nucleolus. C/D box snoRNAs associate with several proteins, including fibrillarin, which is the methyl transferase that is involved in the 2'-O-methylation of particular ribonucleotides, and H/ACA box snoRNAs associate with proteins such as the pseudouridine synthase dyskerin. Antisense sequences within the C/D box and H/ACA box snoRNAs guide the snoRNP complex to the appropriate nucleotide within the target RNA (most often ribosomal RNA). In a minority of cases both C/D-associated and C'D'-associated antisense sequences within the same C/D box snoRNA can act as guides for 2'-O-methylation of the target RNA. The eukaryotic H/ACA box snoRNAs contain two hairpin domains with complementary regions flanking the uridine to be converted in the target rRNA, at a position 14–16 nucleotides upstream of the conserved H and/or ACA box. Most mammalian snoRNAs are encoded within the introns of genes producing 5' terminal oligopyrimidine (5'TOP) RNAs. **B.** Organization of snoRNA genes in representative eukaryotic genomes **C.** Small nucleolar RNAs (snoRNAs) in vertebrate are predominantly located in introns. Following splicing, debranching and trimming, mature snoRNAs are either exported, in which case they function in ribosomal RNA (rRNA) processing, or remain in the nucleus, where they are involved in alternative splicing and additional yet unknown functions.

SnoRNA42 (SNORA42) is located on chromosome 1q22 which is a commonly frequent amplified genomic region in lung cancer and overexpression of SNORA42 is frequently and remarkably found in NSCLC cells [141]. In addition, SNORA42 exhibited close correlations between its increases of copy number and expression level, suggesting that SNORA42 overexpression could be activated through its amplification. Importantly, engineered repression of SNORA42 caused marked repression of lung cancer growth in vitro and in vivo and it is associated with increased apoptosis by a p53-dependent pathway. Although not exhibiting apoptosis, p53 null and mutant p53 cancer cells with reduced levels of SNORA42 also show inhibited proliferation and growth, suggesting that SNORA42 knockdown can inhibit cell proliferation in p53-dependent or -independent manner. These independent studies on U50 and SNORA42 provide evidence for the functional importance of snoRNAs in cancer, and they show that snoRNAs can promote, as well as suppress, tumour development. In 2002, Wu and coworkers demonstrated that the expression of snoRNAs 5S was differentially displayed in different tissues and noticeably was highly expressed in normal brain, but its expression drastically decreased in meningioma [142]. Recently, genome-wide approaches identified six snoRNAs (SNORD33, SNORD66, SNORD73B, SNORD76, SNORD78, and SNORA42) that were statistically differently expressed between the non small cell lung cancer tumor and paired noncancerous samples [143]. Specifically, all these snoRNAs displayed a strong up-regulation in lung tumor specimens and the majority of them is located in commonly frequent genomic amplified regions in lung cancer: SNORD33 is located in chromosome 19q13.3 that contain potential oncogenes in lung cancer, while SNORD66 and SNORD76 are situated in chromosomal regions 3q27.1 and 1q25.1, respectively 3q27.1 and 1q25.1 are two of the most frequently amplified chromosomal segments in solid tumors, particularly NSCLC [143].

As well as the initial evidence that snoRNAs are involved in cancer development, there are some preliminary data showing that the genes that host snoRNAs might also contribute to the aetiology of this disease. A research screening for potential tumor-suppressor genes identified that Growth arrest-specific transcript 5 (gas5) gene as almost undetectable in actively growing cells but highly expressed in cells undergoing serum starvation or density arrest [144-145]. Gas5 is a multi-snoRNA host gene which encodes 9 (in mouse) or 10 (in human) snoRNAs and like all known snoRNA host genes exhibit characteristics which belong to the class of genes encoding 5' terminal oligopyrimidine (5'TOP) mRNAs [146]. The first and stronger evidence that GAS5 is related to cancer is the identification that GAS5 transcript levels are significantly reduced in breast cancer samples relative to adjacent unaffected normal breast epithelial tissues and some, but not all, GAS5 transcripts sensitize mammalian cells to apoptosis inducers [147]. Other studies have also showed that GAS5 reduced expression is associated with poor prognosis in both breast cancer and head and neck squamous cell carcinoma [148]. Of note, GAS5 has been also identified as a novel partner of the BCL6 in a patient with diffuse large B-cell lymphoma, harboring the t(1;3)(q25;q27) [149]. Another example of a mature spliced transcript that harbors C/D-box snoRNAs and can function independently of the snoRNAs is represented by the transcript Zfas1 [150]. This gene intronically hosts three C/D box snoRNAs (Snord12, Snord12b, and Snord12c) and has been identified as one of the most differentially expressed gene during mouse mammary development. siRNA-mediated downregulation of Zfas1 mRNA in a mouse mammary cell line increased proliferation and differentiation without substantially affecting the levels of the snoRNA hosted within its intron. The human homologue, ZFAS1 (also known as ZNFX1-AS1), which is predicted to share secondary structural features with mouse Zfas1, is expressed at high levels in the mammary gland and is downregulated in breast cancer. Taken together, these findings indicates that snoRNA host genes might have important functions in regulating cellular homeostasis and, potentially, cancer biology but more studies are needed to understand their involvement in molecular basis of disease and classify them as sources of potential biomarkers and therapeutic targets.

Another important aspect of the association between snoRNAs and tumorigenesis is represented by the involvement of their associated proteins in cancer. A point mutations in the DKC1 gene is the cause of a rare X-linked recessive disease, the dyskeratosis congenita (DC) [151-152]. Individuals with DC display features of premature aging, as well as nail dystrophy, mucosal leukoplakia, interstitial fibrosis of the lung, and increased susceptibility to cancer. DKC1 codes for dyskerin, a putative pseudouridine synthase, which carries out two separate functions, both fundamental for proliferating cells. One function is the pseudo-uridylation of ribosomal RNA (rRNA) molecules as a part of the H/ACA ribonucleoprotein complex, and the other is the stabilization of the telomerase RNA component necessary for telomerase activity. Dkc1 mutant mice recapitulate the major features of DC, including an increased susceptibility to tumor formation. Early generation (G1 and G2) of Dkc1 mutant mice showed a full spectrum of DC and presented alterations in rRNA modification, whereas defects in telomere length were not evident until G4 mice, suggesting that deregulated ribosome function is important for the initiation of DC and that impairment in telomerase activity in Dkc1 mutant mice may modify and/or exacerbate the disease in later generations. To this regard, DKC1 was identified as one of only seventy genes that, collectively, constitute a gene expression profile that strongly correlates with the development of aneuploidy and is associated with poor clinical prognosis in a variety of human cancers. Therefore, one hypothesis is that an alteration of physiologic dyskerin function, irrespective of the mechanism, may perturb mitosis and contribute to tumorigenesis but this idea will require more detailed investigation. Another possibility is related to the strong effect of dyskerin loss on H/ACA accumulation. Recent finding in fact have shown that some H/ACA box and C/D box can be processed to produce small RNAs, at least some of which can function like miRNAs [153]. Such processing may be of crucial importance, as miRNAs have important roles in the development of many cancers as previously discussed. To date, Xiao and colleagues have recently reported that an H/ACA box snoRNA- derived miRNA, miR-605, has a key role in stress-induced stabilization of the p53 tumour suppressor protein [154]. p53 transcriptionally activates its negative regulator, MDM2, in addition to miR-605. miR-605 counteracts MDM2 through post-transcriptional repression; under conditions of stress, this snoRNA-derived miRNA offsets the MDM2 negative-feedback loop, generating a positive-feedback loop to enable the rapid accumulation of p53. However, whether this regulation of p53 by miR-605 is relevant to cancer biology has not yet been addressed. Like dyskerin, NHP2 and NOP10 proteins, both components of the H/ACA snoRNPs, are also significantly up-regulated in sporadic cancers and high levels may be associated with poor clinical prognosis. Moreover, germline NHP2 and NOP10 mutations give rise to autosomal recessive forms of dyskeratosis congenita, and cancer susceptibility is also a feature of these genetic forms of the disease. Since the functions of several snoRNAs have not yet been identified (orphan snoRNAs), it is possible that disruption of snoRNP biogenesis by any mechanism may affect an array of important cellular processes, and could potentiate cancer development and/or progression.

7.2. piRNAs: Guardians of the genome

Piwi-interacting RNAs (piRNAs) are germline-specific small silencing RNAs of 24–30 nt in length, that suppress transposable elements (TE) activity and maintain genome integrity during germline development, a role highly conserved across animal species [155-156]. TEs are genomic parasites that threaten the genomic integrity of the host genome: they are able to move to new sites by insertion or transposition and thereby disrupt genes and alter the genome [157]. In animals, endogenous siRNAs also silence TEs, but the piRNA pathway is at the forefront of defense against transposons in germ cells [158]. piRNAs specifically associate with PIWI proteins, which are germline-specific members of the AGO protein family, AGO3, Aubergine (Aub) and Piwi, and form a piRNA-induced silencing complex (piRISC) which will guide the TE silencing [159-162]. Any mutations in each of the three members of the PIWI family lead to transposon derepression in the germline, indicating that they act non-redundantly during TE silencing. Initial screening of piRNA sequences revealed that there are hundreds of thousands, if not millions, of individual piRNA sequences [163-165]. Furthermore, they are characterized by the absence of specific sequence motifs or secondary structures such as miRNA precursors. Despite their large diversity, most piRNAs can be mapped to a relatively small number of genomic regions called piRNA clusters. Each cluster extends from several to more than 200 kilobases, it contains multiple sequences that generate piRNAs and some piRNAs map to both genomic strands, suggesting bidirectional transcription [163-165] Indeed, analysis of piRNA clusters in different *Drosophila* species has shown that, although the clusters locations are conserved, their sequence content has evolved very quickly suggesting adjustments in the piRNAs patrimony in order to suppress new active transposons invading the species. Therefore, piRNA clusters may be considered as repositories of information, enabling production of many mature piRNAs that target diverse TEs. Two main pathways, highly conserved in many animal species, have been discovered to be responsible for the biogenesis of the piRNAs: the primary pathways and the Ping-Pong amplification (**Figure 3**) [166-168]. First, the primary piRNA biogenesis pathway provides an initial pool of piRNAs that target multiple TEs. Next, the Ping-Pong cycle further shapes the piRNA population by amplifying sequences that target active transposons. It is currently unclear how primary piRNAs are produced from piRNA clusters but it is likely that piRNA precursors are single-stranded and therefore do not require Dicer for their processing. Interestingly, piRNAs that associate with each member of the PIWI protein family have a distinct size, suggesting that PIWI proteins can act as 'rulers' that define the size of mature piRNAs. Several additional proteins (e.s. Zucchini, Armitage and Yb) have also been identified that are involved in primary piRNA biogenesis and mutations in and/or depletion of any of these three proteins eliminates primary piRNAs associated with PIWI proteins. In some cell types, such as somatic follicle cells of the *D. melanogaster* ovary, primary piRNA biogenesis is the only mechanism that generates piRNAs. However, in germline cells of the *D. melanogaster* ovary and in the pre-meiotic spermatogonia in mice, there is another mechanism called the Ping-Pong cycle that amplifies specific sequences generated by the primary biogenesis pathway

[163,169]. Mainly the Ping-Pong pathway engages AGO3 and Aubergine, both of which are accumulated in perinuclear structures located at the cytoplasmic face of the nuclear envelope in animal germline cells, named "nuage". The pathway depends on the endoribonuclease or Slicer activity of AGO3 and Aubergine, which act catalytically one after the other, leading to a cleavage of the target RNAs between their tenth and eleventh nucleotides relative to the 'guide' small RNAs. This process results in the generation of repeated rounds of piRNA production having exactly the same sequence of the original primary piRNA. The ping-pong pathway amplifies piRNAs in *D. melanogaster* testes, especially those originating from TEs. Non-TE-derived piRNAs seem to be barely amplified by the amplification loop. This two steps of piRNA biogenesis can be compared with the function of the adaptive immune system in protecting against pathogens. The primary piRNA biogenesis pathway resembles the initial generation of the hypervariable antibody repertoire, whereas the amplification loop is analogous to antigen-directed clonal expansion of antibody-producing lymphocytes during the acute immune response. An emerging number of studies highlight the role of piRNAs or PIWI proteins in the regulation of tumorigenesis. First examples of the piRNA involvement in cancer is represented by the up-regulation of HIWI, one of the four human Piwi homologues, in about 60 % of seminomas [170]. In fact, HIWI maps to a locus known as a germ cell tumor susceptibility locus (12aq24.33). HIWI overexpression has also been found in somatic cells such as soft-tissue sarcomas or ductal pancreas adenocarcinoma, and strongly correlates with bad prognosis and high incidence of tumor-related death, providing an example for a potential tumorigenic role of a piRNA-related protein in somatic cells [171,172]. In some cancers, PIWIL2 overexpression has been suggested to induced resistance in cells to cisplatin, which might arise because of increased chromatin condensation that prevents the normal process of DNA repair [173]. Furthermore, new high-throughput sequencing data revealed the presence of piRNAs in somotic cells, such as HeLa cells. These somatic piRNAs appear located in the nucleolus and in the cytoplasmic area surrounding the nuclear envolope and in contrast with the large population of known piRNAs in male germ cells, this population of piRNAs is dramatically smaller [174]. Another recent study demonstrated that the level of piR-651 is significantly higher in several cancer histotype including lung, mesothelium, breast, liver, and cervical cancer compared to non-cancerous adjacent tissues and inhibition of piR-651 induced block of gastric cancer cells at the G2/M phase [175,176]. Another example is represented by the downregulation of piR-823 in gastric cancer tissues; its enforced expression inhibited gastric cancer cell growth in vitro and in vivo, suggesting a tumor suppressive properties for piR-823 [177]. Interestingly, piRNAs not are only involved in direct regulation by degradation of TE but they have also been linked to DNA methylation of the retrotraspon regions, extending piRNA functions beyond post-transcriptional silencing. In fact, CpG DNA methylation, which is required for efficient transcriptional silencing of LINE and LTR retrotransposons in the genome, is decreased in the male germ line of mice with defective PIWI proteins. Specifically, mice with defective PIWI proteins fail to establish de novo methylation of TE sequences during spermatogenesis, leading to the hypothesis that the piRISC can also guide the *de novo* methylation machinery to TE loci. In this scenerio, piRNAs may present a perfect guide for discriminating TE sequences from normal protein-coding genes and marking them for DNA methylation; however, the biochemical details of how these two mechanisms of piRNA

action might be linked have not yet been revealed [178,179]. All together, these data revealed that PIWI-associated RNAs and PIWI pathway has a more profound function outside germline cells than was originally thought but many more studies are needed to clarify their specific role in tumorigenesis.

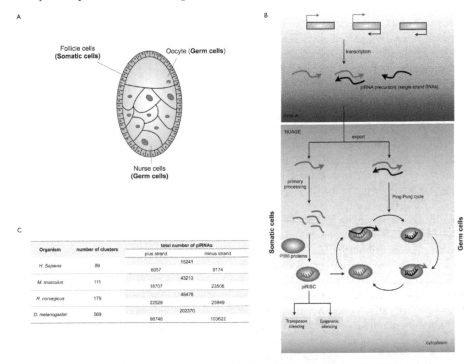

Organism	number of clusters	total number of piRNAs	
		plus strand	minus strand
H. Sapiens	89	15241	
		6057	9174
M. musculus	111	43213	
		18707	23506
R. norvegicus	179	48478	
		22529	25949
D. melanogaster	569	202370	
		98748	103622

Figure 3. piRNAs. A, schematic representation of the Drosophila egg chamber. **B,**piRNAs (which are 24–32 nt in length) are processed from single-stranded RNA precursors that are transcribed largely from mono- or bidirectional intergenic repetitive elements known as piRNA clusters. Unlike miRNAs and siRNAs, piRNAs do not require Dicer for their processing. First, primary piRNAs are produced through the primary processing pathway and are amplified through the ping-pong pathway, which requires Slicer activity of PIWI proteins. Subsequently, additional piRNAs are produced through a PIWI-protein-catalysed amplification loop (called the 'ping-pong cycle') via sense and antisense intermediates. Primary piRNA processing and loading onto mouse PIWI proteins might occur in the cytoplasm. The PIWI ribonucleoprotein (piRISC) complex functions in transposon repression through target degradation and epigenetic silencing. **C,** total number of piRNA clusters in different animal species according to the piRNA Database (http://pirnabank.ibab.ac.in/).

8. The emergence of long non-coding RNAs

Over the last decade, advances in genome-wide analyses of the eukaryotic transcriptome have revealed that most of the human genome is transcribed, generating a large repertoire of (>200 nt) long non-coding RNAs (lncRNA or lincRNA, for long intergenic ncRNA) that map to intronic and intergenic regions [181,181]. Given their unexpected abundance, lncRNAs were initially thought to be spurious transcriptional noise resulting from low RNA polymerase fidelity [182]. However, the restricted expression of many long ncRNAs to particular developmental contexts, the often exhibiting precise subcellular localization and the binding of transcription factors to non-coding loci, suggested that a significant portion of ncRNAs fulfills functional roles beyond transcriptional remodelling [183-187]. lncRNA typically refers to a polyadenylated long ncRNA that is transcribed by RNA polymerase II and is associated with epigenetic signatures common to protein-coding genes, such as trimethylation of histone 3 lysine 4 (H3K4me3) at the transcriptional start site (TSS) and trimethylation of histone 3 lysine 36 (H3K36me3) throughout the gene body [188-189]. lncRNAs also commonly exhibit splicing of multiple exons into a mature transcript, and their transcription occurs from an independent gene promoter and is not coupled to the transcription of a nearby or associated parental gene. RNA-Seq studies now suggest that several thousand uncharacterized lncRNAs are present in any given cell type [188-189], and that the human genome may harbor nearly as many lncRNAs as protein-coding genes (perhaps ~15,000 lncRNAs), although only a fraction is expressed in a given cell type. One main characteristic of the lncRNAs is their very low sequence conservation that had fueled the idea that they are not functional. This assertion needs to be carefully considered and takes in consideration several points. First, a recent study identified the presence of 1,600 lncRNAs that show a strong evolutionary conservation and function ranging from from embryonic stem cell pluripotency to cell proliferation [189]. In contrast to the protein coding genes, long ncRNAs can exhibit shorter stretches of sequence that are conserved to maintain functional domains and structures. Indeed, many long ncRNAs with a known function, such as *Xist*, only exhibit high conservation over short sections of their length [190]. Third, rather than being indicative of non-functionality, low sequence conservation can also be explained by high rates of primary sequence evolution if long ncRNAs have, like promoters and other regulatory elements, more plastic structure–function constraints than proteins [190]. The diverse selection pressures acting on long ncRNAs probably reflect the wide range of their functions which can be regrouped in three major subclasses: chromatin remodeling, transcriptional modulation and nuclear architecture/subnuclear localization.

long ncRNAs can mediate epigenetic changes by recruiting chromatin remodelling complexes to specific genomic loci resolving the paradox of how a small repertoire of chromatin remodelling complexes are able To specify the large array of chromatin modifications without any apparent specificity for the genomic loci [191,192]. A recent study found that 20% of 3300 human long non coding RNAs are bound by Polycomb Repressive Complex 2 (PRC2) [193]. Although the specific molecular mechanisms are not defined, there are several examples that can illustrate the silencing potential of lncRNAs (**Figure 4**). The first most known example is represented by the X-chromosome inactivation which is carried out by a number of lncRNAs including Xist and RepA, which bind PRC2 complex, and the antagonist of Xist, Tsix [194]. In pre-X-inactivation cells, Tsix competes with RepA for the binding of PRC2 complex; when the X-inactivation starts Tsix is downregulated and PRC2 becomes available to RepA which can actively induced the transcription of Xist. The up-regulated Xist in turn preferentially binds to PRC2 and spreads across the chromosome X inducing PCR2-mediated trimethylated histone H3 lysine27. Another important example is represented by the hundreds of long ncRNAs which are sequentially expressed along the temporal and spatial developmental axes of the human homeobox (Hox) loci, where they define chromatin domains of differential histone methylation and RNA polymerase accessibility [195]. One of these ncRNAs, Hox transcript antisense RNA (HOTAIR), originates from the HOXC locus and silences transcription across 40 kb of the HOXD locus in trans by inducing a repressive chromatin state, which is proposed to occur by recruitment of the Polycomb chromatin remodelling complex PRC2 by HOTAIR (**Figure 4**). Recently, it has been proposed that HOTAIR has the ability to bind other histone-modifying enzymes such as the demethylase LSD1 [196]. In fact, knockdown of HOTAIR induces a rapid loss of LSD1 or PRC2 at hundreds of gene loci with the corresponding increase in expression. This model fits other chromatin modifying complexes, such as Mll, PcG, and G9a methyltransferase, which can be similarly directed by their associated ncRNAs [196]. As modulator of epigenetic landmark, it has been shown that HOTAIR has a profound effect on tumorigenesis. In fact, HOTAIR is upregulated in breast carcinoma and colon cancer and its correlates with metastasis and poor prognosis [197] Enforced expression of HOTAIR consistently changed the pattern of occupancy of Polycomb proteins from the typical epithelial mammary cells pattern to that of embryonic fibroblasts [198]. Another important effect of lncRNAs on chromatin modification that can highlight their impact on cancer is the relationship between the lncRNA ANRIL and the INK4b/ARF/INK4a locus, encoding for three tumor-suppressor genes highly deleted or silenced in a large cohort of tumors [199]. ANRIL, which is transcribed antisense to the protein coding genes of the locus, controls the epigenetic status of the locus by interacting with subunits of PRC1 and PRC2. High expression of ANRIL is found in some cancer tissues and is associated to a high levels of PCR-mediated trimethylated histone H3 lysine27. Inhibition of ANRIL releases PRC1 and PRC2 complexes from the locus, decreases the histone methylation status with the following increase of the protein coding gene transcription. Many other tumor suppressor genes that are frequently silenced by epigenetic mechanisms in cancer also have antisense partners, which can affect gene expression with different other mechanism. First, antisense ncRNAs can mask key cis-elements in mRNA by the formation of RNA duplexes, as in the case of the Zeb2 antisense RNA, which complements the 5' splice site of an intron of Zeb2 mRNA [200]. Expression of the ncRNA prevents the splicing of the intron that contains an internal ribosome entry site required for efficient translation and expression of the ZEB2 protein with a further efficient translation (**Figure 4**). In this context, it has been evaluated that the prevalence of lncRNAs are antisense to introns, hypothesizing their role in the regulation of splicing or capable of generating mRNA duplexes that fuel the RISC machinery to silence gene expression. One major emergent theme is the involvement of the lncRNAs in the assembly or activity of transcription factors functioning as a scaffold for the docking of many proteins, mimicking functional DNA elements or modulation of PolII itself. The first example is represented by the suppression of CCND1 mediated by the lncRNAs through the recruitment and integration of the RNA binding protein TLS into a transcriptional programme. DNA damage signals induce the expression of long ncRNAs associated with the cyclin D1 gene promoter, where they act cooperatively to recruit the RNA binding

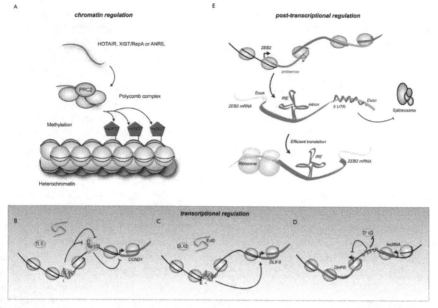

Figure 4. lncRNAs. Schematic representation of the control operated on protein coding gene by the lncRNAs at the level of chromatin remodelling, transcriptional control and post-transcriptional processing. **A**, lncRNAs (Xist, HOTAIR, ANRIL, etc) can recruit chromatin modifying complexes to specific genomic loci to localize their catalytic activity. In this case, the lncRNA recruits the Polycomb complex by inducing trimethylation of the lysine 27 residues (me3K27) of histone H3 to produce heterochromatin formation and repress gene expression. **B, C, D**, lncRNAs can regulate the transcriptional process through a range of mechanisms. First, lncRNAs tethered to the promoter of the cyclin D1 gene recruit the RNA binding protein TLS to modulate the histone acetyltransferase activity of CREB binding protein (CBP) and p300 to repress gene transcription. Second, an ultraconserved enhancer is transcribed as a long ncRNA, Evf2, which subsequently acts as a co-activator to the transcription factor DLX2, to regulate the Dlx6 gene transcription. Third, a lncRNA transcribed from the DHFR minor promoter form a triplex at the major promoter to reduce the access of the general transcription factor TFIID, and thereby suppress DHFR gene expression. **E**, a lncRNA is antisense to Zeb2 mRNA and mask the 5′ splice site resulting in intron retention. This retention results in an efficient Zeb2 translation related to the presence of an internal ribosome entry site (IRE) in the retained intron.

protein TLS. The modified and promoter-docked TLS inhibits the histone acetyltransferase activities of CReB binding protein and p300 inducing the silencing of cyclin D1 expression (Figure 4) [201]. A different co-activator activity mediated by lncRNAs is also evident in the regulation of Dlx genes, important modulators of neuronal development and patterning [202]. Dlx5-6 expression is regulated by two ultraconserved enhancers one of which is transcribed in a lncRNA, named Evf-2. Evf2 forms a stable complex with the homodomein protein DLX-2 which in turn acts as a transcriptional enhancer of Dxl5-6 gene (Figure 4). In some cases, lncRNAs can also affect RNA polymerase activity by influencing the initiation complex in the choice of the promoter. For example, in humans, a ncRNA transcribed from an upstream region of the dihydrofolate reductase (DHFR) locus forms a triplex in the major promoter of DHFR to prevent the binding of the transcriptional co-factor TFIID (Figure 4). This could be a widespread mechanism for controlling promoter usage as thousands of triplex structures exist in eukaryotic chromosomes. Recently, lncRNAs have also shown their tumorigenic potential by modulating the transcriptional program of p53 [203]. An 3kb lncRNAs, linc-RNA-p21, transcriptionally activated by p53, has been shown to collaborate with p53 in order to control the gene expression in response to DNA damage. Specifically, silencing of lincRNA-p21 derepresses the expression of hundred of genes which are also derepressed following p53 knockdown. It has also been discovered that lincRNA-p21 interacts with hnRNPK and this binding is essential for the modulation of p53 activity.

The final category of lncRNAs is represented by those molecules capable to generate the formation of compartmentalized nuclear organelles, subnuclear membraneless nuclear bodies whose funtion is relative unknown. One of them is represented by cell-cycle regulated nuclear foci, named paraspeckles. In addition to protein components, two lncRNAs, NEAT1 and Men epsilon, have been detected as essential part of the paraspeckles. While depletion of NEAT or Men epsilon disrupts the paraspeckles, their overexpression strongly increases their number. There is a number of different lncRNAs that localize to different nuclear regions [204]. Metastasis-associated lung adenocarcinoma transcript 1 (MALAT1) localizes to the splicing speckles, Xist and Kcnq1ot1 both, localize to the perinucleolar region during the S phase of the cell cycle, a class of repeat-associated lncRNAs (es SatIII) are associated to nuclear stress bodies which are produced on specifc pericentromeric heterochromatic domains containing SatIII gene itself.

9. Conclusions

Alterations in microRNAs and other short or long non-coding RNA (ncRNA) are involved in the initiation, progression, and metastasis of human cancer. Over the last decade, a growing number of non-coding transcripts have been found to have roles in gene regulation and RNA processing. The most well known small non-coding RNAs are the microRNAs, but the network of long and short non-coding transcripts is complex and is likely to contain as yet unidentified classes of molecules that form transcriptional regulatory networks. The field of small and long non coding RNAs is rapidly advancing toward in vivo delivery for therapeutic purposes. Advanced molecular therapies aimed at downmodulating or upmodulating the level of a given miRNA in model organisms have been successfully established. RNA-based gene therapy can be used to treat cancer by using RNA or DNA molecules as therapy against the mRNA of genes involved in cancer pathogenesis or by directly targeting the ncRNAs that participate in pathogenesis. The use of miRNAs is still being evaluated preclinically; no clinical or toxicologic studies have been published but the future is promising. Kota and collegues reported that systemic administration of this miRNA in a mouse model of HCC using adeno-associated virus (AAV) results in inhibition of cancer cell proliferation, induction of tumor-specific apoptosis, and dramatic protection from disease progression without toxicity (116). Recently, Pineau et al. (117) identified DNA damage-inducible transcript 4 (DDIT4), a modulator of the mTor pathway, as a bona fide target of miR-221. They introduced into liver cancer cells, by lipofection, LNA-modified oligonucleotides specifically designed for miR-221 (antimiR-221) and miR-222 (antimiR-222) knockdown. Treatment by antagomiRs, but not scrambled oligonucleotide, reduced cell growth in liver cancer cell lines that overexpressed miR-221 and miR-222 by 35% and 22%, respectively. Thus the use of synthetic inhibitors of miR-221 may prove to be a promising approach to liver cancer treatment (117). Despite recent progress in silencing of miRNAs in rodents, the development of effective and safe approaches for sequence-specific antagonism of miRNAs in vivo remains a significant scientific and therapeutic challenge. Recently, Elmen and collaborators (118) showed for the first time, that the simple systemic delivery of an unconjugated, PBS-formulated LNA-antimiR effectively antagonizes the liver-expressed miR-122 in nonhuman primates. Administration by intravenous injections of LNA-antimiR into African green monkeys resulted in the formation of stable heteroduplexes between the LNA-antimiR and miR-122, accompanied by depletion of mature miR-122 and dose-dependent lowering of plasma cholesterol. These findings demonstrate the utility of systemically administered LNA-antimiRs in exploring miRNA functions in primates and show the impressive potential of this strategy to overcome a major hurdle for clinical miRNA therapy. In conclusion, the discovery of small RNAs and their functions has revitalized the prospect of controlling expression of specific genes in vivo, with the ultimate hope of building a new class of gene-specific medical therapies. Just how significant are the ncRNAs? They appear to be doing something important and highly sophisticated; there are so many of them, their sequences are so highly conserved, their expression is tissue specific, and they have recognition sites on more than 30% of the entire transcriptome. It seems that ncRNAs were overlooked in the past simply because researchers were specifically looking for RNAs that code proteins. The above discussed data highlight that the complexity of genomic control operated by the ncRNAs is somewhat greater than previously imagined, and that they could represent a total new order of genomic control. In this scenario, understanding the precise roles of ncRNAs is a key challenge. The targeting of other ncRNAs, in addition to miRNAs, is still in its infancy, but new important developments are expected in this area. Therefore, small RNAs could become powerful therapeutic tools in the near future.

Author details

Gianpiero Di Leva and Michela Garofalo*
The Ohio State University, Department of Molecular Immunology, Virology and Medical Genetics. Columbus, OH, USA

10. References

[1] Matsubara K, Okubo K. (1993). Identification of new genes by systematic analysis of cDNAs and database construction. Curr Opin Biotechnol. 4:672-677.

[2] Liang F, Holt I, Pertea G, Karamycheva S, Salzberg SL, Quackenbush J. (2000). Gene index analysis of the human genome estimates approximately 120,000 genes. Nat Genet. 25:239-240.

---

* Corresponding Author

[3]   Lander ES, Linton LM, Birren B, Nusbaum C, Zody MC, Baldwin J, Devon K, Dewar K,
      Doyle M, FitzHugh W, Funke R, Gage D, Harris K, Heaford A, Howland J, Kann L,
      Lehoczky J, LeVine R, McEwan P, McKernan K, Meldrim J, Mesirov JP, Miranda C,
      Morris W, Naylor J, Raymond C, Rosetti M, Santos R, Sheridan A, Sougnez C, Stange-
      Thomann N, Stojanovic N, Subramanian A, Wyman D, Rogers J, Sulston J, Ainscough
      R, Beck S, Bentley D, Burton J, Clee C, Carter N, Coulson A, Deadman R, Deloukas P,
      Dunham A, Dunham I, Durbin R, French L, Grafham D, Gregory S, Hubbard T,
      Humphray S, Hunt A, Jones M, Lloyd C, McMurray A, Matthews L, Mercer S, Milne S,
      Mullikin JC, Mungall A, Plumb R, Ross M, Shownkeen R, Sims S, Waterston RH,
      Wilson RK, Hillier LW, McPherson JD, Marra MA, Mardis ER, Fulton LA, Chinwalla
      AT, Pepin KH, Gish WR, Chissoe SL, Wendl MC, Delehaunty KD, Miner TL,
      Delehaunty A, Kramer JB, Cook LL, Fulton RS, Johnson DL, Minx PJ, Clifton SW,
      Hawkins T, Branscomb E, Predki P, Richardson P, Wenning S, Slezak T, Doggett N,
      Cheng JF, Olsen A, Lucas S, Elkin C, Uberbacher E, Frazier M, Gibbs RA, Muzny DM,
      Scherer SE, Bouck JB, Sodergren EJ, Worley KC, Rives CM, Gorrell JH, Metzker ML,
      Naylor SL, Kucherlapati RS, Nelson DL, Weinstock GM, Sakaki Y, Fujiyama A, Hattori
      M, Yada T, Toyoda A, Itoh T, Kawagoe C, Watanabe H, Totoki Y, Taylor T,
      Weissenbach J, Heilig R, Saurin W, Artiguenave F, Brottier P, Bruls T, Pelletier E, Robert
      C, Wincker P, Smith DR, Doucette-Stamm L, Rubenfield M, Weinstock K, Lee HM,
      Dubois J, Rosenthal A, Platzer M, Nyakatura G, Taudien S, Rump A, Yang H, Yu J,
      Wang J, Huang G, Gu J, Hood L, Rowen L, Madan A, Qin S, Davis RW, Federspiel NA,
      Abola AP, Proctor MJ, Myers RM, Schmutz J, Dickson M, Grimwood J, Cox DR, Olson
      MV, Kaul R, Raymond C, Shimizu N, Kawasaki K, Minoshima S, Evans GA,
      Athanasiou M, Schultz R, Roe BA, Chen F, Pan H, Ramser J, Lehrach H, Reinhardt R,
      McCombie WR, de la Bastide M, Dedhia N, Blöcker H, Hornischer K, Nordsiek G,
      Agarwala R, Aravind L, Bailey JA, Bateman A, Batzoglou S, Birney E, Bork P, Brown
      DG, Burge CB, Cerutti L, Chen HC, Church D, Clamp M, Copley RR, Doerks T, Eddy
      SR, Eichler EE, Furey TS, Galagan J, Gilbert JG, Harmon C, Hayashizaki Y, Haussler D,
      Hermjakob H, Hokamp K, Jang W, Johnson LS, Jones TA, Kasif S, Kaspryzk A,
      Kennedy S, Kent WJ, Kitts P, Koonin EV, Korf I, Kulp D, Lancet D, Lowe TM,
      McLysaght A, Mikkelsen T, Moran JV, Mulder N, Pollara VJ, Ponting CP, Schuler G,
      Schultz J, Slater G, Smit AF, Stupka E, Szustakowski J, Thierry-Mieg D, Thierry-Mieg J,
      Wagner L, Wallis J, Wheeler R, Williams A, Wolf YI, Wolfe KH, Yang SP, Yeh RF,
      Collins F, Guyer MS, Peterson J, Felsenfeld A, Wetterstrand KA, Patrinos A, Morgan
      MJ, de Jong P, Catanese JJ, Osoegawa K, Shizuya H, Choi S, Chen YJ. (2001).
      International Human Genome Sequencing Consortium. Initial sequencing and analysis
      of the human genome. Nature. 409:860-921.
[4]   Guttman M, Amit I, Garber M, French C, Lin MF, Feldser D, Huarte M, Zuk O, Carey
      BW, Cassady JP, Cabili MN, Jaenisch R, Mikkelsen TS, Jacks T, Hacohen N, Bernstein
      BE, Kellis M, Regev A, Rinn JL, Lander ES. (2009). Chromatin signature reveals over a
      thousand highly conserved large non-coding RNAs in mammals. Nature. 458:223–227
[5]   Guttman M, Garber M, Levin JZ, Donaghey J, Robinson J, Adiconis X, Fan L, Koziol MJ,
      Gnirke A, Nusbaum C, Rinn JL, Lander ES, Regev A. (2010). Ab initio reconstruction of

cell type-specific transcriptomes in mouse reveals the conserved multi-exonic structure of lincRNAs. Nat. Biotechnol. 28:503–510.

[6] Marques AC, Ponting CP. (2009). Catalogues of mammalian long noncoding RNAs: modest conservation and incompleteness. Genome Biol.10:R124.

[7] Cech TR. (2009). Crawling out of the RNA world. Cell. 136:599-602.

[8] Kapranov P, Cheng J, Dike S, Nix DA, Duttagupta R, Willingham AT, Stadler PF, Hertel J, Hackermüller J, Hofacker IL, Bell I, Cheung E, Drenkow J, Dumais E, Patel S, Helt G, Ganesh M, Ghosh S, Piccolboni A, Sementchenko V, Tammana H, Gingeras TR. (2007). RNA maps reveal new RNA classes and a possible function for pervasive transcription. Science. 316:1484–1488.

[9] Crick FH, Barnett L, Brenner S, Watts-Tobin RJ. (1961). General nature of the genetic code for proteins. Nature. 192:1227–1232.

[10] Mercer TR, Dinger ME, Mattick JS. (2009) Long non-coding RNAs insight into functions. Nature Rev. Genet. 10:155–159.

[11] He L, Hannon GJ. (2004). MicroRNAs: small RNAs with a big role in gene regulation. Nature Rev. Genet. 5:522–531.

[12] Mendell JT. (2005). MicroRNAs: critical regulators of development, cellular physiology and malignancy. Cell Cycle 4:1179–1184.

[13] Esquela-Kerscher A, Slack FJ. (2006). OncomiRs — microRNAs with a role in cancer. Nature Rev. Cancer 6:259–269.

[14] Hammond SM. (2007). MicroRNAs as tumor suppressors. Nature Genet. 39:582–583.

[15] Croce CM. (2009). Causes and consequences of microRNA dysregulation in cancer. Nature Rev. Genet. 10:704–714.

[16] Nicoloso M S, Spizzo R, Shimizu M, Rossi S, Calin GA. (2009). MicroRNAs — the micro steering wheel of tumour metastases. Nature Rev. Cancer. 9:293–302.

[17] Carninci P, Kasukawa T, Katayama S, Gough J, Frith MC, Maeda N, Oyama R, Ravasi T, Lenhard B, Wells C, Kodzius R, Shimokawa K, Bajic VB, Brenner SE, Batalov S, Forrest AR, Zavolan M, Davis MJ, Wilming LG, Aidinis V, Allen JE, Ambesi-Impiombato A, Apweiler R, Aturaliya RN, Bailey TL, Bansal M, Baxter L, Beisel KW, Bersano T, Bono H, Chalk AM, Chiu KP, Choudhary V, Christoffels A, Clutterbuck DR, Crowe ML, Dalla E, Dalrymple BP, de Bono B, Della Gatta G, di Bernardo D, Down T, Engstrom P, Fagiolini M, Faulkner G, Fletcher CF, Fukushima T, Furuno M, Futaki S, Gariboldi M, Georgii-Hemming P, Gingeras TR, Gojobori T, Green RE, Gustincich S, Harbers M, Hayashi Y, Hensch TK, Hirokawa N, Hill D, Huminiecki L, Iacono M, Ikeo K, Iwama A, Ishikawa T, Jakt M, Kanapin A, Katoh M, Kawasawa Y, Kelso J, Kitamura H, Kitano H, Kollias G, Krishnan SP, Kruger A, Kummerfeld SK, Kurochkin IV, Lareau LF, Lazarevic D, Lipovich L, Liu J, Liuni S, McWilliam S, Madan Babu M, Madera M, Marchionni L, Matsuda H, Matsuzawa S, Miki H, Mignone F, Miyake S, Morris K, Mottagui-Tabar S, Mulder N, Nakano N, Nakauchi H, Ng P, Nilsson R, Nishiguchi S, Nishikawa S, Nori F, Ohara O, Okazaki Y, Orlando V, Pang KC, Pavan WJ, Pavesi G, Pesole G, Petrovsky N, Piazza S, Reed J, Reid JF, Ring BZ, Ringwald M, Rost B, Ruan Y, Salzberg SL, Sandelin A, Schneider C, Schönbach C, Sekiguchi K, Semple CA, Seno S, Sessa L, Sheng Y, Shibata Y, Shimada H, Shimada K, Silva D, Sinclair B, Sperling S, Stupka E, Sugiura K, Sultana R, Takenaka Y, Taki K, Tammoja K, Tan SL, Tang S, Taylor MS, Tegner J,

Teichmann SA, Ueda HR, van Nimwegen E, Verardo R, Wei CL, Yagi K, Yamanishi H, Zabarovsky E, Zhu S, Zimmer A, Hide W, Bult C, Grimmond SM, Teasdale RD, Liu ET, Brusic V, Quackenbush J, Wahlestedt C, Mattick JS, Hume DA, Kai C, Sasaki D, Tomaru Y, Fukuda S, Kanamori-Katayama M, Suzuki M, Aoki J, Arakawa T, Iida J, Imamura K, Itoh M, Kato T, Kawaji H, Kawagashira N, Kawashima T, Kojima M, Kondo S, Konno H, Nakano K, Ninomiya N, Nishio T, Okada M, Plessy C, Shibata K, Shiraki T, Suzuki S, Tagami M, Waki K, Watahiki A, Okamura-Oho Y, Suzuki H, Kawai J, Hayashizaki Y; FANTOM Consortium; RIKEN Genome Exploration Research Group and Genome Science Group (Genome Network Project Core Group).(2005). The transcriptional landscape of the mammalian genome. Science. 309:1559–1563.

[18] Gibb EA, Brown CJ, Lam WL. (2011). The functional role of long non-coding RNA in human carcinomas. Mol Cancer 10:38.

[19] Taft RJ, Pang KC, MErcer TR, Dinger M, Mattick JS. (2010) Non-coding RNAs: regulators of disease. J Pathol.220:126-39.

[20] Di Leva G, Croce CM. (2010). Roles of small RNAs in tumor formation. Trends Mol Med.16:257-67.

[21] Garofalo M, Croce CM. (2011). microRNAs: Master regulators as potential therapeutics in cancer. Annu Rev Pharmacol Toxicol. 51:25-43.

[22] ENCODE Project Consortium, Birney E, Stamatoyannopoulos JA, Dutta A, Guigó R, Gingeras TR, Margulies EH, Weng Z, Snyder M, Dermitzakis ET, Thurman RE, Kuehn MS, Taylor CM, Neph S, Koch CM, Asthana S, Malhotra A, Adzhubei I, Greenbaum JA, Andrews RM, Flicek P, Boyle PJ, Cao H, Carter NP, Clelland GK, Davis S, Day N, Dhami P, Dillon SC, Dorschner MO, Fiegler H, Giresi PG, Goldy J, Hawrylycz M, Haydock A, Humbert R, James KD, Johnson BE, Johnson EM, Frum TT, Rosenzweig ER, Karnani N, Lee K, Lefebvre GC, Navas PA, Neri F, Parker SC, Sabo PJ, Sandstrom R, Shafer A, Vetrie D, Weaver M, Wilcox S, Yu M, Collins FS, Dekker J, Lieb JD, Tullius TD, Crawford GE, Sunyaev S, Noble WS, Dunham I, Denoeud F, Reymond A, Kapranov P, Rozowsky J, Zheng D, Castelo R, Frankish A, Harrow J, Ghosh S, Sandelin A, Hofacker IL, Baertsch R, Keefe D, Dike S, Cheng J, Hirsch HA, Sekinger EA, Lagarde J, Abril JF, Shahab A, Flamm C, Fried C, Hackermüller J, Hertel J, Lindemeyer M, Missal K, Tanzer A, Washietl S, Korbel J, Emanuelsson O, Pedersen JS, Holroyd N, Taylor R, Swarbreck D, Matthews N, Dickson MC, Thomas DJ, Weirauch MT, Gilbert J, Drenkow J, Bell I, Zhao X, Srinivasan KG, Sung WK, Ooi HS, Chiu KP, Foissac S, Alioto T, Brent M, Pachter L, Tress ML, Valencia A, Choo SW, Choo CY, Ucla C, Manzano C, Wyss C, Cheung E, Clark TG, Brown JB, Ganesh M, Patel S, Tammana H, Chrast J, Henrichsen CN, Kai C, Kawai J, Nagalakshmi U, Wu J, Lian Z, Lian J, Newburger P, Zhang X, Bickel P, Mattick JS, Carninci P, Hayashizaki Y, Weissman S, Hubbard T, Myers RM, Rogers J, Stadler PF, Lowe TM, Wei CL, Ruan Y, Struhl K, Gerstein M, Antonarakis SE, Fu Y, Green ED, Karaöz U, Siepel A, Taylor J, Liefer LA, Wetterstrand KA, Good PJ, Feingold EA, Guyer MS, Cooper GM, Asimenos G, Dewey CN, Hou M, Nikolaev S, Montoya-Burgos JI, Löytynoja A, Whelan S, Pardi F, Massingham T, Huang H, Zhang NR, Holmes I, Mullikin JC, Ureta-Vidal A, Paten B, Seringhaus M, Church D, Rosenbloom K, Kent WJ, Stone EA; NISC Comparative Sequencing Program; Baylor College of Medicine Human Genome Sequencing Center; Washington University

Genome Sequencing Center; Broad Institute; Children's Hospital Oakland Research Institute, Batzoglou S, Goldman N, Hardison RC, Haussler D, Miller W, Sidow A, Trinklein ND, Zhang ZD, Barrera L, Stuart R, King DC, Ameur A, Enroth S, Bieda MC, Kim J, Bhinge AA, Jiang N, Liu J, Yao F, Vega VB, Lee CW, Ng P, Shahab A, Yang A, Moqtaderi Z, Zhu Z, Xu X, Squazzo S, Oberley MJ, Inman D, Singer MA, Richmond TA, Munn KJ, Rada-Iglesias A, Wallerman O, Komorowski J, Fowler JC, Couttet P, Bruce AW, Dovey OM, Ellis PD, Langford CF, Nix DA, Euskirchen G, Hartman S, Urban AE, Kraus P, Van Calcar S, Heintzman N, Kim TH, Wang K, Qu C, Hon G, Luna R, Glass CK, Rosenfeld MG, Aldred SF, Cooper SJ, Halees A, Lin JM, Shulha HP, Zhang X, Xu M, Haidar JN, Yu Y, Ruan Y, Iyer VR, Green RD, Wadelius C, Farnham PJ, Ren B, Harte RA, Hinrichs AS, Trumbower H, Clawson H, Hillman-Jackson J, Zweig AS, Smith K, Thakkapallayil A, Barber G, Kuhn RM, Karolchik D, Armengol L, Bird CP, de Bakker PI, Kern AD, Lopez-Bigas N, Martin JD, Stranger BE, Woodroffe A, Davydov E, Dimas A, Eyras E, Hallgrímsdóttir IB, Huppert J, Zody MC, Abecasis GR, Estivill X, Bouffard GG, Guan X, Hansen NF, Idol JR, Maduro VV, Maskeri B, McDowell JC, Park M, Thomas PJ, Young AC, Blakesley RW, Muzny DM, Sodergren E, Wheeler DA, Worley KC, Jiang H, Weinstock GM, Gibbs RA, Graves T, Fulton R, Mardis ER, Wilson RK, Clamp M, Cuff J, Gnerre S, Jaffe DB, Chang JL, Lindblad-Toh K, Lander ES, Koriabine M, Nefedov M, Osoegawa K, Yoshinaga Y, Zhu B, de Jong PJ. Identification and analysis of functional elements in 1% of the human genome by the ENCODE pilot project.(2007). Nature.447:799-816.

[23] Siomi MC, Sato K, Pezic D, Aravin AA. (2011). PIWI-interacting small RNAs: the vanguard of genome defence. Nat Rev Mol Cell Biol.12:246-58.

[24] Faulkner GJ, Kimura Y, Daub CO, Wani S, Plessy C, Irvine KM, Schroder K, Cloonan N, Steptoe AL, Lassmann T, Waki K, Hornig N, Arakawa T, Takahashi H, Kawai J, Forrest AR, Suzuki H, Hayashizaki Y, Hume DA, Orlando V, Grimmond SM, Carninci P. (2009). The regulated retrotransposon transcriptome of mammalian cells. Nat Genet. 41:563-71.

[25] Huarte M, Rinn JL. (2010). Large non-coding RNAs: missing links in cancer? Hum Mol Genet. 19:R152-61.

[26] Pauli A, Rinn JL, Schier AF. (2011). Non-coding RNAs as regulators of embryogenesis. Nat Rev Genet.12:136–49.

[27] Calin GA, Liu CG, Ferracin M, Hyslop T, Spizzo R, Sevignani C, Fabbri M, Cimmino A, Lee EJ, Wojcik SE, Shimizu M, Tili E, Rossi S, Taccioli C, Pichiorri F, Liu X, Zupo S, Herlea V, Gramantieri L, Lanza G, Alder H, Rassenti L, Volinia S, Schmittgen TD, Kipps TJ, Negrini M, Croce CM. (2007). Ultraconserved regions encoding ncRNAs are altered in human leukemias and carcinomas. Cancer Cell. 12:215-29.

[28] Poliseno L, Salmena L, Zhang J, Carver B, Haveman WJ, Pandolfi PP. (2010). A coding-independent function of gene and pseudogene mRNAs regulates tumour biology. Nature. 465:1033-8.

[29] He Y, Vogelstein B, Velculescu VE, Papadopoulos N, Kinzler KW. (2008). The antisense transcriptomes of human cells. Science. 322:1855-7.

[30] Kim TK, Hemberg M, Gray JM, Costa AM, Bear DM, Wu J, Harmin DA, Laptewicz M, Barbara-Haley K, Kuersten S, Markenscoff-Papadimitriou E, Kuhl D, Bito H, Worley PF,

Kreiman G, Greenberg ME. (2010). Widespread transcription at neuronal activity-regulated enhancers. Nature. 465:182-7.

[31] Lee RC, Feinbaum RL, Ambros V. (1993). The C. elegans heterochronic gene lin-4 encodes small RNAs with antisense complementarity to lin-14. Cell. 75:843–54.

[32] Kim VN. 2005. MicroRNA biogenesis: coordinated cropping and dicing. Nat. Rev. Mol. Cell Biol. 6:376–85.

[33] Rodriguez A, Griffiths-Jones S, Ashurst JL, Bradley A. (2004). Identification of mammalian microRNA host genes and transcription units. Genome Res. 14:1902–10.

[34] Lagos-Quintana M, Rauhut R, Yalcin A, Meyer J, Lendeckel W, Tuschl T. (2002). Identification of tissue-specific microRNAs from mouse. Curr Biol. 12: 735–739.

[35] Altuvia Y, Landgraf P, Lithwick G, Elefant N, Pfeffer S, Aravin A, Brownstein MJ, Tuschl T, Margalit H.(2005). Clustering and conservation patterns of human microRNAs. Nucleic Acids Res 33: 2697–2706.

[36] Borchert GM, Lanier W, Davidson BL. (2006). RNA polymerase III transcribes human microRNAs. Nat Struct Mol Biol. 13: 1097–1101.

[37] Han J, Lee Y, Yeom KH, Nam JW, Heo I, Rhee JK, Sohn SY, Cho Y, Zhang BT, Kim VN. (2006). Molecular basis for the recognition of primary microRNAs by the Drosha-DGCR8 complex. Cell 125: 887–901.

[38] Saetrom P, Snove O, Nedland M, Grunfeld TB, Lin Y, Bass MB, Cannon JR. (2006). Conserved microRNA characteristics in mammals. Oligonucleotides. 16:115-44.

[39] Gregory RI, Yan KP, Amuthan G, Chendrimada T, Doratotaj B, Cooch N, Shiekhattar R. (2004). The Microprocessor complex mediates the genesis of microRNAs. Nature 432:235–40.

[40] Han J, Lee Y, Yeom KH, Kim YK, Jin H, Kim VN. (2004). The Drosha-DGCR8 complex in primary microRNA processing. Genes Dev. 18:3016–27.

[41] Yi R, Qin Y, Macara IG, Cullen BR. (2003). Exportin-5 mediates the nuclear export of pre-microRNAs and short hairpin RNAs. Genes Dev. 17:3011–3016.

[42] Lund E, Guttinger S, Calado A, Dahlberg JE, Kutay U. (2004). Nuclear export of microRNA precursors. Science. 303:95–98.

[43] Bohnsack MT, Czaplinski K, Gorlich D. (2004). Exportin 5 is a RanGTP-dependent dsRNA-binding protein that mediates nuclear export of pre-miRNAs. RNA. 10:185–191.

[44] Maniataki E, Mourelatos Z. (2005). A human, ATP-independent, RISC assembly machine fueled by pre-miRNA. Genes Dev. 19:2979–2990.

[45] Lee Y, Hur I, Park SY, Kim YK, Suh MR, Kim VN. (2006). The role of PACT in the RNA silencing pathway. EMBO J. 25:522–532.

[46] Haase AD, Jaskiewicz L, Zhang H, Laine S, Sack R, Gatignol A, Filipowicz W. (2005). TRBP, a regulator of cellular PKR and HIV-1 virus expression, interacts with Dicer and functions in RNA silencing. EMBO Rep 6: 961–967.

[47] Gregory RI, Chendrimada TP, Cooch N, Shiekhattar R. (2005). Human RISC couples microRNA biogenesis and posttranscriptional gene silencing. Cell. 123:631–640.

[48] Forstemann K, Tomari Y, Du T, Vagin VV, Denli AM, Bratu DP, Klattenhoff C, Theurkauf WE, Zamore PD. (2005). Normal microRNA maturation and germ-line stem cell maintenance requires Loquacious, a double-stranded RNA-binding domain protein. PLoS Biol. 3:e236.

[49] Chendrimada TP, Gregory RI, Kumaraswamy E, Norman J, Cooch N, Nishikura K,Nishikura K, Shiekhattar R. (2005). TRBP recruits the Dicer complex to Ago2 for microRNA processing and gene silencing. Nature. 436: 740–744.

[50] Castanotto D, Sakurai K, Lingeman R, Li H, Shively L, Aagaard L, Soifer H, Gatignol A, Riggs A, Rossi JJ. (2007). Combinatorial delivery of small interfering RNAs reduces RNAi efficacy by selective incorporation into RISC. Nucleic Acids Res. 35:5154-64.

[51] Rand TA, Petersen S, Du F, Wang X. (2005). Argonaute2 cleaves the anti-guide strand of siRNA during RISC activation. Cell. 123:621–29.

[52] Leuschner PJ, Ameres SL, Kueng S, Martinez J. (2006). Cleavage of the siRNA passenger strand during RISC assembly in human cells. EMBO Rep. 7:314–20.

[53] Martinez J, Patkaniowska A, UrlaubH, Luhrmann R, Tuschl T. (2002). Single-stranded antisense siRNAs guide target RNA cleavage in RNAi. Cell. 110:563–74.

[54] Zamore PD, Tuschl T, Sharp PA, Bartel DP. (2000). RNAi: double-stranded RNA directs the ATP-dependent cleavage of mRNA at 21 to 23 nucleotide intervals. Cell. 101: 25–33.

[55] Yekta S, Shih IH, Bartel DP. (2004). MicroRNA-directed cleavage of HOXB8 mRNA. Science. 304: 594–596.

[56] Wu L, Fan J, Belasco JG. (2006). MicroRNAs direct rapid deadenylation of mRNA. Proc Natl Acad Sci USA. 103: 4034–4039.

[57] Bagga S, Bracht J, Hunter S, Massirer K, Holtz J, Eachus R, Pasquinelli AE. (2005). Regulation by let-7 and lin-4 miRNAs results in target mRNA degradation. Cell. 122: 553–563.

[58] Reinhart BJ, Slack FJ, Basson M, Pasquinelli AE, Bettinger JC, Rougvie AE, Horvitz HR, Ruvkun G. (2000). The 21-nucleotide let-7 RNA regulates developmental timing in Caenorhabditis elegans. Nature 403: 901–906.

[59] Olsen PH, Ambros V. (1999). The lin-4 regulatory RNA controls developmental timing in Caenorhabditis elegans by blocking LIN-14 protein synthesis after the initiation of translation. Dev Biol. 216: 671–680.

[60] Pillai RS, Bhattacharyya SN, Filipowicz W. (2007). Repression of protein synthesis by miRNAs: how many mechanisms? Trends Cell Biol. 17:118–26.

[61] Garzon R, Fabbri M, Cimmino A, Calin GA, Croce CM. (2006). MicroRNA expression and function in cancer. Trends Mol. Med. 12:580-587.

[62] Wu W, Sun M, Zou GM, Chen J. (2007). MicroRNA and cancer: Current status and prospective. Int. J. Cancer.120: 953-960.

[63] Boettger T, Braun T. (2012). A New Level of Complexity: The Role of MicroRNAs in Cardiovascular Development. Circ Res.110:1000-1013.

[64] Han R, Kan Q, Sun Y, Wang S, Zhang G, Peng T, Jia Y. (2012). MiR-9 promotes the neural differentiation of mouse bone marrow mesenchymal stem cells via targeting zinc finger protein 521. Neurosci Lett. Ahead of print.

[65] D'Urso PI, D'Urso OF, Storelli C, Mallardo M, Gianfreda CD, Montinaro A, Cimmino A, Pietro C, Marsigliante S. (2012). miR-155 is up-regulated in primary and secondary glioblastoma and promotes tumour growth by inhibiting GABA receptors. Int J Oncol. doi: 10.3892/ijo.2012.1420.

[66] Garofalo M, Romano G, Di Leva G, Nuovo G, Jeon YJ, Ngankeu A, Sun J, Lovat F, Alder H, Condorelli G, Engelman JA, Ono M, Rho JK, Cascione L, Volinia S, Nephew KP,

Croce CM. (2011). EGFR and MET receptor tyrosine kinase-altered microRNA expression induces tumorigenesis and gefitinib resistance in lung cancers. Nat Med.18:74-82.

[67] Frank D, Gantenberg J, Boomgaarden I, Kuhn C, Will R, Jarr KU, Eden M, Kramer K, Luedde M, Mairbäurl H, Katus HA, Frey N. (2012). MicroRNA-20a inhibits stress-induced cardiomyocyte apoptosis involving its novel target Egln3/PHD3. J Mol Cell Cardiol. 52:711-717.

[68] Calin GA, DumitruCD, ShimizuM,BichiR, Zupo S, Noch E, Aldler H, Rattan S, Keating M, Rai K, Rassenti L, Kipps T, Negrini M, Bullrich F, Croce CM. (2002). Frequent deletions and down-regulation of micro-RNA genes miR15 and miR16 at 13q14 in chronic lymphocytic leukemia. Proc. Natl. Acad. Sci. USA. 99:15524–29

[69] Calin GA, Croce CM. (2006). MicroRNA signatures in human cancers. Nat Rev Cancer. 6:857–866.

[70] Cai X, Hagedorn CH, Cullen BR. (2004). Human microRNAs are processed from capped, polyadenylated transcripts that can also function as mRNAs. RNA. 10:1957–1966.

[71] Cai X, Hagedorn CH, Cullen BR. (2004). Human microRNAs are processed from capped, polyadenylated transcripts that can also function as mRNAs. RNA. 10:1957–1966.

[72] Chan JA, Krichevsky AM, Kosik KS. 2005. MicroRNA-21 is an antiapoptotic factor in human glioblastoma cells. Cancer Res. 65:6029–6033.

[73] Zhu S, Wu H, Wu F, Nie D, Sheng S, Mo YY. (2008). MicroRNA-21 targets tumor suppressor genes in invasion and metastasis. Cell Res. 18:350–359.

[74] Zhu Q, Wang Z, Hu Y, Li J, Li X, Zhou L, Huang Y. (2012). miR-21 promotes migration and invasion by the miR-21-PDCD4-AP-1 feedback loop in human hepatocellular carcinoma. Oncol Rep.27:1660-1668.

[75] Medina PP, Nolde M, Slack FJ. (2010). OncomiR addiction in an in vivo model of microRNA-21-induced pre-B-cell lymphoma. Nature. 467:86-90.

[76] Metzler M, Wilda M, Busch K, Viehmann S, Borkhardt A. (2004). High expression of precursor microRNA-155/BIC RNA in children with Burkitt lymphoma. Genes Chromosom. Cancer. 39:167–169.

[77] Kluiver J, Poppema S, de Jong D, Blokzijl T, Harms G, Jacobs S, Kroesen BJ, van den Berg A. (2005). BIC and miR-155 are highly expressed in Hodgkin, primary mediastinal and diffuse large B cell lymphomas. J. Pathol. 207:243–249.

[78] Calin GA, Ferracin M, Cimmino A, Di Leva G, Shimizu M, Wojcik SE, Iorio MV, Visone R, Sever NI, Fabbri M, Iuliano R, Palumbo T, Pichiorri F, Roldo C, Garzon R, Sevignani C, Rassenti L, Alder H, Volinia S, Liu CG, Kipps TJ, Negrini M, Croce CM.(2005). A microRNA signature associated with prognosis and progression in chronic lymphocytic leukemia. N. Engl. J. Med. 353:1793–1801.

[79] Garzon R, Volinia S, Liu CG, Fernandez-Cymering C, Palumbo T, Pichiorri F, Fabbri M, Coombes K, Alder H, Nakamura T, Flomenberg N, Marcucci G, Calin GA, Kornblau SM, Kantarjian H, Bloomfield CD, Andreeff M, Croce CM. (2008). MicroRNA signatures associated with cytogenetics and prognosis in acute myeloid leukemia. Blood. 111:3183–3189.

[80] Volinia S, Calin GA, Liu CG, Ambs S, Cimmino A, Petrocca F, Visone R, Iorio M, Roldo C, Ferracin M, Prueitt RL, Yanaihara N, Lanza G, Scarpa A, Vecchione A, Negrini M, Harris CC, Croce CM. (2006). A microRNA expression signature of human solid tumors defines cancer gene targets. Proc. Natl. Acad. Sci. USA. 103:2257–2261.

[81] Greither T, Grochola LF, Udelnow A, Lautenschlager C, W"url P, Taubert H. (2010). Elevated expression of microRNAs 155, 203, 210 and 222 in pancreatic tumors is associated with poorer survival. Int. J. Cancer. 126:73–80.

[82] Costinean S, Zanesi N, Pekarsky Y, Tili E, Volinia S, Heerema N, Croce CM. (2006). Pre-B cell proliferation and lymphoblastic leukemia/high-grade lymphoma in E(mu)-miR155 transgenic mice. Proc Natl Acad Sci U S A. 103:7024-7029.

[83] Pallante P, Visone R, Ferracin M, Ferraro A, Berlingieri MT, Troncone G, Chiappetta G, Liu CG, Santoro M, Negrini M, Croce CM, Fusco A. (2006). MicroRNA deregulation in human thyroid papillary carcinomas. Endocr. Relat. Cancer. 13:497–508.

[84] Fornari F, Gramantieri L, Ferracin M, Veronese A, Sabbioni S, Calin GA, Grazi GL, Giovannini C, Croce CM, Bolondi L, Negrini M. (2008). MiR-221 control CDKN1C/p57 and CDKN1B/p27 expression in human hepatocellular carcinoma. Oncogene. 27:5651–5661.

[85] Di Leva G, Gasparini P, Piovan C, Ngankeu A, Garofalo M, Taccioli C, Iorio MV, Li M, Volinia S, Alder H, Nakamura T, Nuovo G, Liu Y, Nephew KP, Croce CM. (2010). MicroRNA cluster 221–222 and estrogen receptor αinteractions in breast cancer. J. Natl. Cancer Inst. 102:706–721.

[86] Felicetti F, Errico MC, Bottero L, Segnalini P, Stoppacciaro A, Biffoni M, Felli N, Mattia G, Petrini M, Colombo MP, Peschle C, Carè A. (2008). The promyelocytic leukemia zinc finger–microRNA-221/-222 pathway controls melanoma progression through multiple oncogenic mechanisms. Cancer Res. 68:2745–2754.

[87] le Sage C, Nagel R, Egan DA, Schrier M, Mesman E, Mangiola A, Anile C, Maira G, Mercatelli N, Ciafrè SA, Farace MG, Agami R. (2007). Regulation of the p27Kip1 tumor suppressor by miR-221 and miR-222 promotes cancer cell proliferation. EMBO J. 26:3699–3708.

[88] Garofalo M, Quintavalle C, Di Leva G, Zanca C, Romano G, Taccioli C, Liu CG, Croce CM, Condorelli G. (2008). MicroRNA signatures of TRAIL resistance in human non-small cell lung cancer. Oncogene. 27:3845–3855.

[89] Garofalo M, Di Leva G, Romano G, Nuovo G, Suh SS, Ngankeu A, Taccioli C, Pichiorri F, Alder H, Secchiero P, Gasparini P, Gonelli A, Costinean S, Acunzo M, Condorelli G, Croce CM. (2009). miR-221&222 regulate TRAIL resistance and enhance tumorigenicity through PTEN and TIMP3 downregulation. Cancer Cell. 16:498–509.

[90] Petrocca F, Visone R, Onelli MR, Shah MH, Nicoloso MS, de Martino I, Iliopoulos D, Pilozzi E, Liu CG, Negrini M, Cavazzini L, Volinia S, Alder H, Ruco LP, Baldassarre G, Croce CM, Vecchione A. (2008). E2F1-regulated microRNAs impair TGFβ-dependent cell-cycle arrest and apoptosis in gastric cancer. Cancer Cell. 13:272–286.

[91] Ota A, Tagawa H, Karnan S, Tsuzuki S, Karpas A, Kira S, Yoshida Y, Seto M. (2004). Identification and characterization of a novel gene, C13orf25, as a target for 13q31-q32 amplification in malignant lymphoma. Cancer Res. 64:3087–3095.

[92] Hayashita Y, Osada H, Tatematsu Y, Yamada H, Yanagisawa K, Tomida S, Yatabe Y, Kawahara K, Sekido Y, Takahashi T. (2005). A polycistronic microRNA cluster, miR-17-92, is overexpressed in human lung cancers and enhances cell proliferation. Cancer Res. 65:9628–9632.

[93] Ventura A, Young AG, Winslow MM, Lintault L, Meissner A, Erkeland SJ, Newman J, Bronson RT, Crowley D, Stone JR, Jaenisch R, Sharp PA, Jacks T. (2008). Targeted deletion reveals essential and overlapping functions of the miR-17 through 92 family of miRNA clusters. Cell.132:875-886.

[94] Park JK, Lee EJ, Esau C, Schmittgen TD. (2009). Antisense inhibition of microRNA-21 or -221 arrests cell cycle, induces apoptosis, and sensitizes the effects of gemcitabine in pancreatic adenocarcinoma. Pancreas. 38:e190–199.

[95] Inomata M, Tagawa H, Guo YM, Kameoka Y, Takahashi N, Sawada K. (2009). MicroRNA-17-92 downregulates expression of distinct targets in different B-cell lymphoma subtypes. Blood. 113:396–402.

[96] Wang PY, Li YJ, Zhang S, Li ZL, Yue Z, Xie N, Xie SY. (2010). Regulating A549 cells growth by ASO inhibiting miRNA expression. Mol. Cell. Biochem. 339:163–171.

[97] Bandi N, Zbinden S, Gugger M, Arnold M, Kocher V, Hasan L, Kappeler A, Brunner T, Vassella E. (2009). miR-15a and miR-16 are implicated in cell cycle regulation in a Rb-dependent manner and are frequently deleted or down-regulated in non–small cell lung cancer. Cancer Res. 69:5553–5559.

[98] Cimmino A, Calin GA, Fabbri M, Iorio MV, Ferracin M, Shimizu M, Wojcik SE, Aqeilan RI, Zupo S, Dono M, Rassenti L, Alder H, Volinia S, Liu CG, Kipps TJ, Negrini M, Croce CM. (2005). miR-15 and miR-16 induce apoptosis by targeting BCL2. Proc. Natl. Acad. Sci. USA.102:13944–13949.

[99] Klein U, Lia M, Crespo M, Siegel R, Shen Q, Mo T, Ambesi-Impiombato A, Califano A, Migliazza A, Bhagat G, Dalla-Favera R. (2010). The DLEU2/miR-15a/16-1 cluster controls B cell proliferation and its deletion leads to chronic lymphocytic leukemia. Cancer Cell 17:28–40.

[100] Bonci D, Coppola V, Musumeci M, Addario A, Giuffrida R, Memeo L, D'Urso L, Pagliuca A, Biffoni M, Labbaye C, Bartucci M, Muto G, Peschle C, De Maria R. (2008). The miR-15a–miR-16-1 cluster controls prostate cancer by targeting multiple oncogenic activities. Nat. Med. 14:1271–1277.

[101] He X, He L, Hannon GJ. (2007). The guardian's little helper: microRNAs in the p53 tumor suppressor network. Cancer Res.67:11099-11101.

[102] He L, He X, Lim LP, de Stanchina E, Xuan Z, Liang Y, Xue W, Zender L, Magnus J, Ridzon D, Jackson AL, Linsley PS, Chen C, Lowe SW, Cleary MA, Hannon GJ. (2007). A microRNA component of the p53 tumour suppressor network. Nature. 447:1130-1134.

[103] Cole KA, Attiyeh EF, Mosse YP, Laquaglia MJ, Diskin SJ, Brodeur GM, Maris JM. (2008). A functional screen identifies miR-34a as a candidate neuroblastoma tumor suppressor gene. Mol. Cancer Res. 6:735–742.

[104] Siemens H, Jackstadt R, Hünten S, Kaller M, Menssen A, Götz U, Hermeking H. (2011). miR-34 and SNAIL form a double-negative feedback loop to regulate epithelial-mesenchymal transitions. Cell Cycle.10:4256-4271.

[105] Tsai WC, Hsu PW, Lai TC, Chau GY, Lin CW, Chen CM, Lin CD, Liao YL, Wang JL, Chau YP, Hsu MT, Hsiao M, Huang HD, Tsou AP. (2009). MicroRNA-122, a tumor suppressor microRNA that regulates intrahepatic metastasis of hepatocellular carcinoma. Hepatology. 49:1571-1582.

[106] Xu Y, Xia F, Ma L, Shan J, Shen J, Yang Z, Liu J, Cui Y, Bian X, Bie P, Qian C. (2011). MicroRNA-122 sensitizes HCC cancer cells to adriamycin and vincristine through modulating expression of MDR and inducing cell cycle arrest. Cancer Lett. 310:160-169.

[107] Xu J, Zhu X, Wu L, Yang R, Yang Z, Wang Q, Wu F. (2012). MicroRNA-122 suppresses cell proliferation and induces cell apoptosis in hepatocellular carcinoma by directly targeting Wnt/β-catenin pathway. Liver Int. 32:752-760.

[108] Coulouarn C, Factor VM, Andersen JB, Durkin ME, Thorgeirsson SS. (2009). Loss of miR-122 expression in liver cancer correlates with suppression of the hepatic phenotype and gain of metastatic properties. Oncogene. 28:3526-3536.

[109] Hsu SH, Wang B, Kota J, Yu J, Costinean S, Kutay H, Yu L, Bai S, La Perle K, Chivukula RR, Mao H, Wei M, Clark KR, Mendell JR, Caligiuri MA, Jacob ST, Mendell JT, Ghoshal K. (2012). Essential metabolic, anti-inflammatory, and anti-tumorigenic functions of miR-122 in liver. J Clin Invest.122:2871-2883.

[110] Nguyen DX, Bos PD, Massague J. (2009). Metastasis: From dissemination to organ-specific colonization. Nat. Rev. Cancer.9:274–284.

[111] Hanahan D, Weinberg RA. (2000). The hallmarks of cancer. Cell.100:57–70.

[112] Steeg PS. (2006). Tumor metastasis: Mechanistic insights and clinical challenges. Nat. Med.12:895–904.

[113] Ma L, Reinhardt F, Pan E, Soutschek J, Bhat B, Marcusson EG, Teruya-Feldstein J, Bell GW, Weinberg RA. (2010). Therapeutic silencing of miR-10b inhibits metastasis in a mouse mammary tumor model. Nat. Biotechnol.28:341–347

[114] Tavazoie SF, Alarcon C, Oskarsson T, Padua D, Wang Q, Bos PD, Gerald WL, Massagué J. (2008). Endogenous human microRNAs that suppress breast cancer metastasis. Nature. 451:147–52.

[115] Valastyan S, Reinhardt F, Benaich N, Calogrias D, Szász AM, Wang ZC, Brock JE, Richardson AL, Weinberg RA. (2009). A pleiotropically acting microRNA, miR-31, inhibits breast cancer metastasis. Cell. 137:1032–1046.

[116] Ma L, Young J, Prabhala H, Pan E, Mestdagh P, Muth D, Teruya-Feldstein J, Reinhardt F, Onder TT, Valastyan S, Westermann F, Speleman F, Vandesompele J, Weinberg RA. (2010). MiR-9, a MYC/MYCN-activated microRNA, regulates E-cadherin and cancer metastasis. Nat. Cell Biol.12: 247–256.

[117] Gregory, P.A., et al., The miR-200 family and miR-205 regulate epithelial to mesenchymal transition by targeting ZEB1 and SIP1. Nat Cell Biol, 2008. 10(5): p. 593-601.

[118] Gibbons, D.L., et al., Contextual extracellular cues promote tumor cell EMT and metastasis by regulating miR-200 family expression. Genes Dev, 2009. 23(18): p. 2140-51.

[119] Korpal, M., et al., Direct targeting of Sec23a by miR-200s influences cancer cell secretome and promotes metastatic colonization. Nat Med, 2011. 17(9): p. 1101-8.

[120] Kiss-Laszlo, Z., Henry, Y., Bachellerie, J., Caizergues- Ferrer, M. & Kiss, T. (1996). Site-specific ribose methylation of preribosomal RNA: a novel function for small nucleolar RNAs. Cell. 85:1077–1088.

[121] Tollervey, D. & Kiss, T. (1997). Function and synthesis of small nucleolar RNAs. Curr. Opin. Cell Biol. 9:337–342.

[122] Weinstein L. B., Steitz J. A. (1999). Guided tours: from precursor snoRNA to functional snoRNP. Curr. Opin. Cell Biol. 11: 378–384.

[123] Williams GT, Hughes JP, Stoneman V, Anderson CL, McCarthy NJ, Mourtada-Maarabouni M, Pickard M, Hedge VL, Trayner I, Farzaneh F. (2006). Isolation of genes controlling apoptosis through their effects on cell survival. Gene Ther. Mol. Biol.10B:255–261.

[124] Mourtada-Maarabouni M, Hedge VL, Kirkham L, Farzaneh F, Williams GT. (2008). Growth arrest in human T-cells is controlled by the non-coding RNA growth-arrest-specific transcript 5 (GAS5). J. Cell Sci. 121:939–946.

[125] Mourtada-Maarabouni M, Pickard MR, Hedge VL, Farzaneh F, Williams GT. (2009) GAS5, a non-protein-coding RNA, controls apoptosis and is downregulated in breast cancer. Oncogene. 28:195–208.

[126] Dong XY, Guo P, Boyd J, Sun X, Li Q, Zhou W, Dong JT. (2009). Implication of snoRNA U50 in human breast cancer. J. Genet. Genomics 36:447–454.

[127] Dong XY, Rodriguez C, Guo P, Sun X, Talbot JT, Zhou W, Petros J, Li Q, Vessella RL, Kibel AS, Stevens VL, Calle EE, Dong JT. (2008). SnoRNA U50 is a candidate tumor-suppressor gene at 6q14.3 with a mutation associated with clinically significant prostate cancer. Hum. Mol. Genet. 17:1031–1042.

[128] Gee HE, Buffa FM, Camps C, Ramachandran A, Leek R, Taylor M, Patil M, Sheldon H, Betts G, Homer J, West C, Ragoussis J, Harris AL. (2011). The small-nucleolar RNAs commonly used for microRNA normalisation correlate with tumour pathology and prognosis. Br. J. Cancer. 104:1168–1177.

[129] Liao J, Yu L, Mei Y, Guarnera M, Shen J, Li R, Liu Z, Jiang F. (2010). Small nucleolar RNA signatures as biomarkers for non-small-cell lung cancer. Mol. Cancer. 9:198.

[130] Martens-Uzunova ES, Jalava SE, Dits NF, van Leenders GJ, Møller S, Trapman J, Bangma CH, Litman T, Visakorpi T, Jenster G. (2011). Diagnostic and prognostic signatures from the small non-coding RNA transcriptome in prostate cancer. Oncogene. 31:978-991.

[131] Brown JW, Marshall DF, Echeverria M. (2008). Intronic noncoding RNAs and splicing. Trends Plant Sci.13:335–342.

[132] Chanfreau G, Legrain P, Jacquier A. (1998). Yeast RNase III as a key processing enzyme in small nucleolar RNAs metabolism. J. Mol. Biol. 284:975–988.

[133] Petfalski E, Dandekar T, Henry Y, Tollervey D. (1998). Processing of the precursors to small nucleolar RNAs and rRNAs requires common components. Mol. Cell. Biol.18:1181–1189.

[134] Qu LH, Henras A, Lu YL, Zhou H, Zhou WX, Zhu YQ, Zhao J, Henry Y, Caizergues-Ferrer M, Bachellerie JP. (1999). Seven novel methylation guide small nucleolar RNAs are processed from a common polycistronic transcript by Rat1p and RNase III in yeast Mol. Cell. Biol.19:1144–1158.

[135] Nicholls RD, Knepper JL. (2001). Genome organization, function, and imprinting in Prader—Willi and Angelman syndromes Annu. Rev. Genomics Hum. Genet. 2:153–175.

[136] Skryabin BV, Gubar LV, Seeger B, Pfeiffer J, Handel S, Robeck T, Karpova E, Rozhdestvensky TS, Brosius J. (2007). Deletion of the MBII-85 snoRNA gene cluster in mice results in postnatal growth retardation. PLoS Genet. 3:e235.

[137] Gurevich I, Englander MT, Adlersberg M, Siegal NB, Schmauss C. (2002). Modulation of serotonin 2C receptor editing by sustained changes in serotonergic neurotransmission J. Neurosci.22:10529–1053.

[138] Burns CM, Chu H, Rueter SM, Hutchinson LK, Canton H, Sanders-Bush E, Emeson RB. (1997). Regulation of serotonin-2C receptor G-protein coupling by RNA editing Nature. 387:303–308.

[139] Tanaka R, Satoh H, Moriyama M, Satoh K, Morishita Y, Yoshida S, Watanabe T, Nakamura Y, Mori S. (2000). Intronic U50 small-nucleolar-RNA (snoRNA) host gene of no protein-coding potential is mapped at the chromosome breakpoint t(3;6) (q27;q15) of human B-cell lymphoma. Genes Cells. 5:277–287.

[140] Dong XY, Rodriguez C, Guo P, Sun X, Talbot JT, Zhou W, Petros W, Li Q, Vessella RL, Kibel AS, Stevens VL, Calle EE, Dong DJ. (2008). SnoRNA U50 is a candidate tumor-suppressor gene at 6q14.3 with a mutation associated with clinically significant prostate cancer Hum. Mol. Genet.17:1031-1042.

[141] Mei YP, Liao JP, Shen JP, Yu L, Liu BL, Liu L, Li RY, Ji L, Dorsey SG, Jiang ZR, Katz RL, Wang JY, Jiang F. (2011). Small nucleolar RNA 42 acts as an oncogene in lung tumorigenesis. Oncogene.(doi:10.1038/onc.2011.449).

[142] Chang LS, Lin S Y, Lieu AS, Wu TL. (2002). Differential expression of human 5S snoRNA genes. Biochem. Biophys. Res. Commun. 299:196–200.

[143] Liao J, Yu L, Mei Y, Guarnera M, Shen J. (2010). Small nucleolar RNA signatures as biomarkers for non-small-cell lung cancer. Mol. Cancer. 9:198.

[144] Li R, Wang H, Bekele BN, Yin Z, Caraway NP, Katz RL, Stass SA, Jiang F.(2006). Identification of putative oncogenes in lung adenocarcinoma by a comprehensive functional genomic approach. Oncogene.18:2628–2635.

[145] Schneider C, King RM, Philipson L. Genes specifically expressed at growth arrest of mammalian cells. Cell. 1988;54:787–793.

[146] Amaldi F, Pierandrei-Amaldi P. (1997). TOP genes: a translationaly controlled class of genes including those coding for ribosomal proteins. In: Jeanteur P, editor. Progress in molecular and subcellular biology. Vol. 18. Springer-Verlag; Berlin, Germany: pp. 1–17.

[147] Mourtada-Maarabouni M, Pickard MR, Hedge VL, Farzaneh F, Williams GT. (2009). GAS5, a non-protein-coding RNA, controls apoptosis and is downregulated in breast cancerGAS5 regulates apoptosis. Oncogene. 28:195-208.

[148] Gee HE, Buffa FM, Camps C, Ramachandran A, Leek R, Taylor M, Patil M, Sheldon H, Betts G, Homer J, West C, Ragoussis J, Harris AL. (2011). The small-nucleolar RNAs commonly used for microRNA normalisation correlate with tumour pathology and prognosis. Br. J. Cancer. 104, 1168–1177.

[149] Nakamura Y, Takahashi N, Kakegawa E, Yoshida K, Ito Y, Kayano H, Niitsu N, Jinnai I, Bessho M. (2008). The GAS5 (growth arrest-specific transcript 5) gene fuses to BCL6 as

a result of t(1;3)(q25;q27) in a patient with B-cell lymphoma. Cancer Genetics and Cytogenetics.182:144-149.

[150] Askarian-Amiri ME, Crawford J, French JD, Smart CE, Smith MA, Clark MB, Ru K, Mercer TR, Thompson ER, Lakhani SR, Vargas AC, Campbell IG, Brown MA, Dinger ME, Mattick JS. (2011). SNORD-host RNA Zfas1 is a regulator of mammary development and a potential marker for breast cancer RNA. 17:878-891.

[151] Gupta V, Kumar A. (2010). Dyskeratosis congenita. Adv Exp Med Biol.685:215-219.

[152] Ruggero D, Grisendi S, Piazza F, Rego E, Mari F, Rao PH, Cordon-Cardo C, Pandolfi PP. (2003). Dyskeratosis congenita and cancer in mice deficient in ribosomal RNA modification. Science. 299:259-62.

[153] Ono M, Scott MS, Yamada K, Avolio F, Barton GJ, Lamond AI. (2011). Identification of human miRNA precursors that resemble box C/D snoRNAs. Nucleic Acids Res.39:3879-3891.

[154] Xiao J, Lin H, Luo X, Luo X, Wang Z. (2011). miR-605 joins p53 network to form a p53:miR-605:Mdm2 positive feedback loop in response to stress. EMBO J.30:5021.

[155] Siomi MC, Sato K, Pezic D, Aravin AA. (2011). PIWI-interacting small RNAs: the vanguard of genome defence. Nat Rev Mol Cell Biol.12:246-258.

[156] Ishizu H, Nagao A, Siomi H. (2011). Gatekeepers for Piwi-piRNA complexes to enter the nucleus. Curr Opin Genet Dev. 21:484-490.

[157] Kazazian HH Jr. (2004). Mobile elements: drivers of genome evolution. Science 303:1626–1632.

[158] Saito K, Siomi MC. (2010). Small RNA-mediated quiescence of transposable elements in animals. Dev. Cell. 19:687–697.

[159] Vagin VV, Klenov MS, Kalmykova AI, Stolyarenko AD, Kotelnikov RN, Gvozdev VA. (2004). The RNA interference proteins and vasa locus are involved in the silencing of retrotransposons in the female germline of Drosophila melanogaster. RNA Biol. 1:54–58.17.

[160] Kalmykova AI, Klenov MS, Gvozdev VA. (2005). Argonaute protein PIWI controls mobilization of retrotransposons in the Drosophila male germline. Nucleic Acids Res. 33:2052–2059.

[161] Savitsky M, Kwon D, Georgiev P, Kalmykova A, Gvozdev V. (2006). Telomere elongation is under the control of the RNAi-based mechanism in the Drosophila germline. Genes Dev. 20:345–354.

[162] Li C, Vagin VV, Lee S, Xu J, Ma S, Xi H, Seitz H, Horwich MD, Syrzycka M, Honda BM, Kittler EL, Zapp ML, Klattenhoff C, Schulz N, Theurkauf WE, Weng Z, Zamore PD. (2009). Collapse of germline piRNAs in the absence of Argonaute3 reveals somatic piRNAs in flies. Cell. 137:509–521.

[163] Aravin A, Gaidatzis D, Pfeffer S, Lagos-Quintana M, Landgraf P, Iovino N, Morris P, Brownstein MJ, Kuramochi-Miyagawa S, Nakano T, Chien M, Russo JJ, Ju J, Sheridan R, Sander C, Zavolan M, Tuschl T. (2006). A novel class of small RNAs bind to MILI protein in mouse testes. Nature. 442:203–207.

[164] Girard A, Sachidanandam R, Hannon GJ, Carmell MA. (2006) A germline-specific class of small RNAs binds mammalian Piwi proteins. Nature. 442:199–202.

[165] Brennecke J, Aravin AA, Stark A, Dus M, Kellis M, Sachidanandam R, Hannon GJ. (2007). Discrete small RNA-generating loci as master regulators of transposon activity in Drosophila. Cell. 128:1089–1103.

[166] Lau NC, Seto AG, Kim J, Kuramochi-Miyagawa S, Nakano T, Bartel DP, Kingston RE. (2006). Characterization of the piRNA complex from rat testes. Science 313, 363–367

[167] Houwing S, Berezikov E, Ketting RF. (2008). Zili is required for germ cell differentiation and meiosis in zebrafish. EMBO J. 27:2702–2711.

[168] Robine N, Lau NC, Balla S, Jin Z, Okamura K, Kuramochi-Miyagawa S, Blower MD, Lai EC. (2009) A broadly conserved pathway generates 3'UTR-directed primary piRNAs. Curr. Biol. 19:2066–2076.

[169] Aravin AA, Sachidanandam R, Bourc'his D, Schaefer C, Pezic D, Toth KF, Bestor T, Hannon GJ. (2008). A piRNA pathway primed by individual transposons is linked to de novo DNA methylation in mice. Mol. Cell. 31:785–799.

[170] Qiao D, Zeeman AM, Deng W, Looijenga LH, Lin H. (2002). Molecular characterization of hiwi, a human member of the piwi gene family whose overexpression is correlated to seminomas. Oncogene.21:3988-3999.

[171] Taubert H, Würl P, Greither T, Kappler M, Bache M, Bartel F, Kehlen A, Lautenschläger C, Harris LC, Kaushal D, Füssel S, Meye A, Böhnke A, Schmidt H, Holzhausen HJ, Hauptmann S. (2007). Stem cell-associated genes are extremely poor prognostic factors for soft-tissue sarcoma patients. Oncogene. 26:7170-7174.

[172] Taubert H, Greither T, Kaushal D, Würl P, Bache M, Bartel F, Kehlen A, Lautenschläger C, Harris L, Kraemer K, Meye A, Kappler M, Schmidt H, Holzhausen HJ, Hauptmann S. (2007) Expression of the stem cell self-renewal gene Hiwi and risk of tumour-related death in patients with soft-tissue sarcoma. Oncogene.26:1098-1100.

[173] Wang QE, Han C, Milum K, Wani AA. (2011). Stem cell protein Piwil2 modulates chromatin modifications upon cisplatin treatment. Mutat Res.708:59-68.

[174] Lu Y, Li C, Zhang K, Sun H, Tao D, Liu Y, Zhang S, Ma Y. (2010). Identification of piRNAs in Hela cells by massive parallel sequencing. BMB Rep.43:635-41.

[175] Cui L, Lou Y, Zhang X, Zhou H, Deng H, Song H, Yu X, Xiao B, Wang W, Guo J. (2011). Detection of circulating tumor cells in peripheral blood from patients with gastric cancer using piRNAs as markers. Clin Biochem. 44:1050-1057.

[176] Cheng J, Guo JM, Xiao BX, Miao Y, Jiang Z, Zhou H, Li QN. (2011). piRNA, the new non-coding RNA, is aberrantly expressed in human cancer cells. Clin Chim Acta. 412:1621-1625.

[177] Cheng J, Deng H, Xiao B, Zhou H, Zhou F, Shen Z, Guo J. (2012). piR-823, a novel non-coding small RNA, demonstrates in vitro and in vivo tumor suppressive activity in human gastric cancer cells. Cancer Lett. 315:12-17

[178] Reuter M, Chuma S, Tanaka T, Franz T, Stark A, Pillai RS. (2009). Loss of the Mili-interacting Tudor domain-containing protein-1 activates transposons and alters the Mili-associated small RNA profile. Nature Struct. Mol. Biol. 16:639–646.

[179] Shoji M, Tanaka T, Hosokawa M, Reuter M, Stark A, Kato Y, Kondoh G, Okawa K, Chujo T, Suzuki T, Hata K, Martin SL, Noce T, Kuramochi-Miyagawa S, Nakano T, Sasaki H, Pillai RS, Nakatsuji N, Chuma S. (2009) The TDRD9-MIWI2 complex is

essential for piRNA-mediated retrotransposon silencing in the mouse male germline. Dev. Cell 17:775–787.

[180] Struhl, K. (2007). Transcriptional noise and the fidelity of initiation by RNA polymerase II. Nature Struct. Mol. Biol. 14:103–105.

[181] Amaral PP, Mattick JS. (2008). Noncoding RNA in development. Mamm. Genome. 19:454–492.

[182] Dinger ME, Amaral PP, Mercer TR, Pang KC, Bruce SJ, Gardiner BB, Askarian-Amiri ME, Ru K, Soldà G, Simons C, Sunkin SM, Crowe ML, Grimmond SM, Perkins AC, Mattick JS. (2008). Long noncoding RNAs in mouse embryonic stem cell pluripotency and differentiation. Genome Res. 18:1433–1445.

[183] Mercer TR, Dinger ME, Sunkin SM, Mehler MF, Mattick JS. (2008). Specific expression of long noncoding RNAs in the adult mouse brain. Proc. Natl Acad. Sci. USA. 105:716–721.

[184] Cawley S, Bekiranov S, Ng HH, Kapranov P, Sekinger EA, Kampa D, Piccolboni A, Sementchenko V, Cheng J, Williams AJ, Wheeler R, Wong B, Drenkow J, Yamanaka M, Patel S, Brubaker S, Tammana H, Helt G, Struhl K, Gingeras TR. (2004). Unbiased mapping of transcription factor binding sites along human chromosomes 21 and 22 points to widespread regulation of noncoding RNAs. Cell.116:499–509.

[185] Ponjavic J, Ponting CP, Lunter G. (2007). Functionality or transcriptional noise? Evidence for selection within long noncoding RNAs. Genome Res. 17:556–565.

[186] Faulkner GJ, Kimura Y, Daub CO, Wani S, Plessy C, Irvine KM, Schroder K, Cloonan N, Steptoe AL, Lassmann T, Waki K, Hornig N, Arakawa T, Takahashi H, Kawai J, Forrest AR, Suzuki H, Hayashizaki Y, Hume DA, Orlando V, Grimmond SM, Carninci P. (2009). The regulated retrotransposon transcriptome of mammalian cells. Nat Genet. 41:563–71.

[187] Guttman M, Amit I, Garber M, French C, Lin MF, Feldser D, Huarte M, Zuk O, Carey BW, Cassady JP, Cabili MN, Jaenisch R, Mikkelsen TS, Jacks T, Hacohen N, Bernstein BE, Kellis M, Regev A, Rinn JL, Lander ES. (2009). Chromatin signature reveals over a thousand highly conserved large non-coding RNAs in mammals. Nature.458:223–227.

[188] Pang KC, Frith MC, Mattick JS. (2006). Rapid evolution of noncoding RNAs: lack of conservation does not mean lack of function. Trends Genet. 22:1–5.

[189] Cheng LL, Carmichael GG. (2010). Decoding the function of nuclear long non-coding RNAs. Curr Opinion in Cell Biology. 22:357-364.

[190] Kugel JF, Goodrich JA. (2012). Non-coding RNAs: key regulators of mammalian transcription. Trends in Biochemical Sciences. 37:144-151.

[191] Khalil AM, Guttman M, Huarte M. Garber M Ray A. Rivea Morales D. Thomas K, Presser A. (2009). Many human large intergenic noncoding RNAs associated with chromatin-modifying complexes and affect gene expression. Proc Natl Acad Sci USA. 106:11667-11672.

[192] Zhao J, Sun BK, Erwin JA, Song JJ, Lee JT. (2008). Polycomb proteins targeted by a short repeat RNA to the mouse X chromosome. Science 322:750-756.

[193] Rinn JL, Kertesz M, Wang JK, Squazzo SL, Xu X, Brugmann SA, Goodnough LH, Helms JA, Farnham PJ, Segal E, Chang HY.(2007) Functional demarcation of active and silent chromatin domains in human HOX loci by noncoding RNAs. Cell 129, 1311–1323.

[194] Tsai MC, Manor O, Wan Y, Mosammaparast N, Wang JK, Lan F, Shi Y, Segal E, Chang HY. (2010). Long noncoding RNA as modular scaffold of histone modification complexes. Sciences. 329:689-693.

[195] Morris KV, Santoso S, Turner AM, Pastori C, Hawkins PG. (2008). Bidirectional transcription directs both transcriptional gene activation and suppression in human cells. PLoS Genet. 4:e1000258.

[196] Nagano T, Mitchell JA, Sanz LA, Pauler FM, Ferguson-Smith AC, Feil R, Fraser P. (2008).The Air noncoding RNA epigenetically silences transcription by targeting G9a to chromatin. Science. 322:1717–1720.

[197] Gupta RA, Shah N, Wang KC, Kim J, Horlings HM, Wong DJ, Tsai MC, Hung T, Argani P, Rinn JL, Wang Y, Brzoska P, Kong B, Li R, West RB, van de Vijver MJ, Sukumar S, Chang HY. (2010). Long non-coding RNA HOTAIR reprograms chromatin state to promote cancer metastasis. Nature. 464:1071-1076.

[198] Kogo R, Shimamura T, Mimori K, Kawahara K, Imoto S, Sudo T, Tanaka F, Shibata K, Suzuki A, Komune S, Miyano S, Mori M. (2011). Long non-coding RNA HOTAIR regulates Polycomb-dependent chromatin modification and is associated with poor prognosis in colorectal cancers. Cancer Res.71: 6320-6326.

[199] Yap KL, Li S, Muñoz-Cabello AM, Raguz S, Zeng L, Mujtaba S, Gil J, Walsh MJ, Zhou MM. (2010). Molecular interplay of the non coding RNA ANRIL and methylated histone H3 lysine 27 by polycomb CBX7 in transcriptional silencing of INK4a. Mol Cell. 38:662-674.

[200] Beltran M, Puig I, Peña C, García JM, Alvarez AB, Peña R, Bonilla F, de Herreros AG. (2008). A natural antisense transcript regulates Zeb2/Sip1 gene expression during Snail1-induced epithelial–mesenchymal transition. Genes Dev. 22:756–769.

[201] Wang X, Arai S, Song X, Reichart D, Du K, Pascual G, Tempst P, Rosenfeld MG, Glass CK, Kurokawa R. (2008). Induced ncRNAs allosterically modify RNA-binding proteins in cis to inhibit transcription. Nature. 454:126–130.

[202] Feng J, Bi C, Clark BS, Mady R, Shah P, Kohtz JD. (2006). The Evf-2 noncoding RNA is transcribed from the Dlx-5/6 ultraconserved region and functions as a Dlx-2 transcriptional coactivator. Genes Dev. 20:1470–1484.

[203] Huarte M, Guttman M, Feldser D, Garber M, Koziol MJ, Kenzelmann-Broz D, Khalil AM, Zuk O, Amit I, Rabani M, Attardi LD, Regev A, Lander ES, Jacks T, Rinn JL. (2010). A large intergenic noncoding RNA induced by p53 mediates global gene repression in the p53 response. Cell. 142:409-419.

[204] Bond CS, Fox AH. (2009). Paraspeckles: nuclear bodies built on long noncoding RNA. J Cell Biol. 186:637-644.

Chapter 2

MiRNA and Proline Metabolism in Cancer

Wei Liu and James M. Phang

Additional information is available at the end of the chapter

1. Introduction

Tumor metabolism and bioenergetics are important areas for cancer research and present promising targets for anticancer therapy. Growing tumors alter their metabolic profiles to meet the bioenergetic and biosynthetic demands of increased cell growth and proliferation. These alterations include the well-known aerobic glycolysis, the Warburg effect, which has been considered as the central tenet of cancer cell metabolism for more than 80 years [1]. Interest in cancer cell metabolism has been refueled by recent advances in the study of signaling pathways involving known oncogene and tumor suppressor genes, which reveal their close interaction with metabolic pathways [2-4]. For example, recent studies document an important role of glutamine catabolism in tumor stimulated by the oncogenic transcriptional factor c-MYC (herein termed MYC) which has been previously shown to stimulate glycolysis [5, 6]. Although glucose and glutamine serve as the main metabolic substrate for tumor cells, proline as a microenvironmental stress substrate has attracted lots of attention due to its unique metabolic system, its availability in tumor microenvironments and its responses to various stresses.

1.1. Special features of proline metabolism

Proline is the only proteinogenic secondary amino acid, and it has special functions in biology [7-11]. Proline metabolism is distinct from that of primary amino acids. The inclusion of an alpha-nitrogen within its pyrrolidine ring precludes its being the substrate for the usual amino acid-metabolizing enzymes, such as, the decarboxylases, aminotransferases, and racemases. Instead, proline metabolism has its own family of enzymes with their tissue and subcellular localization and their own regulatory mechanisms. As shown in the schematic of proline metabolic pathway (Figure 1), these enzymes include proline dehydrogenase/oxidase (PRODH/POX) and pyrroline-5-carboxylate reductase (PYCR) catalyzing the interconversion of proline and Δ^1-pyrroline-5-carboxylate (P5C), P5C dehydrogenase (P5CDH) and P5C synthase (P5CS) mediating the

interconversion of P5C and glutamate, and ornithine aminotransferase (OAT) catalyzing the
interconversion of P5C and ornithine. Glutamate can be converted to α-ketoglutarate (α-KG)
entering the tricarboxylic acid (TCA) cycle, which is also the main pathway of glutamine
catabolism. Ornithine can be converted to arginine entering the urea cycle. Thus proline
metabolism is closely related with glutamine metabolism, TCA cycle, and urea cycle, the
main metabolic pathways in human body.

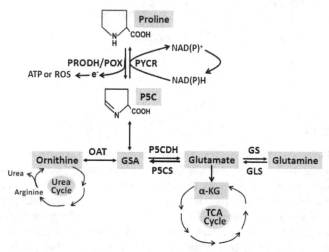

Figure 1. Proline metabolic pathway. Proline metabolism is closely related with glutamine
metabolism, TCA cycle, urea cycle and pentose phosphate pathway (PPP). Abbreviations: P5C, Δ1 -
pyrroline-5-carboxylate; GSA, glutamic-gamma-semialdehyde; PRODH/POX, proline
dehydrogenase/oxidase; PYCR, P5C reductase; P5CDH, P5C dehydrogenase; GS, glutamine synthase;
GLS, glutaminase; P5CS, P5C Synthase; OAT, ornithine aminotransferase. The interconversion between
P5C and GSA is spontaneous.

Importantly, the interconversion between proline and P5C, catalyzed by PRODH/POX and
PYCR, respectively, forms the "proline cycle" in the cytosol and mitochondria as shown in
Figure 2, which acts as a redox shuttle transferring reducing and oxidizing potential. In the
mitochondria, during the degradation of proline to P5C, PRODH/POX, the flavin adenine
dinucleotide-containing enzyme tightly bound to mitochondrial inner membranes, donates
electrons through its intervening flavine adenine dinucleotide into the electron transport
chain (ETC) to generate ATP or ROS [7, 12, 13]. This characteristic of PRODH/POX serves as
the basis of its function in human cancers, which will be discussed in detail in the following
sections. P5C produced from the oxidation of proline, emerges from mitochondria and is
converted back to proline in the cytosol using NADPH or NADH as cofactor, which
interlock with the pentose phosphate pathway (Figure 1) or other metabolic pathways.

Proline metabolism has been shown to play an important role in various human physiologic
and pathologic situations. For example, in the early 1970s, P5C, the immediate product of
proline catabolism was found to be also the immediate biosynthetic precursor [7]. And in

the 1980s, the conversion of P5C to proline was recognized to regulate redox homeostasis as mentioned above [8, 14, 15]. A variety of evidence has shown the inborn errors of the proline metabolic pathway in several human genetic diseases and their potential roles [11, 16], such as familial hyperprolinemias [11, 17], mutations of PRODH/POX in neuropsychiatric diseases [18, 19], mutations of PYCR1 in cutis laxa [20], mutations of P5CS in hyperammonemia [21, 22], and so on. During the last decade, our understanding of the roles of proline metabolism as represented by the regulation and functions of PRODH/POX in tumorigenesis and tumor progression has made significant advances, which will be main focus in this chapter.

1.2. Proline availability in tumor microenvironment

Proline is one of the most abundant amino acids in the cellular microenvironment. Together with hydroxyproline, proline constitutes more than 25% of residues in collagen, the predominant protein (80%) in the extracellular matrix (ECM) of the human body. Although proline can be obtained from the dietary proteins, an important source of proline is from the degradation of collagen in the ECM by sequential enzymatic catalysis of matrix metalloproteinases (MMPs) and prolidase [9, 23]. The upregulation of MMPs in tumors has been considered a critical step for tumor progression and invasion [24-26]. A number of reports have shown that proline concentration is increased in various tumors, which may result from the upregulated MMPs degrading collagen. Previous work from our lab showed that glucose depletion activated MMP-2 and MMP-9 in cancer cells, which accompanied an increase in intracellular proline levels [27].

Autophagy-induced degradation of the intracellular protein, which has been shown to regulate cancer development and progression as a survival strategy of cancer cells [28, 29], may also provide an important source of free proline. Furthermore, proline can be biosynthesized from either glutamate or ornithine as shown in Figure 1 and Figure 2. Our latest finding showed that a large part of products from glutamine catabolism stimulated by MYC is proline [30], suggesting proline biosynthesis might serve as an additional source of proline availability in cancer. Taken together, the ample sources of proline in tumor microenvironment ensure its availability as an important stress substrate for metabolism in human cancers.

2. PRODH/POX as a mitochondrial tumor suppressor

2.1. PRODH/POX induces apoptosis through ROS generation

PRODH, the gene encoding PRODH/POX was discovered to be a p53-induced gene in a screening study in 1997 [31]. Importantly, the p53-initiated apoptosis was later found to depend on the induction of PRODH/POX [32]. To further study the function of PRODH/POX, we developed a DLD1-POX colorectal cancer cell line (designated as DLD1-POX tet-off cell line), which was stably transfected with the *PRODH* gene under the control of a tetracycline-controllable promoter [33]. When doxycycline (DOX) was removed from the culture medium and the expression of PRODH/POX was induced, apoptotic cell death was initiated.

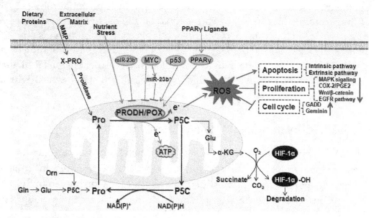

Figure 2. Proline metabolism in cancer. 1. Proline cycle: Interconversion of proline and P5C forms the proline cycle in the cytosol and mitochondria. Proline cycle acts as a redox shuttle transferring reducing potential generated by the pentose phosphate pathway or other metabolic pathway into mitochondria for the production of either ROS or ATP responding to different stresses. 2. Proline availability in human tumor microenvironment: dietary proteins, glutamate and ornithine catabolism, and degradation of extracellular matrix by matrix metalloproteinases (MMPs) are all important sources of proline, especially the last one. 3. The central enzyme of proline metabolism, PRODH/POX, localized in the mitochondrial inner membrane, function as a mitochondrial tumor suppressor. PRODH/POX is induced by p53, PPARγ and its ligands, and suppressed by miR-23b* and oncogenic protein MYC. PRODH/POX overexpression could initiate apoptosis, inhibit proliferation and induce G2 cell cycle arrest through ROS generation, and suppress HIF-1 signaling through increasing α-KG production. Abbreviations: X-PRO, x-prolyl dipeptide; Pro, proline; Orn, ornithine; Gln, glutamine; Glu, glutamate.

ROS, which include superoxide radical ($O_2^-\cdot$), hydroxyl radicals (OH·) and the non-radical hydrogen peroxide (H_2O_2), play an important role in the induction of apoptosis [34]. PRODH/POX could donate electron to the ETC to generate ROS. In cells overexpressing PRODH/POX, the addition of proline increased ROS generation in a concentration-dependent manner, and the proline-dependent ROS increased with PRODH/POX expression [35]. N-acetyl cysteine (NAC), a widely used antioxidant agent, dramatically reduced PRODH/POX-induced apoptosis, indicating PRODH/POX induces apoptosis through ROS generation [13]. By introducing the recombinant adenoviruses containing different antioxidant enzymes, such as manganese superoxide dismutase (MnSOD), Cu/Zn superoxide dismutase (CuZnSOD) or catalase (CAT) into the DLD1-POX tet-off cells, we found that only the expression of MnSOD, which localizes in the mitochondria, inhibited PRODH/POX-induced apoptosis, suggesting that it is superoxide as the form of ROS initially mediating PRODH/POX-induced apoptosis [13].

Further investigation on the molecular signaling involved in PRODH/POX-induced apoptosis showed that PRODH/POX activated both intrinsic and extrinsic apoptotic pathways [35, 36]. The DLD-1-POX cells overproducing PRODH/POX exhibited the mitochondria (intrinsic pathway) and death receptor (extrinsic pathway)-mediated apoptotic responses in a proline-dependent manner [35]. Intrinsic pathway induced by PRODH/POX includes the release of cytochrome c, activation of caspase-9, chromatin condensation, DNA fragmentation, and cell shrinkage. Extrinsic pathway induced by PRODH/POX involves the stimulation of the expression of tumor necrosis factor-related apoptosis inducing ligand (TRAIL), and death receptor 5 (DR5) and then cleavage of caspase-8 [36]. Both pathways culminate in the activation of caspase-3 and cleavage of substrates. NFATc1, a member of the nuclear factor of activated T cells (NFAT) family of transcription factors is partially responsible for the TRAIL activity stimulated by PRODH/POX [36]. All of these effects mediated by PRODH/POX could be partially reversed by MnSOD, further confirming the role of ROS/superoxides in PRODH/POX-induced apoptosis [36].

Parallel studies showed that peroxisome proliferator activated receptor gamma (PPARγ) is another critical regulator of PRODH/POX, besides p53. PPARγ belongs to the nuclear hormone receptor superfamily and functions as a ligand-dependent transcription factor [37]. It is widely expressed in many malignant tissues, and its ligands can induce terminal differentiation, apoptosis, and cell growth inhibition in a variety of cancer cells [38-40]. Using a *PRODH*-promoter luciferase construct [41], we found that PPARγ was the most potent effector activating the *PRODH* promoter. PRODH/POX contributes greatly to apoptosis induced by the pharmacologic ligands of PPARγ through ROS signaling in human colorectal cancer cells and non-small cell lung carcinoma cells [41, 42].

More recently, we found that PRODH/POX was upregulated to contribute to ATP production under nutrient stress, such as glucose deprivation [27]. Under hypoxic conditions [43] or high levels of oxidized low-density lipoproteins (oxLDLs) [44], ROS produced by PRODH/POX contributes to autophagy as a survival signal. These effects seem paradoxical with PRODH/POX-induced apoptosis, but they can be well understood considering the temporal and spatial development of the evolving tumor, like the "two faces" of tumor suppressor p53 [45]. A detailed description of this point can be found in our recent review [9].

2.2. PRODH/POX inhibits tumor cell growth through ROS generation

In addition to initiating apoptosis, PRODH/POX also inhibits tumor cell growth and proliferation. In DLD1-POX tet-off cells, soft agar colony formation assays showed that the cells readily formed clones when PRODH/POX expression was inhibited by DOX, whereas the cloning ability of the cells was totally blocked when POX was overexpressed [46].

Several signaling pathways associated with tumor growth are downregulated by PRODH/POX. First, PRODH/POX suppresses the phosphorylation of three major subtypes of the mitogen-activated protein kinase (MAPK) pathways, including MEK/ERK, JNK, p38 [36]. In fact, MAPK pathways play an important role in a variety of cellular responses, including proliferation, differentiation, development, transformation, and apoptosis. The inhibition of MEK/ERK pathway is involved in PRODH/POX-induced apoptosis. Secondly,

PRODH/POX markedly reduces the expression of cyclooxygenase-2 (COX-2), and thus suppresses the production of prostaglandin E_2 (PGE$_2$) [47]. The addition of PGE$_2$ partially reverses the apoptosis and inhibits tumor growth induced by PRODH/POX. Cyclooxygenase is an enzyme that catalyzes the key step of the conversion of free arachidonic acid to prostaglandins. It has been widely accepted that elevated COX2/PGE$_2$ signaling plays a critical role in the initiation and development of various solid tumors, especially colorectal cancer [48-50]. Thirdly, PRODH/POX inhibits the phosphorylation of epidermal growth factor receptor (EGFR). Activating mutants and overexpression of EGFR signaling contributes to carcinogenesis of various tumors by inducing cell proliferation and counteracting apoptosis [51]. Fourthly, Wnt/β-catenin signaling is decreased by PRODH/POX [47]. Constitutive activation of this signaling pathway is found in many human cancers, which regulates proliferation, differentiation and cell fate [52]. Phosphorylation of β-catenin by GSK-3β leads to its ubiquitination and proteasomal degradation. PRODH/POX decreases phosphorylation of GSK-3β and thereby increases phosphorylation of β-catenin, resulting in the reduced activity of Wnt/ β-catenin signaling. All of aforementioned changes induced by PRODH/POX are partially reversed by MnSOD, further indicating the critical role of ROS/superoxides in PRODH/POX-mediated effects.

Furthermore, PRODH/POX induces G2 cell cycle arrest through affecting the regulators of cell cycle, such as geminin, cyclin-dependent kinase (CDC), and growth arrest and DNA damage inducible proteins (GADDs) [46]. Geminin is a nuclear protein that inhibits DNA replication, and has been used as a marker for G2 phase [53]. Its expression is up-regulated by PRODH/POX. CDC2 normally drives cells into mitosis and is the ultimate target of pathways that mediate rapid G2 arrest in response to DNA damage [54]. Although total CDC2 did not change with PRODH/POX expression, the phosphorylated CDC2 at tyrosine 15 increased, whereas phosphorylation at threonine 161 decreased when PRODH/POX was overexpressed, indicating that CDC2 is in an inactive status. CDC25C, the phosphatase that removes the inhibitory phosphates from CDC2 and activates cyclinB-CDC2, is downregulated by PRODH/POX. Additionally, the most important regulators of G2 cell cycle arrest, GADDs [55] also play a role in PRODH/POX-induced G2 cell cycle arrest, including GADD34, GADD45a, GADDh, GADDg [46].

2.3. PRODH/POX inhibits HIF signaling mainly through increasing α-KG production

The above described PRODH/POX-mediated induction of apoptosis together with the suppression of cell growth suggests that PRODH/POX could function as a tumor suppressor. PRODH/POX protein is located in the mitochondrial inner membrane, and has an anaplerotic role through glutamate and α-KG for the TCA cycle (Fig.1). The identification of several mitochondrial tumor suppressors has demonstrated that one of the critical ways they exert their antitumor effects is through hypoxia inducible factor-1 (HIF-1) signaling, which mediates the transcriptional response to hypoxia as a transcriptional factor and plays an important role in angiogenesis and tumor growth [56, 57]. Similarly, PRODH/POX also downregulates HIF-1 signaling including its downstream gene VEGF in both normoxic and hypoxic conditions [46]. This is another mechanism, along with those described above, by which PRODH/POX exerts its tumor-suppressing role. However, unlike the effects of PRODH/POX on other signaling pathways, its effect on HIF-1 signaling could not be reversed by MnSOD, suggesting ROS is not the mediator for HIF inhibition.

The stability and transcriptional activity of HIF-1α are regulated through oxygen-sensitive modifications. Briefly, the posttranslational hydroxylation of specific prolyl and asparaginal residues in its α-subunits of HIF-1, catalyzed by prolyl hydroxylases (PHD), results in the degradation of HIF-1 through ubiquitinal and proteasomal degradation systems [58]. As an important substrate of PHD, the members of the 2-oxoglutarate (α-KG) dioxygenase family could increase the hydroxylation and degradation of HIF-1α [58]. HPLC analysis showed that α-KG was increased by overexpression of PRODH/POX [46]. When PRODH/POX expression is high, P5C, glutamate and α-KG are sequentially produced from proline, forming an important link between proline and the TCA cycle. The widely used cell-permeating α-KG analogue, dimethyloxalylglycine, was shown to block the inhibition of HIF-1 signaling by PRODH/POX, suggesting the pivotal role of α-KG in the down-regulation of HIF by PRODH/POX.

In addition, several TCA cycle intermediates and glycolytic metabolites, such as succinate and fumarate, have been revealed to inhibit PHD activity and stabilize HIF-1 signaling [58-61]. PRODH/POX expression could decrease succinate, fumarate and lactate as measured by gas chromatography-mass spectrometry (GC-MS) [46], which may also contribute to the impaired HIF-1 signaling.

2.4. PRODH/POX suppresses tumor formation *in vivo* and is downregulated in human tumors

The inhibitory effects of PRODH/POX on tumor cell growth are corroborated in a human colon cancer mouse xenograft model [46]. DLD-1 POX Tet-off cells were injected into immunodeficient mice. The expression of PRODH/POX was controlled by giving mice doxycycline in their drinking water. When PRODH/POX was suppressed by doxycycline, tumors readily formed in all the mice within a few days. By contrast, when PRODH/POX was overexpressed by removal of doxycycline in their drinking water, tumor development was greatly reduced and none of the mice developed tumors.

Further investigation on a variety of cancer tissues along with normal tissue counterparts including kidney, bladder, stomach, colon and rectum, liver, pancreas, breast, prostate, ovary, brain, lung, skin, etc., showed that 61% of all tumors had decreased expression of PRODH/POX compared to normal tissues, especially the tumor from kidney and digestive tract [46, 47, 62], suggesting tumor could eliminate the tumor suppressor roles of PRODH/POX. Suppression of PRODH/POX was more significant in kidney and digestive tract. More interestingly, PRODH/POX protein levels showed more striking decrease than mRNA levels in renal cancers, implicating that PRODH/POX might be regulated at the post-transcriptional level.

Sequencing the *PRODH* gene showed no somatic mutation or functionally significant single nucleotide polymorphisms (SNP) in tumor tissues. Hypermethylation analysis also didn't show any differences of PRODH genomic DNA between tumor and normal tissues. Therefore, PRODH does not satisfy the canonical requisite for tumor suppressor genes which often show genetic or epigenetic mutations in human cancers. With the discovery of microRNAs (miRNAs), a new mechanism to regulate protein expression has been revealed. Considering the inconsistency between PRODH/POX mRNA and protein expression and the importance of miRNAs in cancer, the regulation of miRNAs on PRODH/POX represented a very promising hypothesis.

3. MiRNA in cancer

3.1. Biogenesis and function of miRNAs

3.1.1. Discovery of miRNAs

MiRNAs are a class of post-transcriptional regulators. They are conserved, endogenously expressed, non-coding small RNAs of 18-25 nucleotides in length. MiRNAs were first discovered in 1993 by Lee RC *et al.* [63] and Wightman R *et al.* [64] in the nematode *Caenorhabditis elegans (C. elegans)* as a regulator of developmental timing regarding the gene lin-14. They found that the lin-14 could be regulated by the small RNA products from lin-4, a gene that does not code for any protein but instead produces a pair of small RNAs. These lin-4 RNAs had antisense complementarity to multiple sites in the 3′ UTR of the lin-14 mRNA. However, it did not attract substantial attention until seven years later when let-7 was discovered to repress the expression of several mRNAs including lin-14 during transition in developmental stages in *C. elegans* [65]. Since then over 4000 miRNAs have been identified in eukaryotes including mammals, fungi and plants. More than 700 miRNAs have been found in humans.

3.1.2. Processing and biogenesis of miRNAs

In mammals, miRNA genes are usually transcribed as long primary transcripts (pri-miRNAs) by RNA polymerase II from DNA [66]. The pri-miRNAs then are cropped into the hairpin-shaped miRNA precursors (pre-miRNAs) by the RNase III enzyme Drosha [67, 68]. A single pri-miRNA may contain one to six pre-miRNAs which are composed of about 70 nucleotides. They are exported from the nucleus to the cytoplasm by exportin-5 (XPO5), a member of the Ran-dependent nuclear transport receptor family [69-71]. In cytoplasm, the pre-miRNA hairpin is subsequently cleaved by the endonuclease Dicer [72] into an imperfect miRNA:miRNA* duplex. Usually, only one strand of the duplex is incorporated into the RNA induced silencing complex (RISC) where the miRNA and its mRNA target interact. The thermodynamic stability, strength of base-pairing and the position of the stem-loop determine which strand becomes mature miRNA to incorporate into the RISC [73-75]. The other strand is normally degraded and is denoted with an asterisk (*) due to its lower levels in the steady state. However, recent evidence indicates that both strands of duplex are viable and become functional miRNA that target different mRNA populations [62, 76-78].

RISC is a multiprotein complex that incorporates mature miRNA to recognize complementary target mRNA. Once binding to target mRNA, miRNAs inhibit their target genes with the help of RISC. The key component of the RISC complex is the Argonaute (Ago) proteins, which are consistently found in RISC complexes from a variety of organisms [79]. Ago proteins directly interact with the miRNA [80, 81]. They are needed for miRNA-induced silencing and contain two conserved RNA binding domains: a PAZ domain, that can bind the single stranded 3' end of the mature miRNA, and a PIWI domain, that structurally resembles ribonuclease-H (RNaseH) and functions in slicer activity through interacting with the 5' end of the guide strand [82]. Most eukaryotes contain multiple Ago family members, with different Ago often specialized for distinct functions [83]. The human genome encodes four Ago proteins and Ago2 is the only Ago capable of endonuclease cleavage of target transcripts directly [84, 85].

Additional components of RISC involved in miRNA processing include the Vasa intronic gene (VIG) protein, the fragile X mental retardation protein (FMRP), human immunodeficiency virus transactivating response RNA binding protein (TARBP), protein activator of the interferon induced protein kinase (PACT), the SMN complex, Gemin3 and DICER1, and so on [86-92]. However their generality or precise function in miRNA silencing remains to be determined.

3.1.3. Stability of miRNAs

Turnover of mature miRNA is needed for rapid changes in miRNA expression profiles. Besides inducing the cleavage of the target mRNAs, Ago proteins have been recently reported to regulate the stability of miRNAs [93-98]. Mature miRNAs are stabilized after incorporation into Ago proteins, and release from this complex leaves miRNAs vulnerable to decay by exonucleases [94, 95]. Ectopic overexpression of Ago proteins prevents degradation of miRNAs, and loss of Ago2 significantly reduces miRNA stability and differentially regulates miRNAs production [93, 96].

In addition to taking refuge in protein complexes, mature miRNAs can undergo protective modifications [97]. For example, as indicated by work in the model organism *Arabidopsis thaliana*, mature plant miRNAs appear to be stabilized by the addition of methyl groups at the 3' end which prevents uridylation of miRNAs [99]. The addition of adenines to 3' end of miRNAs detected in many different plant and animal miRNAs also has a stabilizing effect on miRNAs [100-104].

3.1.4. Function of miRNAs

MiRNAs inhibit the expression of their target genes through three different mechanisms [105, 106]. The first one is direct endonucleolytic cleavage of mRNAs supported by the slicer activity of specific Ago proteins present within RISC. As mentioned above, Ago2 is the only one of the four mammalian Ago proteins capable of directing cleavage [84, 85]. This mechanism is generally favored by a complete match of the so called seed-sequence of the miRNA (nucleotides 2-7 of 5' end of miRNAs) and target mRNA [107], although some mismatches can be tolerated and still allow cleavage to occur [108, 109]. The complementarity of the seed region defines the targets of the miRNA because the seed region binds to the mRNA as governed by binding of complementary nucleotides. The second mechanism is by inhibiting protein translation but without degradation of the mRNA [110-112]. It seems to be the most prevalent in mammals [113]. In this mechanism, the seed region of the miRNA does not need to be fully complementary; yet, efficient translation repression by miRNAs often requires multiple miRNA-binding sites, as suggested by the observations that the identified mRNA targets of miRNAs contained multiple sites for miRNA binding, either the same miRNA or a combination of several different miRNAs [114, 115]. However, many predicted mRNA targets of miRNAs contain only a single miRNA-binding site in their 3'UTR [107], indicating that such single sites may lead to fine "tuning" of mRNA function [116]. Distinct from the slicer activity of the specific Ago in the first manner, translation repression by miRNAs is common to all members of the Ago protein family. The third mechanism is called mRNA decay independent of slicer [117, 118]. In this manner, miRNAs either promote mRNAs decapping and 5' to 3' degradation, or target mRNAs by an unknown decay pathway. In the former way, the protecting poly-A-tail and "cap" of the mRNAs are removed, resulting in their rapid destruction by RNA splicing enzymes.

MiRNAs are now known to target thousands of genes. Bioinformatics analyses estimated that up to 30% of known human genes are under miRNAs' control [107], whereas later reports increased this number to 74~92% [119]. A key issue in miRNAs function is the specificity of their interactions with their target mRNAs and how each interaction leads to discrete downstream consequences. Some miRNAs regulate specific individual targets, while others can function as master regulators of a process. Key miRNAs regulate the expression levels of hundreds of genes simultaneously, and many types of miRNAs regulate their targets cooperatively. Because of their potent and wide action on gene expression, miRNAs become critical regulators of cellular functions. They are involved in modulating a variety of biological processes, including cellular proliferation, differentiation, metabolic signaling, apoptosis and development. The aberrant expression or alteration of miRNAs has been linked to a range of human diseases, especially cancers.

3.2. Dysregulation of miRNA in cancer

In 2002, Calin *et al.* first demonstrated that miR-15 and miIR-16 are frequently deleted or down-regulated in chronic lymphocytic leukemia [120]. Subsequently, aberrant miRNA expression, and amplification or deletion of miRNAs are observed in various human tumors [121, 122]. MiRNAs are differentially expressed in cancer cells, in which they form distinct and unique miRNA expression patterns [123]. These properties make miRNAs become potential biomarkers for cancer diagnosis, in particular for the early detection of cancer [124]. The control of gene expression by miRNAs is seen in virtually all cancer cells. Their target genes are usually important proteins such as oncogenic factors (i.e., MYC, RAS), tumor suppressors (i.e., p53), or proteins regulating the cell cycle (i.e., the cyclin family). Even small changes in these crucial proteins can have profound effects on tumorigenesis or tumor development. Conversely, miRNAs are often critical downstream effectors of classic oncogene/tumor suppressor networks, such as MYC and p53 described below.

miRNAs can act as oncogenes or tumor suppressor genes in tumorigenesis depending on the targets they regulate. Oncogenic miRNAs repress known tumor suppressors, whereas tumor-suppressor miRNAs often negatively regulate protein-coding oncogenes (this has been reviewed in detail by others [125-127]). Oncogenic miRNAs are overexpressed in various human cancers. For example, the miR-17-92 cluster miRNAs which are transcribed as a polycistronic unit, are highly expressed in B-cell lymphoma and various solid cancer, such as breast, colon, lung, pancreas, prostate and stomach [128-130]. They function as oncogenes to promote proliferation, inhibit apoptosis, induce tumor angiogenesis, and augment the oncogenic effects of MYC [131-134]. Their effects on cell cycle and proliferation are at least in part through its regulation of E2F transcription factors [130, 135], and anti-apoptotic effects are through their inhibition of BIM, PTEN and p21 [135]. MiR-221 and miR-222 are frequently overexpressed in lung, liver and ERα- breast cancers. Their overexpression has been demonstrated to enhance tumorigenicity through suppressing the expression of different tumor suppressors, such as CDKN1B/C, BIM, PTEN, TIMP3 and FOXO3 [136, 137]. Overexpression of miR-504 promotes tumorgenicity of colon cancer *in vivo*, which directly targets tumor suppressor p53 and functions in apoptosis and cell cycle [138].

On the other hand, miRNAs that act as tumor suppressors are often found to be deleted or mutated in various human cancers. For example, Let-7 family miRNAs are frequently down-regulated in various cancers, including lung and colorectal cancers [139]. They can directly suppress the expression of oncogenes, including RAS and MYC, and therefore show tumor suppressive functions [139, 140]. MiR-15a and miR-16-1 are often deleted or down-regulated in B-cell chronic lymphocytic leukemia (B-CLL). They negatively regulate anti-apoptotic protein BCL2. Therefore, decreased expression of miR-15a and miR-16-1 up-regulates BCL2 levels and reduces apoptosis, contributing to malignant transformation [141].

Based on the critical role of miRNAs in tumorigenesis, recent research efforts are directed towards translating these basic discoveries into clinical applications in diagnosis, prognosis and therapy through identifying and targeting dysregulated miRNAs. Both silencing the oncogenic miRNAs and restoring the expression of silenced tumor-suppressor miRNAs have yielded positive results in mouse models of cancer and thus becomes promising therapeutic strategy for cancer [142, 143]. The silencing of oncogenic miRNAs can be achieved by using antisense oligonucleotides (antagomirs or anti-miRs), sponges or locked nucleic acid (LNA) constructs [144]. By contrast, the restoration of tumor-suppressor miRNA expression can be achieved by the use of synthetic miRNA mimics, adenovirus vectors, and pharmacological agents [144]. Although the drug delivery, proper drug composition and off-target effects are still the current challenges in the clinical application of miRNAs, the future is bright for miRNA-based therapy.

3.3. MiRNAs regulated by transcriptional factors, genetic and epigenetic changes

3.3.1. MiRNAs regulated by oncogenic transcriptional factor MYC

MiRNAs can be dysregulated by multiple transcription factors in cancer. Oncogenic transcriptional factor MYC regulates a variety of gene expression affecting a series of cellular processes in cancer including cell growth and proliferation, metabolism, cell-cycle, differentiation, apoptosis, angiogenesis and metastasis [145-147]. Recently, it was found that MYC is also an important regulator of miRNAs. Consistent with their ability to potently influence cancer phenotypes, the regulation of miRNAs by MYC affects virtually all aspects of the MYC oncogenic program.

MYC directly activates the transcription of miR-17-92 polycistronic cluster though binding to an E-box within the first intron of the gene encoding the miR-17-92 primary transcript [148, 149]. Given its oncogenic role, the inhibition of key targets of miR-17-92 contributes to MYC-induced tumorigenesis. MiR-9 could also be activated directly by MYC, which regulates E-cadherin and cancer metastasis [150]. In contrast, MYC activity also results in repression of numerous miRNAs [151]. This repression involves the downregulation of miRNAs with antiproliferative, antitumorigenic and pro-apoptotic activity, such as let-7, miR-15a/16-1, miR-26a miR-29 or miR-34 family members [143, 151-153]. MiR-23a/b is an additional important example to be directly suppressed by MYC, which targets glutaminase to enhance glutamine catabolism [5]. MYC-driven reprogramming of miRNA expression patterns was shown to be a contributing factor in hepatoblastoma (HB), a rare embryonal neoplasm derived from liver progenitor cells [154]. Like an embryonic stem cell expression profile, undifferentiated aggressive HBs overexpress the miR-371-3 cluster with concomitant down-regulation of the miR-100/let-7a-2/miR-125b-1 cluster, which exerts antagonistic effects on cell proliferation and tumorigenicity. Chromatin immunoprecipitation (ChIP) and MYC inhibition assays in hepatoma cells demonstrated that both miR clusters are regulated by MYC in an opposite manner.

Although further investigation is necessary, the current studies have indicated that MYC uses both transcriptional and post-transcriptional mechanisms to modulate miRNA expression [151, 155]. Primary transcript mapping and ChIP revealed that MYC associates directly with evolutionarily conserved promoter regions upstream of several miRNAs [151], such as the direct activation of miR-17-92 cluster and direct suppression of miR-23a/b described above. MYC is also able to modulate the maturation of specific miRNAs without affecting transcription of the pri-miRNAs. For example, MYC activity results in repression of mature let-7 miRNAs while the expression of let-7 primary transcripts is unchanged [151, 156]. This phenomenon could be due to Lin28A and Lin28B being the direct target of MYC, which interacts with let-7 pre-miRNA stem-loops and may regulate let-7 at multiple levels including Drosha and Dicer processing [156, 157]. Additionally, interaction of Lin28A and Lin28B recruits the 3' terminal uridylyl transferase 4 (TUT4) to pre-let-7, resulting in uridylation and subsequent decay of the pre-miRNA [158, 159].

3.3.2. MiRNAs regulated by tumor suppressor p53

The tumor suppressor p53 is another transcription factor that regulate the expression of a group of miRNAs mediating a variety of anti-proliferative processes [160]. The miR-34 family, which consists of miR-34a, miR-34b and miR-34c, was initially reported to be induced directly by p53 [161] and mediate some of the p53 effects. ChIP and luciferase assays showed that p53 binds to p53 response elements (REs) in miR-34 promoters and activates their transcription [162]. MiR-34 family members directly repress the expression of several targets involved in the regulation of cell cycle and in the promotion of cell proliferation and survival. These targets include cyclin E2, cyclin-dependent kinases 4 and 6 (CDK4 and CDK6), BCL2 and hepatocyte growth factor receptor c-Met [161]. Later on, p53 was reported to directly regulate the transcriptional expression of several additional miRNAs, including miR-145, miR-107, miR-192 and miR215, miR-149* [160, 163]. MiR-145 negatively regulates oncogene *MYC*, which accounts partially for the miR-145-mediated inhibition of tumor cell growth both *in vitro* and *in vivo* [164]. MiR-107 contributes to the role of p53 in the regulation of hypoxia signaling and anti-angiogenesis through repressing the expression of HIF-1β, which interacts with HIF-1α subunits to form a HIF-1 complex, a key player in tumor formation. MiR-192 and miR-215 induce cell cycle arrest and reduce tumor cell growth through targeting a number of regulators of DNA synthesis and cell cycle checkpoints, such as CDC7, MDA2L1 and CUL5 [165]. MiRNA-149* targets glycogen synthase kinase-3α, resulting in increased expression of Mcl-1 and resistance to apoptosis in melanoma cells [163].

Moreover, p53 also enhances the post-transcriptional maturation of miRNAs. In response to doxorubicin, P53 interacts with the Drosha processing complex through the association with DEAD box RNA helicases p68 (also known as DDX5) and p72 (also known as DDX17), and facilitates the Drosha-mediated processing of pri-miRNAs to pre-miRNAs. These miRNAs include miR-16-1, miR-143 and miR-145 with growth-suppressive functions. Transcriptionally inactive p53 mutants interfere with a functional assembly between Drosha complex and p68, leading to attenuation of miRNA processing activity [166].

3.3.3. MiRNAs regulated by other transcription factors

Estrogen receptor alpha (ERα), a member of the nuclear receptor superfamily of transcription factors, was found to negatively regulate expression of miR-221 and miR-222 by promoter binding and recruiting the corepressors NCoR and SMRT [137]. Overexpression of miR-221 and miR-222 conversely suppresses the expression of ERα, conferring estrogen-independent growth. They also suppress the expression of different tumor suppressors, such as CDKN1B, CDKN1C, BIM, PTEN, TIMP3, DNA damage-inducible transcript 4, and FOXO3, to promote high proliferation [137]. Transcription factor c-Jun could also activate miR-221 and miR-222 [136].

Microarray-based expression profiles reveal that a specific spectrum of miRNAs is induced in response to low oxygen, at least some via a HIF-dependent mechanism, such as miR-210, miR-26a-2, miR-24 and miR-181c [167]. Of these, miR-210 as a direct transcriptional target of HIF-1α has emerged as a critical element of the cellular hypoxia response in a broad variety of cell types ranging from cancer cell lines to human umbilical vein endothelial cells [168-170]. MiR-210 has diverse functions, including modulating angiogenesis [171], stem cell survival [172], and hypoxia-induced cell cycle arrest [173]. MiR-143 and miR-145 could be repressed by RAS-responsive element-binding protein 1 (RREB1), a zinc finger transcription factor which binds to RAS-responsive elements (RREs) of their promoters. Thus these two miRNAs are embedded in KRAS oncogenic network [174].

In general, miRNAs can be dysregulated by transcription factors and, therefore, genetic or epigenetic alterations that result in the dysregulation of transcription factors can cause miRNA dysregulation. Importantly, miRNAs can also be directly regulated by genetic or epigenetic alterations.

3.3.4. MiRNAs regulated by genetic and epigenetic changes

MiRNAs are frequently located in fragile regions of the chromosomes, such as common chromosomal-breakpoints that are associated with the development of cancer [175, 176]. These fragile regions are often missing, amplified or mutated in cancer cells, resulting in the genetic alterations of miRNAs. The genetic alterations can affect the production of the primary miRNA transcript, their processing to mature miRNAs and/or interactions with mRNA targets. The dysregulation of miR-15 and miR-16 in most B cell chronic lymphocytic leukemias, one of the first observations between miRNAs and cancer development, is the result from chromosome 13q14 deletion [120]. Interestingly, somatic translocations in miRNA target sites can also occur, representing a drastic means of altering miRNA function [177, 178].

In addition to the structural genetic alterations, dysregulation of miRNAs in cancer can occur through epigenetic changes, such as methylation of the CpG islands of their promoters, the modification of histone [179-181]. As the example, miR-127 is silenced by promoter methylation, which leads to the overexpression of BCL6, an oncogene involved in the development of diffuse large B cell lymphoma [179]. The expression of miR-127 could be restored by using hypomethylating agents such as azacytidine. MiRNA-200 family could serve as another example. The miR-200 family can be shifted to hypermethylated or unmethylated 5'-CpG island status corresponding to the epithelial-mesenchymal transition (EMT) and mesenchymal-epithelial transition (MET) phenotypes, respectively, which contributes to the evolving and adapting phenotypes of human tumors [181].

4. miR-23b* targets PRODH/POX

Although numerous targets of miRNAs have been identified, miRNA regulators of critical cancer proteins and pathways remain largely unknown. As described above, PRODH/POX is frequently reduced in a variety of human cancers, including renal cancer, and PRODH/POX protein but not mRNA level is markedly down-regulated in renal cancers [46, 62]. The fact that miRNAs are critical post-transcriptional regulators, and miRNAs function as oncogenes to inhibit the expression of tumor suppressors raises attractive possibility that some specific miRNAs may regulate PRODH/POX and proline catabolism. Target-prediction algorithms have been used to identify the protein targets of miRNAs or miRNAs regulators of known protein, followed by experimental validation to eliminate false positives [141]. The bioinformatic analysis according to target-prediction algorithms predicted that 91 potential miRNAs could target PRODH/POX mRNA 3′UTR [62]. In miRNA microarrays, 10 miRNAs showed an increased expression in renal cancer cells relative to normal cells. However, only miR-23b* was shown to significantly inhibit

PRODH/POX protein expression, but not mRNA level. This is consistent with many previous reports, that is, in mammals, miRNAs more often inhibit protein translation of the target mRNA, other than inducing its degradation [113]. Subsequently, miR-23b* directly binding to PRODH/POX mRNA 3'UTR was experimentally confirmed through luciferase assays by co-transfecting the mimic miR-23b* and the luciferase reporter containing 3'UTR of PRODH/POX mRNA. Functional analysis showed that this miRNA impaired PRODH/POX functions, including PRODH/POX-mediated ROS generation, apoptosis, and PRODH/POX-inhibited HIF-1 signaling [62]. In contrast, the inhibitory antagomir of miR-23b* increased the expression of PRODH/POX protein in renal cancer cells. As a result, ROS production, the percentage of cells undergoing apoptosis increased, and HIF-1 signaling decreased.

The clinical relevance of these *in vitro* findings was substantiated by the data obtained in human renal carcinoma tissues *in vivo* [62]. There were statistical significant differences in both miR-23b* and PRODH/POX protein expression between carcinoma tissues and corresponding normal tissues, but not PRODH/POX mRNA levels. A negative correlation between miR-23b* and PRODH/POX protein was found.

In summary, PRODH/POX is subject to the negative regulation of miR-23b*, which is a novel mechanism for cells to regulate PRODH/POX protein level and functions. The increased miR-23b* might contribute to renal oncogenesis and progression by downregulating tumor suppressor PRODH/POX. This provides a possible strategic opening to inhibit tumor growth by decreasing the levels of miR-23b* or by blocking its function.

5. Regulation of miR-23b* in cancer

5.1. MiR-23b* regulation by oncogenic protein MYC

Recently, the oncogenic transcription factor MYC has been reported to transcriptionally suppress miR-23b to stimulate mitochondrial glutaminase expression and glutamine metabolism in lymphoma cells [5]. MiR-23b and miR-23b* are sibling miRNAs processed from the same transcript. Thus, this finding attracted our attention and compelled us to seek the potential effect of MYC on miR-23b* and related PRODH/POX expression and proline metabolism. As described above, MYC is a critical regulator of miRNAs expression at both transcriptional and post-transcriptional levels. Furthermore, proline and glutamine metabolism are closely related: not only their interconversions, but also both can be anaplerotic in the TCA cycle as an important energy source, as mentioned above. These facts strengthened our hypothesis that MYC may regulate the expression of miR-23b*, thereby PRODH/POX, and link proline and glutamine metabolism.

Using human Burkitt lymphoma model P493 cells that bear a tetracycline-repressible *MYC* construct, we found that MYC upregulated the expression of miR-23b* [30]. In PC3 prostate cancer cells which overexpress MYC, the same result was obtained, i.e., MYC knockdown by siRNA resulted in the decrease of miR-23b* expression. These results are distinct from the previous report which showed MYC directly bound to the transcriptional unit encompassing miR-23b, and regulated its expression at the transcriptional level [5]. Re-examination of the expression of miR-23b*, miR-23b, and their primary transcript (pri-miR23b) showed that pri-miR23b increased about 50% with MYC suppression by tetracycline and then decreased on MYC re-induction in P493 cells [30]. Similarly, in PC3 prostate cancer cells, with MYC knockdown by siRNA, miR-23b* decreased 68%, while miR-23b and Pri-miR-23b increased 51% and 70%, respectively [30]. Thus, the level of miR-23b* is higher than miR-23b in cells without MYC knockdown. These results support previous work that MYC suppresses miR-23b expression at the transcriptional level. Considering the fact that MYC enhances the expression of miR-23b*, the sibling of miR-23b, we hypothesized that differential effects of MYC on the sibling miRNAs may be due to their differential stabilization and/or degradation mediated by MYC. As a consequence, even if MYC suppressed the expression of miR-23b primary transcript, its effects on miR-23b* stabilization and/or degradation could account for net higher levels of miR-23b* as observed in this report.

The mechanisms responsible for stabilized miRNA expression have been largely elusive. As mentioned above, Ago proteins, the key players in miRNA processing and function, recently have been shown to regulate miRNA stability [93-96]. Ago2 differentially regulates miRNAs expression [93, 96]. Not surprisingly, MYC significantly upregulated the expression of Ago2 [30]. Knockdown of Ago2 in P493 MYC-overexpressed cells, the expression of miR-23b* and miR-23b were differentially decreased (76% vs. 42%, respectively), but not Pri-23b. Although the differential effects on miR-23b* and miR-23b resulted from Ago2 regulation by MYC do not completely account for the observed differential effects of MYC, they do support our hypothesis that MYC may regulate miRNA levels by differential effects on the stabilization of miRNAs, which can serve as a model for the effects on sibling miRNAs.

Since a large number of RISC components are involved in the miRNA processing [86]. It is likely that MYC with its multitude of target genes may affect many proteins like Ago2 and differentially affect miR-23b* and miR-23b expression. In fact, several reports have described the regulation of MYC on other RISCs or accessory RISCs, such as the upregulation of XPO5 and DEAD box protein 5 (DDX5) [86, 182, 183], and the aforementioned Lin28A and Lin28B regulation by MYC which affects the expression of mature let-7 miRNAs at multiple levels including their processing and modification [151, 156-159], but further studies are needed to elucidate how they affect the final expression of mature miRNAs and their interaction.

5.2. miR-23b* regulation by other factors

As mentioned above, PRODH/POX is encoded by a p53-induced gene [31]. Maxwell SA et al. reported that reduced expression of PRODH/POX mRNA in renal cancer was due to a p53 mutation [184]. On the other hand, p53 is a critical regulator of miRNAs. Thus, the possibility exists that wild-type p53 may regulate the expression of PRODH/POX by both direct and indirect (miR-23b*-dependent) mechanism. Interestingly, the experiment showed that ectopic expression of p53 in p53-mutant renal cancer cell line TK10 increased the expression of miR-23b* [62]. This suggests that the upregulation of miR-23b* by p53 may counteract the direct induction of p53 on PRODH/POX gene expression in clear cell renal cell carcinoma. This interaction might also account for discrepancies between PRODH/POX mRNA and protein expression.

In addition, current evidence suggests that miR-23b* could be regulated by factors other than p53 and MYC. For example, as discussed above, several reports have shown the link between upregulation of miR-23b and hypoxia [167, 185, 186]. As miR-23b and miR-23b* share the same precursor, miR-23b* could also be regulated by HIF. In renal cell carcinoma, the constitutive expression of HIF due to VHL deficiency may link this regulation of miR-23b* with VHL. The fact that HIF-1 negatively regulates mitochondrial biogenesis by inhibiting MYC activity in VHL-deficient renal carcinoma cells [187] further increases the possibility that miR-23b* could be regulated by VHL, HIF, thereby affecting the expression of PRODH/POX. These regulatory interactions are of great interest and worth to be pursued.

6. Regulation of proline metabolism by MYC

6.1. MYC suppresses PRODH/POX primarily through miR-23b*

In view of the above findings, it is not surprising that MYC suppresses the expression of PRODH/POX through upregulating miR-23b*. First, PRODH/POX protein increased in a time-dependent fashion with diminished MYC expression and then decreased on MYC recovery in P493 cells. PRODH/POX mRNA expression also showed a significant increase with suppressed MYC expression, but the increase was far less than that of protein levels, raising the likelihood that miRNA mediates the effect of MYC on PRODH/POX at the post-transcriptional level. MYC knockdown in PC3 prostate cancer cells by siRNA resulted in the inhibition of PRODH/POX expression with a pattern similar to the P493 cells. Secondly, the inhibition of miR-23b* by its antagomirs in the P493 cells with MYC overexpression increased PRODH/POX protein level [30]. By contrast, the transfection of mimic miR-23b* into the P493 cells under MYC inhibition by tetracycline resulted in a marked decrease of PRODH/POX protein expression. However, the decrease of PRODH/POX still was not comparable with that without tetracycline treatment, indicating that MYC could suppress PRODH/POX expression through pathways other than miRNA, such as the regulation at the transcriptional level, which also is supported by the decrease of PRODH/POX mRNA by MYC. Thirdly, the luciferase assays in PC cells showed that knockdown of MYC increased the luciferase activity of the luciferase reporter containing POX 3'UTR with the binding site of miR-23b*, indicating the decrease of miR-23b* by siMYC. Without MYC knockdown, the luciferase activity of this reporter was much lower than that of the original reporter without POX 3'UTR, due to high levels of miR-23b* binding to PRODH/POX mRNA 3'UTR, thereby suppressing luciferase expression.

By transfecting the PRODH promoter/luciferase reporter construct containing PRODH promoter region in PC3 prostate cancer cells, knockdown of MYC resulted in the increase of PRODH promoter activity, which confirmed that MYC regulates PRODH/POX at the transcriptional level [41]. Analysis of PRODH promoter nucleotide sequence revealed one canonical MYC binding site 5'-CACGTG-3' (E-box) and one noncanonical binding site (5'-ACGGTG-3') at -2808 to -2813bp and -637 to -642bp of the PRODH promoter region, respectively. However, ChIP assay showed none of these PRODH promoter regions had significant PCR amplification, suggesting that MYC does not directly interact with the

PRODH gene, and the decreased PRODH/POX mRNA expression may be mediated through other transcription factors regulated by MYC [30].

6.2. Suppression of proline catabolism is essential for MYC-mediated cancer cell proliferation and survival

In addition to PRODH/POX, MYC also inhibits the expression of another enzyme in proline catabolism, P5CDH [30], but the mechanism remains unclear. However, the suppression of proline catabolism reflected by PRODH/POX inhibition by MYC has been shown to be essential for MYC-induced proliferation and cell survival. First, knockdown of PRODH/POX in P493 cells with MYC suppressed by tetracycline consistently reduced the production of ROS at different time points [30], although the suppression of MYC itself by tetracycline also decreased the accumulation of ROS at late stage which implicates the different effects of various MYC regulated genes on ROS production at various stages [188-190]. Correspondingly, the apoptosis assay by flow cytometry showed that PRODH/POX knockdown decreased the percentage of apoptotic and dead cells occurring with MYC suppression. In contrast, PRODH/POX siRNA significantly rescued 30~40% of the diminished growth rates resulting from MYC suppression by tetracycline [30]. These results indicated that PRODH/POX suppression is critical for MYC-mediated cancer cell proliferation and survival. The same assays performed in PC3 prostate cancer cells confirmed these results [30].

To summarize, oncogenic transcription factor MYC inhibits PRODH/POX expression and thereby inhibits its tumor suppressor function. When MYC is suppressed, the increase of PRODH/POX promotes proline catabolism to generate ROS, leading to the initiation of apoptosis and the decrease of cell proliferation and growth. MYC-induced suppression of PRODH/POX contributes to MYC-mediated changes of cell behavior including proliferation and metabolic reprogramming, which in turn may contribute to tumorigenesis and tumor progression. These findings further indicate the critical roles of proline catabolism catalyzed by PRODH/POX in human cancers.

6.3. MYC increases the biosynthesis of proline from glutamine

Since MYC plays an important role in glutamine metabolism which is closely related with proline metabolism due to the interconversion of proline and glutamate, we not only investigated the effect of MYC on proline catabolism catalyzed by PRODH/POX as shown above, but also examined proline biosynthesis, especially from glutamine. Western blots showed that MYC robustly increased the expression of GLS, P5CS and PYCR1 in the pathway from glutamine to proline biosynthesis [30]. PC3 prostate cancer cells displayed the same correlation between MYC and glutamine and proline metabolism. The measurement of the intracellular proline levels showed that MYC dramatically increased the intracellular levels of proline. Consistently, using $[^{13}C,^{15}N]$-Glutamine as a tracer, the direct production of proline from glutamine induced by MYC was confirmed by GC-MS and NMR analysis [30]. Thus, MYC not only suppresses proline catabolism and stimulates glutamine oxidation to glutamate, but also markedly enhances proline biosynthesis from glutamine.

Both normal and tumor cells depend on glucose and glutamine consumption as sources of metabolic energy, and as precursors for biosynthesis of macromolecules [6, 191]. MYC oncogene is considered a master regulator of tumor cell metabolism and proliferation. It not only promotes glucose uptake and induces aerobic glycolysis, but also enhances glutamine uptake and stimulates glutamine catabolism. Although glutamine catabolism is linked to biosynthesis of protein, nucleotides and lipids, redox homeostasis and energy metabolism, the report from Wise *et al.* suggests that little of the glutamine uptake stimulated by MYC is used for macromolecular synthesis [6]. MYC-induced glutamine catabolism is involved in reprogramming mitochondrial metabolism to sustain cellular viability and TCA cycle anapleurosis [6]. More recent findings reported by Le *et al.* [192] and Wang *et al.* [193] emphasized the metabolic reprogramming controlled by MYC in tumor cells and activated T cells. The latter showed that glutamine catabolism driven by MYC coupled with multiple biosynthetic pathways, especially ornithine and polyamine biosynthesis [193]. However, the importance of the biosynthesis of the ornithine and polyamine from glutamine is understood only in part. Similarly, the metabolic advantage afforded by the increased conversion of glutamine to proline and how biosynthetic pathway fits into the MYC-driven metabolic reprogramming also remain unclear. The connection between the conversion of P5C to proline, the last step of proline biosynthesis and pentose phosphate pathway through the oxidation-reduction reactions of NADPH and $NADP^+$ [8, 14, 15] provides us a clue to understand the importance of proline biosynthesis induced by MYC in cancer, since proline synthesis from P5C could also oxidize NADH to NAD^+ to maintain glucose metabolism, glycolysis. In fact, our unpublished data showed that the blockade of proline biosynthesis by knocking down P5CS or PYCR1 markedly decreased glycolysis, which supports our hypothesis.

It's noteworthy that glutamine may be not the only source of proline biosynthesis promoted by MYC, since the increase of PYCR1 is much greater than that of P5CS and GLS [30], and ornithine could also be converted to proline by ornithine aminotransferase and PYCR1 (see Figure 1). This possibility and its importance in MYC-induced metabolic reprogramming are also worth pursuing.

7. Conclusion

Proline, the unique proteinogenic secondary amino acid, is metabolized by its own family of enzymes. Early studies showed that proline metabolism is linked with TCA cycle, pentose phosphate pathway and urea cycle. During the conversion of proline to P5C, the central enzyme of proline metabolism, PRODH/POX, donates electron to ETC to generate ROS or ATP depending on context. As a tumor suppressor, PRODH/POX is induced by p53, PPARγ and its ligands, and contributes to the initiation of apoptosis and the inhibition of tumor growth through ROS generation (Figure 2). On the other hand, PRODH/POX is suppressed by miR-23b* and oncogene MYC. MYC not only suppresses proline catabolism, but increases proline biosynthesis from glutamine (Figure 3). Thus, these recent studies reveal a new link in human cancer between MYC, miRNA regulation, proline metabolism, glutamine metabolism, TCA cycle, and even glycolysis. These metabolic links emphasizes the complexity of tumor metabolism. Further studies of proline metabolism in tumor microenvironment will provide a deeper understanding of tumor metabolism and novel therapeutic strategies in cancer.

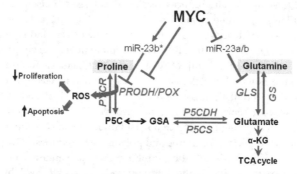

Figure 3. MYC regulation of proline and glutamine metabolism. MYC suppresses proline catabolism through its inhibition of the expression of PRODH/POX and P5CDH. MYC inhibits the expression of PRODH/POX at both transcriptional and post-transcriptional levels (upregulation of miR-23b*), which is essential for MYC-induced proliferation and cell survival. On the other hand, MYC stimulates glutamine catabolism through miR-23a/b-mediated glutaminase (GLS) upregulation. Furthermore, MYC not only suppresses proline catabolism, but also enhances proline biosynthesis from glutamine. Proline and glutamine metabolism are connected by MYC and miRNA regulation.

Author details

Wei Liu and James M. Phang*
Metabolism and Cancer Susceptibility Section, Basic Research Laboratory, Frederick National Laboratory for Cancer Research, NIH. Frederick, MD

Acknowledgement

The work was supported by the Intramural Research Program of the NIH, National Cancer Institute, Center for Cancer Research. This project also has been funded in part with Federal funds from the National Cancer Institute, NIH, under contract no. HHSN27612080001. The content of this review does not necessarily reflect the views or policies of the Department of Health and Human Services, nor does mention of trade names, commercial products, or organizations imply endorsement by the U.S. government. We thank Dr. Ziqiang Zhu for his reading of the manuscript.

8. References

[1]   Warburg O (1956) On the origin of cancer cells, Science 123, 309-314.

* Corresponding Author

[2]   Vander Heiden MG, Cantley LC, & Thompson CB (2009) Understanding the Warburg effect: the metabolic requirements of cell proliferation, Science 324, 1029-1033.

[3]   Fogal V, Richardson AD, Karmali PP, Scheffler IE, Smith JW, & Ruoslahti E (2010) Mitochondrial p32 protein is a critical regulator of tumor metabolism via maintenance of oxidative phosphorylation, Mol Cell Biol 30, 1303-1318.

[4]   Dang CV (2010) Rethinking the Warburg effect with Myc micromanaging glutamine metabolism, Cancer Res 70, 859-862.

[5]   Gao P, Tchernyshyov I, Chang TC, Lee YS, Kita K, Ochi T, et al. (2009) c-Myc suppression of miR-23a/b enhances mitochondrial glutaminase expression and glutamine metabolism, Nature 458, 762-765.

[6]   Wise DR, DeBerardinis RJ, Mancuso A, Sayed N, Zhang XY, Pfeiffer HK, et al. (2008) Myc regulates a transcriptional program that stimulates mitochondrial glutaminolysis and leads to glutamine addiction, Proc Natl Acad Sci U S A 105, 18782-18787.

[7]   Adams E (1970) Metabolism of proline and of hydroxyproline, Int Rev Connect Tissue Res 5, 1-91.

[8]   Phang JM (1985) The regulatory functions of proline and pyrroline-5-carboxylic acid, Curr Top Cell Regul 25, 91-132.

[9]   Phang JM, Liu W, & Zabirnyk O (2010) Proline metabolism and microenvironmental stress, Annu Rev Nutr 30, 441-463.

[10] Phang JM & Liu W (2012) Proline metabolism and cancer, Front Biosci 17, 1835-1845.

[11] Phang JM, Hu CA, & Valle D (2001) Disorders of proline and hydroxyproline metabolism. In: Scriver CR, Beaudet AL, Sly WS, Valle D, editors. In Metabolic and Molecular Bases of Inherited Disease, New York: McGraw-Hill. pp. 1821-1838.

[12] Adams E & Frank L (1980) Metabolism of proline and the hydroxyprolines, Annu Rev Biochem 49, 1005-1061.

[13] Liu Y, Borchert GL, Donald SP, Surazynski A, Hu CA, Weydert CJ, et al. (2005) MnSOD inhibits proline oxidase-induced apoptosis in colorectal cancer cells, Carcinogenesis 26, 1335-1342.

[14] Phang JM, Downing SJ, Yeh GC, Smith RJ, Williams JA, & Hagedorn CH (1982) Stimulation of the hexosemonophosphate-pentose pathway by pyrroline-5-carboxylate in cultured cells, J Cell Physiol 110, 255-261.

[15] Yeh GC, Roth EF, Jr., Phang JM, Harris SC, Nagel RL, & Rinaldi A (1984) The effect of pyrroline-5-carboxylic acid on nucleotide metabolism in erythrocytes from normal and glucose-6-phosphate dehydrogenase-deficient subjects, J Biol Chem 259, 5454-5458.

[16] Hu CA, Bart Williams D, Zhaorigetu S, Khalil S, Wan G, & Valle D (2008) Functional genomics and SNP analysis of human genes encoding proline metabolic enzymes, Amino Acids 35, 655-664.

[17] Schafer IA, Scriver CR, & Efron ML (1962) Familial hyperprolinemia, cerebral dysfunction and renal anomalies occuring in a family with hereditary nephropathy and deafness, N Engl J Med 267, 51-60.

[18] Willis A, Bender HU, Steel G, & Valle D (2008) PRODH variants and risk for schizophrenia, Amino Acids 35, 673-679.

[19] Bender HU, Almashanu S, Steel G, Hu CA, Lin WW, Willis A, *et al.* (2005) Functional consequences of PRODH missense mutations, Am J Hum Genet 76, 409-420.

[20] Reversade B, Escande-Beillard N, Dimopoulou A, Fischer B, Chng SC, Li Y, *et al.* (2009) Mutations in PYCR1 cause cutis laxa with progeroid features, Nat Genet 41, 1016-1021.

[21] Baumgartner MR, Hu CA, Almashanu S, Steel G, Obie C, Aral B, *et al.* (2000) Hyperammonemia with reduced ornithine, citrulline, arginine and proline: a new inborn error caused by a mutation in the gene encoding delta(1)-pyrroline-5-carboxylate synthase, Hum Mol Genet 9, 2853-2858.

[22] Baumgartner MR, Rabier D, Nassogne MC, Dufier JL, Padovani JP, Kamoun P, *et al.* (2005) Delta1-pyrroline-5-carboxylate synthase deficiency: neurodegeneration, cataracts and connective tissue manifestations combined with hyperammonaemia and reduced ornithine, citrulline, arginine and proline, Eur J Pediatr 164, 31-36.

[23] Dixit SN, Seyer JM, & Kang AH (1977) Covalent structure of collagen: amino-acid sequence of chymotryptic peptides from the carboxyl-terminal region of alpha2-CB3 of chick-skin collagen, Eur J Biochem 81, 599-607.

[24] Stallings-Mann M & Radisky D (2007) Matrix metalloproteinase-induced malignancy in mammary epithelial cells, Cells Tissues Organs 185, 104-110.

[25] Deryugina EI & Quigley JP (2006) Matrix metalloproteinases and tumor metastasis, Cancer Metastasis Rev 25, 9-34.

[26] Kakkad SM, Solaiyappan M, O'Rourke B, Stasinopoulos I, Ackerstaff E, Raman V, *et al.* (2010) Hypoxic tumor microenvironments reduce collagen I fiber density, Neoplasia 12, 608-617.

[27] Pandhare J, Donald SP, Cooper SK, & Phang JM (2009) Regulation and function of proline oxidase under nutrient stress, J Cell Biochem 107, 759-768.

[28] Klionsky DJ (2007) Autophagy: from phenomenology to molecular understanding in less than a decade, Nat Rev Mol Cell Biol 8, 931-937.

[29] Mathew R, Karantza-Wadsworth V, & White E (2007) Role of autophagy in cancer, Nat Rev Cancer 7, 961-967.

[30] Liu W, Le A, Hancock C, Lane AN, Dang CV, Fan TW, *et al.* (2012) Reprogramming of proline and glutamine metabolism contributes to the proliferative and metabolic responses regulated by oncogenic transcription factor c-MYC, Proc Natl Acad Sci U S A 109, 8983-8988.

[31] Polyak K, Xia Y, Zweier JL, Kinzler KW, & Vogelstein B (1997) A model for p53-induced apoptosis, Nature 389, 300-305.

[32] Rivera A & Maxwell SA (2005) The p53-induced gene-6 (proline oxidase) mediates apoptosis through a calcineurin-dependent pathway, J Biol Chem 280, 29346-29354.

[33] Donald SP, Sun XY, Hu CA, Yu J, Mei JM, Valle D, *et al.* (2001) Proline oxidase, encoded by p53-induced gene-6, catalyzes the generation of proline-dependent reactive oxygen species, Cancer Res 61, 1810-1815.

[34] Simon HU, Haj-Yehia A, & Levi-Schaffer F (2000) Role of reactive oxygen species (ROS) in apoptosis induction, Apoptosis 5, 415-418.

[35] Hu CA, Donald SP, Yu J, Lin WW, Liu Z, Steel G, *et al.* (2007) Overexpression of proline oxidase induces proline-dependent and mitochondria-mediated apoptosis, Mol Cell Biochem 295, 85-92.

[36] Liu Y, Borchert GL, Surazynski A, Hu CA, & Phang JM (2006) Proline oxidase activates both intrinsic and extrinsic pathways for apoptosis: the role of ROS/superoxides, NFAT and MEK/ERK signaling, Oncogene 25, 5640-5647.

[37] Willson TM, Brown PJ, Sternbach DD, & Henke BR (2000) The PPARs: from orphan receptors to drug discovery, J Med Chem 43, 527-550.

[38] Robbins GT & Nie D (2012) PPAR gamma, bioactive lipids, and cancer progression, Front Biosci 17, 1816-1834.

[39] Reka AK, Goswami MT, Krishnapuram R, Standiford TJ, & Keshamouni VG (2011) Molecular cross-regulation between PPAR-gamma and other signaling pathways: implications for lung cancer therapy, Lung Cancer 72, 154-159.

[40] Phang JM, Pandhare J, Zabirnyk O, & Liu Y (2008) PPARgamma and Proline Oxidase in Cancer, PPAR Res 2008, 542694.

[41] Pandhare J, Cooper SK, & Phang JM (2006) Proline oxidase, a proapoptotic gene, is induced by troglitazone: evidence for both peroxisome proliferator-activated receptor gamma-dependent and -independent mechanisms, J Biol Chem 281, 2044-2052.

[42] Kim KY, Ahn JH, & Cheon HG (2007) Apoptotic action of peroxisome proliferator-activated receptor-gamma activation in human non small-cell lung cancer is mediated via proline oxidase-induced reactive oxygen species formation, Mol Pharmacol 72, 674-685.

[43] Liu W, Glunde K, Bhujwalla ZM, Raman V, Sharma A, & Phang JM (2012) Proline oxidase promotes tumor cell survival in hypoxic tumor microenvironments, Cancer Res 72, 3677-3686.

[44] Zabirnyk O, Liu W, Khalil S, Sharma A, & Phang JM (2010) Oxidized low-density lipoproteins upregulate proline oxidase to initiate ROS-dependent autophagy, Carcinogenesis 31, 446-454.

[45] Smith ML & Kumar MA (2010) The "Two faces" of Tumor Suppressor p53-revisited, Mol Cell Pharmacol 2, 117-119.

[46] Liu Y, Borchert GL, Donald SP, Diwan BA, Anver M, & Phang JM (2009) Proline Oxidase Functions as a Mitochondrial Tumor Suppressor in Human Cancers, Cancer Res 69, 6414-6422.

[47] Liu Y, Borchert GL, Surazynski A, & Phang JM (2008) Proline oxidase, a p53-induced gene, targets COX-2/PGE2 signaling to induce apoptosis and inhibit tumor growth in colorectal cancers, Oncogene 27, 6729-6737.

[48] Greenhough A, Smartt HJ, Moore AE, Roberts HR, Williams AC, Paraskeva C, *et al.* (2009) The COX-2/PGE2 pathway: key roles in the hallmarks of cancer and adaptation to the tumour microenvironment, Carcinogenesis 30, 377-386.

[49] Brown JR & DuBois RN (2004) Cyclooxygenase as a target in lung cancer, Clin Cancer Res 10, 4266s-4269s.

[50] Arun B & Goss P (2004) The role of COX-2 inhibition in breast cancer treatment and prevention, Semin Oncol 31, 22-29.

[51] Henson ES & Gibson SB (2006) Surviving cell death through epidermal growth factor (EGF) signal transduction pathways: implications for cancer therapy, Cell Signal 18, 2089-2097.

[52] Yao H, Ashihara E, & Maekawa T (2011) Targeting the Wnt/beta-catenin signaling pathway in human cancers, Expert Opin Ther Targets 15, 873-887.

[53] Zhu W, Chen Y, & Dutta A (2004) Rereplication by depletion of geminin is seen regardless of p53 status and activates a G2/M checkpoint, Mol Cell Biol 24, 7140-7150.

[54] Stark GR & Taylor WR (2006) Control of the G2/M transition, Mol Biotechnol 32, 227-248.

[55] Liebermann DA & Hoffman B (2008) Gadd45 in stress signaling, J Mol Signal 3, 15.

[56] Gottlieb E & Tomlinson IP (2005) Mitochondrial tumour suppressors: a genetic and biochemical update, Nat Rev Cancer 5, 857-866.

[57] Yamakuchi M, Lotterman CD, Bao C, Hruban RH, Karim B, Mendell JT, et al. (2010) P53-induced microRNA-107 inhibits HIF-1 and tumor angiogenesis, Proc Natl Acad Sci U S A 107, 6334-6339.

[58] Verma A (2006) Oxygen-sensing in tumors, Curr Opin Clin Nutr Metab Care 9, 366-378.

[59] Hewitson KS, Lienard BM, McDonough MA, Clifton IJ, Butler D, Soares AS, et al. (2007) Structural and mechanistic studies on the inhibition of the hypoxia-inducible transcription factor hydroxylases by tricarboxylic acid cycle intermediates, J Biol Chem 282, 3293-3301.

[60] Koivunen P, Hirsila M, Remes AM, Hassinen IE, Kivirikko KI, & Myllyharju J (2007) Inhibition of hypoxia-inducible factor (HIF) hydroxylases by citric acid cycle intermediates: possible links between cell metabolism and stabilization of HIF, J Biol Chem 282, 4524-4532.

[61] Lu H, Dalgard CL, Mohyeldin A, McFate T, Tait AS, & Verma A (2005) Reversible inactivation of HIF-1 prolyl hydroxylases allows cell metabolism to control basal HIF-1, J Biol Chem 280, 41928-41939.

[62] Liu W, Zabirnyk O, Wang H, Shiao YH, Nickerson ML, Khalil S, et al. (2010) miR-23b targets proline oxidase, a novel tumor suppressor protein in renal cancer, Oncogene 29, 4914-4924.

[63] Lee RC, Feinbaum RL, & Ambros V (1993) The C. elegans heterochronic gene lin-4 encodes small RNAs with antisense complementarity to lin-14, Cell 75, 843-854.

[64] Wightman B, Ha I, & Ruvkun G (1993) Posttranscriptional regulation of the heterochronic gene lin-14 by lin-4 mediates temporal pattern formation in C. elegans, Cell 75, 855-862.

[65] Reinhart BJ, Slack FJ, Basson M, Pasquinelli AE, Bettinger JC, Rougvie AE, et al. (2000) The 21-nucleotide let-7 RNA regulates developmental timing in Caenorhabditis elegans, Nature 403, 901-906.

[66] Lee Y, Kim M, Han J, Yeom KH, Lee S, Baek SH, et al. (2004) MicroRNA genes are transcribed by RNA polymerase II, EMBO J 23, 4051-4060.

[67] Lee Y, Ahn C, Han J, Choi H, Kim J, Yim J, et al. (2003) The nuclear RNase III Drosha initiates microRNA processing, Nature 425, 415-419.

[68] Denli AM, Tops BB, Plasterk RH, Ketting RF, & Hannon GJ (2004) Processing of primary microRNAs by the Microprocessor complex, Nature 432, 231-235.

[69] Yi R, Qin Y, Macara IG, & Cullen BR (2003) Exportin-5 mediates the nuclear export of pre-microRNAs and short hairpin RNAs, Genes Dev 17, 3011-3016.

[70] Bohnsack MT, Czaplinski K, & Gorlich D (2004) Exportin 5 is a RanGTP-dependent dsRNA-binding protein that mediates nuclear export of pre-miRNAs, RNA 10, 185-191.

[71] Lund E, Guttinger S, Calado A, Dahlberg JE, & Kutay U (2004) Nuclear export of microRNA precursors, Science 303, 95-98.

[72] Lund E & Dahlberg JE (2006) Substrate selectivity of exportin 5 and Dicer in the biogenesis of microRNAs, Cold Spring Harb Symp Quant Biol 71, 59-66.

[73] Khvorova A, Reynolds A, & Jayasena SD (2003) Functional siRNAs and miRNAs exhibit strand bias, Cell 115, 209-216.

[74] Schwarz DS, Hutvagner G, Du T, Xu Z, Aronin N, & Zamore PD (2003) Asymmetry in the assembly of the RNAi enzyme complex, Cell 115, 199-208.

[75] Lin SL, Chang D, & Ying SY (2005) Asymmetry of intronic pre-miRNA structures in functional RISC assembly, Gene 356, 32-38.

[76] Kim S, Lee UJ, Kim MN, Lee EJ, Kim JY, Lee MY, et al. (2008) MicroRNA miR-199a* regulates the MET proto-oncogene and the downstream extracellular signal-regulated kinase 2 (ERK2), J Biol Chem 283, 18158-18166.

[77] Nass D, Rosenwald S, Meiri E, Gilad S, Tabibian-Keissar H, Schlosberg A, et al. (2009) MiR-92b and miR-9/9* are specifically expressed in brain primary tumors and can be used to differentiate primary from metastatic brain tumors, Brain Pathol 19, 375-383.

[78] Okamura K, Chung WJ, & Lai EC (2008) The long and short of inverted repeat genes in animals: microRNAs, mirtrons and hairpin RNAs, Cell Cycle 7, 2840-2845.

[79] Carmell MA, Xuan Z, Zhang MQ, & Hannon GJ (2002) The Argonaute family: tentacles that reach into RNAi, developmental control, stem cell maintenance, and tumorigenesis, Genes Dev 16, 2733-2742.

[80] Song JJ, Liu J, Tolia NH, Schneiderman J, Smith SK, Martienssen RA, et al. (2003) The crystal structure of the Argonaute2 PAZ domain reveals an RNA binding motif in RNAi effector complexes, Nat Struct Biol 10, 1026-1032.

[81] Ma JB, Ye K, & Patel DJ (2004) Structural basis for overhang-specific small interfering RNA recognition by the PAZ domain, Nature 429, 318-322.

[82] Lingel A & Sattler M (2005) Novel modes of protein-RNA recognition in the RNAi pathway, Curr Opin Struct Biol 15, 107-115.

[83] Okamura K, Ishizuka A, Siomi H, & Siomi MC (2004) Distinct roles for Argonaute proteins in small RNA-directed RNA cleavage pathways, Genes Dev 18, 1655-1666.

[84] Liu J, Carmell MA, Rivas FV, Marsden CG, Thomson JM, Song JJ, et al. (2004) Argonaute2 is the catalytic engine of mammalian RNAi, Science 305, 1437-1441.

[85] Meister G, Landthaler M, Patkaniowska A, Dorsett Y, Teng G, & Tuschl T (2004) Human Argonaute2 mediates RNA cleavage targeted by miRNAs and siRNAs, Mol Cell 15, 185-197.

[86] van Kouwenhove M, Kedde M, & Agami R (2011) MicroRNA regulation by RNA-binding proteins and its implications for cancer, Nat Rev Cancer 11, 644-656.

[87] Melo SA, Ropero S, Moutinho C, Aaltonen LA, Yamamoto H, Calin GA, *et al.* (2009) A TARBP2 mutation in human cancer impairs microRNA processing and DICER1 function, Nat Genet 41, 365-370.

[88] Hill DA, Ivanovich J, Priest JR, Gurnett CA, Dehner LP, Desruisseau D, *et al.* (2009) DICER1 mutations in familial pleuropulmonary blastoma, Science 325, 965.

[89] MacRae IJ, Ma E, Zhou M, Robinson CV, & Doudna JA (2008) In vitro reconstitution of the human RISC-loading complex, Proc Natl Acad Sci U S A 105, 512-517.

[90] Murchison EP & Hannon GJ (2004) miRNAs on the move: miRNA biogenesis and the RNAi machinery, Curr Opin Cell Biol 16, 223-229.

[91] Mourelatos Z, Dostie J, Paushkin S, Sharma A, Charroux B, Abel L, *et al.* (2002) miRNPs: a novel class of ribonucleoproteins containing numerous microRNAs, Genes Dev 16, 720-728.

[92] Caudy AA, Myers M, Hannon GJ, & Hammond SM (2002) Fragile X-related protein and VIG associate with the RNA interference machinery, Genes Dev 16, 2491-2496.

[93] Winter J & Diederichs S (2011) Argonaute proteins regulate microRNA stability: Increased microRNA abundance by Argonaute proteins is due to microRNA stabilization, RNA Biol 8, 1149-1157.

[94] Diederichs S & Haber DA (2007) Dual role for argonautes in microRNA processing and posttranscriptional regulation of microRNA expression, Cell 131, 1097-1108.

[95] O'Carroll D, Mecklenbrauker I, Das PP, Santana A, Koenig U, Enright AJ, *et al.* (2007) A Slicer-independent role for Argonaute 2 in hematopoiesis and the microRNA pathway, Genes Dev 21, 1999-2004.

[96] Zhang X, Graves PR, & Zeng Y (2009) Stable Argonaute2 overexpression differentially regulates microRNA production, Biochim Biophys Acta 1789, 153-159.

[97] Kai ZS & Pasquinelli AE (2010) MicroRNA assassins: factors that regulate the disappearance of miRNAs, Nat Struct Mol Biol 17, 5-10.

[98] Azuma-Mukai A, Oguri H, Mituyama T, Qian ZR, Asai K, Siomi H, *et al.* (2008) Characterization of endogenous human Argonautes and their miRNA partners in RNA silencing, Proc Natl Acad Sci U S A 105, 7964-7969.

[99] Yu B, Yang Z, Li J, Minakhina S, Yang M, Padgett RW, *et al.* (2005) Methylation as a crucial step in plant microRNA biogenesis, Science 307, 932-935.

[100] Li J, Yang Z, Yu B, Liu J, & Chen X (2005) Methylation protects miRNAs and siRNAs from a 3'-end uridylation activity in Arabidopsis, Curr Biol 15, 1501-1507.

[101] Landgraf P, Rusu M, Sheridan R, Sewer A, Iovino N, Aravin A, *et al.* (2007) A mammalian microRNA expression atlas based on small RNA library sequencing, Cell 129, 1401-1414.

[102] Lu S, Sun YH, & Chiang VL (2009) Adenylation of plant miRNAs, Nucleic Acids Res 37, 1878-1885.

[103] Reid JG, Nagaraja AK, Lynn FC, Drabek RB, Muzny DM, Shaw CA, *et al.* (2008) Mouse let-7 miRNA populations exhibit RNA editing that is constrained in the 5'-seed/cleavage/anchor regions and stabilize predicted mmu-let-7a:mRNA duplexes, Genome Res 18, 1571-1581.

[104] Katoh T, Sakaguchi Y, Miyauchi K, Suzuki T, Kashiwabara S, & Baba T (2009) Selective stabilization of mammalian microRNAs by 3' adenylation mediated by the cytoplasmic poly(A) polymerase GLD-2, Genes Dev 23, 433-438.

[105] Valencia-Sanchez MA, Liu J, Hannon GJ, & Parker R (2006) Control of translation and mRNA degradation by miRNAs and siRNAs, Genes Dev 20, 515-524.

[106] Billeter AT, Druen D, Kanaan ZM, & Polk HC, Jr. (2012) MicroRNAs: new helpers for surgeons?, Surgery 151, 1-5.

[107] Lewis BP, Burge CB, & Bartel DP (2005) Conserved seed pairing, often flanked by adenosines, indicates that thousands of human genes are microRNA targets, Cell 120, 15-20.

[108] Mallory AC, Reinhart BJ, Jones-Rhoades MW, Tang G, Zamore PD, Barton MK, et al. (2004) MicroRNA control of PHABULOSA in leaf development: importance of pairing to the microRNA 5' region, EMBO J 23, 3356-3364.

[109] Yekta S, Shih IH, & Bartel DP (2004) MicroRNA-directed cleavage of HOXB8 mRNA, Science 304, 594-596.

[110] Bartel DP (2004) MicroRNAs: genomics, biogenesis, mechanism, and function, Cell 116, 281-297.

[111] Pillai RS, Bhattacharyya SN, Artus CG, Zoller T, Cougot N, Basyuk E, et al. (2005) Inhibition of translational initiation by Let-7 MicroRNA in human cells, Science 309, 1573-1576.

[112] Cimmino A, Calin GA, Fabbri M, Iorio MV, Ferracin M, Shimizu M, et al. (2005) miR-15 and miR-16 induce apoptosis by targeting BCL2, Proc Natl Acad Sci U S A 102, 13944-13949.

[113] Williams AE (2008) Functional aspects of animal microRNAs, Cell Mol Life Sci 65, 545-562.

[114] Zeng Y, Yi R, & Cullen BR (2003) MicroRNAs and small interfering RNAs can inhibit mRNA expression by similar mechanisms, Proc Natl Acad Sci U S A 100, 9779-9784.

[115] Kiriakidou M, Nelson PT, Kouranov A, Fitziev P, Bouyioukos C, Mourelatos Z, et al. (2004) A combined computational-experimental approach predicts human microRNA targets, Genes Dev 18, 1165-1178.

[116] Bartel DP & Chen CZ (2004) Micromanagers of gene expression: the potentially widespread influence of metazoan microRNAs, Nat Rev Genet 5, 396-400.

[117] Eulalio A, Huntzinger E, & Izaurralde E (2008) GW182 interaction with Argonaute is essential for miRNA-mediated translational repression and mRNA decay, Nat Struct Mol Biol 15, 346-353.

[118] Behm-Ansmant I, Rehwinkel J, & Izaurralde E (2006) MicroRNAs silence gene expression by repressing protein expression and/or by promoting mRNA decay, Cold Spring Harb Symp Quant Biol 71, 523-530.

[119] Miranda KC, Huynh T, Tay Y, Ang YS, Tam WL, Thomson AM, et al. (2006) A pattern-based method for the identification of MicroRNA binding sites and their corresponding heteroduplexes, Cell 126, 1203-1217.

[120] Calin GA, Dumitru CD, Shimizu M, Bichi R, Zupo S, Noch E, *et al.* (2002) Frequent deletions and down-regulation of micro- RNA genes miR15 and miR16 at 13q14 in chronic lymphocytic leukemia, Proc Natl Acad Sci U S A 99, 15524-15529.

[121] Caldas C & Brenton JD (2005) Sizing up miRNAs as cancer genes, Nat Med 11, 712-714.

[122] Calin GA & Croce CM (2006) MicroRNAs and chromosomal abnormalities in cancer cells, Oncogene 25, 6202-6210.

[123] Lu J, Getz G, Miska EA, Alvarez-Saavedra E, Lamb J, Peck D, *et al.* (2005) MicroRNA expression profiles classify human cancers, Nature 435, 834-838.

[124] Sandhu S & Garzon R (2011) Potential applications of microRNAs in cancer diagnosis, prognosis, and treatment, Semin Oncol 38, 781-787.

[125] Croce CM (2009) Causes and consequences of microRNA dysregulation in cancer, Nat Rev Genet 10, 704-714.

[126] Nicoloso MS, Spizzo R, Shimizu M, Rossi S, & Calin GA (2009) MicroRNAs--the micro steering wheel of tumour metastases, Nat Rev Cancer 9, 293-302.

[127] Lujambio A & Lowe SW (2012) The microcosmos of cancer, Nature 482, 347-355.

[128] Volinia S, Calin GA, Liu CG, Ambs S, Cimmino A, Petrocca F, *et al.* (2006) A microRNA expression signature of human solid tumors defines cancer gene targets, Proc Natl Acad Sci U S A 103, 2257-2261.

[129] Xiao C, Srinivasan L, Calado DP, Patterson HC, Zhang B, Wang J, *et al.* (2008) Lymphoproliferative disease and autoimmunity in mice with increased miR-17-92 expression in lymphocytes, Nat Immunol 9, 405-414.

[130] Ventura A, Young AG, Winslow MM, Lintault L, Meissner A, Erkeland SJ, *et al.* (2008) Targeted deletion reveals essential and overlapping functions of the miR-17 through 92 family of miRNA clusters, Cell 132, 875-886.

[131] He L, Thomson JM, Hemann MT, Hernando-Monge E, Mu D, Goodson S, *et al.* (2005) A microRNA polycistron as a potential human oncogene, Nature 435, 828-833.

[132] Diosdado B, van de Wiel MA, Terhaar Sive Droste JS, Mongera S, Postma C, Meijerink WJ, *et al.* (2009) MiR-17-92 cluster is associated with 13q gain and c-myc expression during colorectal adenoma to adenocarcinoma progression, Br J Cancer 101, 707-714.

[133] Mu P, Han YC, Betel D, Yao E, Squatrito M, Ogrodowski P, *et al.* (2009) Genetic dissection of the miR-17~92 cluster of microRNAs in Myc-induced B-cell lymphomas, Genes Dev 23, 2806-2811.

[134] Petrocca F, Visone R, Onelli MR, Shah MH, Nicoloso MS, de Martino I, *et al.* (2008) E2F1-regulated microRNAs impair TGFbeta-dependent cell-cycle arrest and apoptosis in gastric cancer, Cancer Cell 13, 272-286.

[135] Mendell JT (2008) miRiad roles for the miR-17-92 cluster in development and disease, Cell 133, 217-222.

[136] Garofalo M, Di Leva G, Romano G, Nuovo G, Suh SS, Ngankeu A, *et al.* (2009) miR-221&222 regulate TRAIL resistance and enhance tumorigenicity through PTEN and TIMP3 downregulation, Cancer Cell 16, 498-509.

[137] Di Leva G, Gasparini P, Piovan C, Ngankeu A, Garofalo M, Taccioli C, *et al.* (2010) MicroRNA cluster 221-222 and estrogen receptor alpha interactions in breast cancer, J Natl Cancer Inst 102, 706-721.

[138] Hu W, Chan CS, Wu R, Zhang C, Sun Y, Song JS, *et al.* (2010) Negative regulation of tumor suppressor p53 by microRNA miR-504, Mol Cell 38, 689-699.

[139] Roush S & Slack FJ (2008) The let-7 family of microRNAs, Trends Cell Biol 18, 505-516.

[140] Bueno MJ, Gomez de Cedron M, Gomez-Lopez G, Perez de Castro I, Di Lisio L, Montes-Moreno S, *et al.* (2011) Combinatorial effects of microRNAs to suppress the Myc oncogenic pathway, Blood 117, 6255-6266.

[141] Calin GA, Cimmino A, Fabbri M, Ferracin M, Wojcik SE, Shimizu M, *et al.* (2008) MiR-15a and miR-16-1 cluster functions in human leukemia, Proc Natl Acad Sci U S A 105, 5166-5171.

[142] Bonci D, Coppola V, Musumeci M, Addario A, Giuffrida R, Memeo L, *et al.* (2008) The miR-15a-miR-16-1 cluster controls prostate cancer by targeting multiple oncogenic activities, Nat Med 14, 1271-1277.

[143] Kota J, Chivukula RR, O'Donnell KA, Wentzel EA, Montgomery CL, Hwang HW, *et al.* (2009) Therapeutic microRNA delivery suppresses tumorigenesis in a murine liver cancer model, Cell 137, 1005-1017.

[144] Garzon R, Marcucci G, & Croce CM (2010) Targeting microRNAs in cancer: rationale, strategies and challenges, Nat Rev Drug Discov 9, 775-789.

[145] Dang CV (1999) c-Myc target genes involved in cell growth, apoptosis, and metabolism, Mol Cell Biol 19, 1-11.

[146] Eilers M & Eisenman RN (2008) Myc's broad reach, Genes Dev 22, 2755-2766.

[147] Dang CV, Le A, & Gao P (2009) MYC-induced cancer cell energy metabolism and therapeutic opportunities, Clin Cancer Res 15, 6479-6483.

[148] Dews M, Homayouni A, Yu D, Murphy D, Sevignani C, Wentzel E, *et al.* (2006) Augmentation of tumor angiogenesis by a Myc-activated microRNA cluster, Nat Genet 38, 1060-1065.

[149] O'Donnell KA, Wentzel EA, Zeller KI, Dang CV, & Mendell JT (2005) c-Myc-regulated microRNAs modulate E2F1 expression, Nature 435, 839-843.

[150] Ma L, Young J, Prabhala H, Pan E, Mestdagh P, Muth D, *et al.* (2010) miR-9, a MYC/MYCN-activated microRNA, regulates E-cadherin and cancer metastasis, Nat Cell Biol 12, 247-256.

[151] Chang TC, Yu D, Lee YS, Wentzel EA, Arking DE, West KM, *et al.* (2008) Widespread microRNA repression by Myc contributes to tumorigenesis, Nat Genet 40, 43-50.

[152] Bui TV & Mendell JT (2010) Myc: Maestro of MicroRNAs, Genes Cancer 1, 568-575.

[153] Klein U, Lia M, Crespo M, Siegel R, Shen Q, Mo T, *et al.* (2010) The DLEU2/miR-15a/16-1 cluster controls B cell proliferation and its deletion leads to chronic lymphocytic leukemia, Cancer Cell 17, 28-40.

[154] Cairo S, Wang Y, de Reynies A, Duroure K, Dahan J, Redon MJ, *et al.* (2010) Stem cell-like micro-RNA signature driven by Myc in aggressive liver cancer, Proc Natl Acad Sci U S A 107, 20471-20476.

[155] Linsley PS, Schelter J, Burchard J, Kibukawa M, Martin MM, Bartz SR, *et al.* (2007) Transcripts targeted by the microRNA-16 family cooperatively regulate cell cycle progression, Mol Cell Biol 27, 2240-2252.

[156] Chang TC, Zeitels LR, Hwang HW, Chivukula RR, Wentzel EA, Dews M, *et al.* (2009) Lin-28B transactivation is necessary for Myc-mediated let-7 repression and proliferation, Proc Natl Acad Sci U S A 106, 3384-3389.

[157] Newman MA, Thomson JM, & Hammond SM (2008) Lin-28 interaction with the Let-7 precursor loop mediates regulated microRNA processing, RNA 14, 1539-1549.

[158] Hagan JP, Piskounova E, & Gregory RI (2009) Lin28 recruits the TUTase Zcchc11 to inhibit let-7 maturation in mouse embryonic stem cells, Nat Struct Mol Biol 16, 1021-1025.

[159] Heo I, Joo C, Kim YK, Ha M, Yoon MJ, Cho J, *et al.* (2009) TUT4 in concert with Lin28 suppresses microRNA biogenesis through pre-microRNA uridylation, Cell 138, 696-708.

[160] Feng Z, Zhang C, Wu R, & Hu W (2011) Tumor suppressor p53 meets microRNAs, J Mol Cell Biol 3, 44-50.

[161] He L, He X, Lim LP, de Stanchina E, Xuan Z, Liang Y, *et al.* (2007) A microRNA component of the p53 tumour suppressor network, Nature 447, 1130-1134.

[162] Raver-Shapira N, Marciano E, Meiri E, Spector Y, Rosenfeld N, Moskovits N, *et al.* (2007) Transcriptional activation of miR-34a contributes to p53-mediated apoptosis, Mol Cell 26, 731-743.

[163] Jin L, Hu WL, Jiang CC, Wang JX, Han CC, Chu P, *et al.* (2011) MicroRNA-149*, a p53-responsive microRNA, functions as an oncogenic regulator in human melanoma, Proc Natl Acad Sci U S A 108, 15840-15845.

[164] Sachdeva M, Zhu S, Wu F, Wu H, Walia V, Kumar S, *et al.* (2009) p53 represses c-Myc through induction of the tumor suppressor miR-145, Proc Natl Acad Sci U S A 106, 3207-3212.

[165] Georges SA, Biery MC, Kim SY, Schelter JM, Guo J, Chang AN, *et al.* (2008) Coordinated regulation of cell cycle transcripts by p53-Inducible microRNAs, miR-192 and miR-215, Cancer Res 68, 10105-10112.

[166] Suzuki HI, Yamagata K, Sugimoto K, Iwamoto T, Kato S, & Miyazono K (2009) Modulation of microRNA processing by p53, Nature 460, 529-533.

[167] Kulshreshtha R, Ferracin M, Wojcik SE, Garzon R, Alder H, Agosto-Perez FJ, *et al.* (2007) A microRNA signature of hypoxia, Mol Cell Biol 27, 1859-1867.

[168] Mutharasan RK, Nagpal V, Ichikawa Y, & Ardehali H (2011) microRNA-210 is upregulated in hypoxic cardiomyocytes through Akt- and p53-dependent pathways and exerts cytoprotective effects, Am J Physiol Heart Circ Physiol 301, H1519-1530.

[169] Hu S, Huang M, Li Z, Jia F, Ghosh Z, Lijkwan MA, *et al.* (2010) MicroRNA-210 as a novel therapy for treatment of ischemic heart disease, Circulation 122, S124-131.

[170] Camps C, Buffa FM, Colella S, Moore J, Sotiriou C, Sheldon H, *et al.* (2008) hsa-miR-210 Is induced by hypoxia and is an independent prognostic factor in breast cancer, Clin Cancer Res 14, 1340-1348.

[171] Fasanaro P, D'Alessandra Y, Di Stefano V, Melchionna R, Romani S, Pompilio G, *et al.* (2008) MicroRNA-210 modulates endothelial cell response to hypoxia and inhibits the receptor tyrosine kinase ligand Ephrin-A3, J Biol Chem 283, 15878-15883.

[172] Kim HW, Haider HK, Jiang S, & Ashraf M (2009) Ischemic preconditioning augments survival of stem cells via miR-210 expression by targeting caspase-8-associated protein 2, J Biol Chem 284, 33161-33168.

[173] Zhang Z, Sun H, Dai H, Walsh RM, Imakura M, Schelter J, *et al.* (2009) MicroRNA miR-210 modulates cellular response to hypoxia through the MYC antagonist MNT, Cell Cycle 8, 2756-2768.

[174] Kent OA, Chivukula RR, Mullendore M, Wentzel EA, Feldmann G, Lee KH, *et al.* (2010) Repression of the miR-143/145 cluster by oncogenic Ras initiates a tumor-promoting feed-forward pathway, Genes Dev 24, 2754-2759.

[175] Calin GA, Sevignani C, Dumitru CD, Hyslop T, Noch E, Yendamuri S, *et al.* (2004) Human microRNA genes are frequently located at fragile sites and genomic regions involved in cancers, Proc Natl Acad Sci U S A 101, 2999-3004.

[176] Zhang L, Huang J, Yang N, Greshock J, Megraw MS, Giannakakis A, *et al.* (2006) microRNAs exhibit high frequency genomic alterations in human cancer, Proc Natl Acad Sci U S A 103, 9136-9141.

[177] Mayr C, Hemann MT, & Bartel DP (2007) Disrupting the pairing between let-7 and Hmga2 enhances oncogenic transformation, Science 315, 1576-1579.

[178] Veronese A, Visone R, Consiglio J, Acunzo M, Lupini L, Kim T, *et al.* (2011) Mutated beta-catenin evades a microRNA-dependent regulatory loop, Proc Natl Acad Sci U S A 108, 4840-4845.

[179] Saito Y, Liang G, Egger G, Friedman JM, Chuang JC, Coetzee GA, *et al.* (2006) Specific activation of microRNA-127 with downregulation of the proto-oncogene BCL6 by chromatin-modifying drugs in human cancer cells, Cancer Cell 9, 435-443.

[180] Cao Q, Mani RS, Ateeq B, Dhanasekaran SM, Asangani IA, Prensner JR, *et al.* (2011) Coordinated regulation of polycomb group complexes through microRNAs in cancer, Cancer Cell 20, 187-199.

[181] Davalos V, Moutinho C, Villanueva A, Boque R, Silva P, Carneiro F, *et al.* (2011) Dynamic epigenetic regulation of the microRNA-200 family mediates epithelial and mesenchymal transitions in human tumorigenesis, Oncogene doi: 10.1038/onc.2011.383.

[182] Guo QM, Malek RL, Kim S, Chiao C, He M, Ruffy M, *et al.* (2000) Identification of c-myc responsive genes using rat cDNA microarray, Cancer Res 60, 5922-5928.

[183] Li Z, Van Calcar S, Qu C, Cavenee WK, Zhang MQ, & Ren B (2003) A global transcriptional regulatory role for c-Myc in Burkitt's lymphoma cells, Proc Natl Acad Sci U S A 100, 8164-8169.

[184] Maxwell SA & Rivera A (2003) Proline oxidase induces apoptosis in tumor cells, and its expression is frequently absent or reduced in renal carcinomas, J Biol Chem 278, 9784-9789.

[185] Kulshreshtha R, Davuluri RV, Calin GA, & Ivan M (2008) A microRNA component of the hypoxic response, Cell Death Differ 15, 667-671.

[186] Guimbellot JS, Erickson SW, Mehta T, Wen H, Page GP, Sorscher EJ, *et al.* (2009) Correlation of microRNA levels during hypoxia with predicted target mRNAs through genome-wide microarray analysis, BMC Med Genomics 2, 15.

[187] Zhang H, Gao P, Fukuda R, Kumar G, Krishnamachary B, Zeller KI, *et al.* (2007) HIF-1 inhibits mitochondrial biogenesis and cellular respiration in VHL-deficient renal cell carcinoma by repression of C-MYC activity, Cancer Cell 11, 407-420.

[188] Vafa O, Wade M, Kern S, Beeche M, Pandita TK, Hampton GM, *et al.* (2002) c-Myc can induce DNA damage, increase reactive oxygen species, and mitigate p53 function: a mechanism for oncogene-induced genetic instability, Mol Cell 9, 1031-1044.

[189] DeNicola GM, Karreth FA, Humpton TJ, Gopinathan A, Wei C, Frese K, *et al.* (2011) Oncogene-induced Nrf2 transcription promotes ROS detoxification and tumorigenesis, Nature 475, 106-109.

[190] Wonsey DR, Zeller KI, & Dang CV (2002) The c-Myc target gene PRDX3 is required for mitochondrial homeostasis and neoplastic transformation, Proc Natl Acad Sci U S A 99, 6649-6654.

[191] Fan TW, Tan JL, McKinney MM, & Lane AN (2011) Stable isotope resolved metabolomics analysis of ribonucleotide and RNA metabolism in human lung cancer cells Metabolomics doi:10.1007/s11306-011-0337-9.

[192] Le A, Lane AN, Hamaker M, Bose S, Gouw A, Barbi J, *et al.* (2012) Glucose-Independent Glutamine Metabolism via TCA Cycling for Proliferation and Survival in B Cells, Cell Metab 15, 110-121.

[193] Wang R, Dillon CP, Shi LZ, Milasta S, Carter R, Finkelstein D, *et al.* (2011) The transcription factor Myc controls metabolic reprogramming upon T lymphocyte activation, Immunity 35, 871-882.

Chapter 3

Post-Transcriptional Regulation of Proto-Oncogene *c-fms* in Breast Cancer

Ho-Hyung Woo and Setsuko K. Chambers

Additional information is available at the end of the chapter

1. Introduction

1.1. *c-fms* and breast cancer

In the development and progression of breast cancers, both the *c-fms* proto-oncogene (which encodes the tyrosine kinase receptor for CSF-1) as well as CSF-1 (colony stimulating factor-1), play an important role. Evidence from transgenic models suggests that *c-fms* encodes for the sole receptor for CSF-1 (Dai *et al*, 2002). We and others have found that *c-fms* and/or CSF-1 are expressed by the tumor epithelium in several human epithelial cancers (Kacinski *et al*, 1988, 1990, 1991; Rettenmier *et al*, 1989; Filderman *et al*, 1992; Ide *et al*, 2002); elevated levels of *c-fms* and CSF-1 are associated with poor prognosis (Kacinski *et al*, 1988; Tang *et al*, 1990; Price *et al*, 1993; Chambers *et al*, 1997, 2009; Scholl *et al*, 1993; Kluger *et al*, 2004; Sapi 2004). In human breast cancer, 94% of *in situ* and invasive lesions express *c-fms* (Kacinski *et al*, 1991; Flick *et al*, 1997), while 36% express both CSF-1 and *c-fms* (Kacinski *et al*, 1991; Scholl *et al*, 1993). Among breast cancer patients, serum levels of CSF-1 are frequently elevated in those with metastases (Kacinski *et al*, 1991). In breast tumors, nuclear CSF-1 staining is associated with poor survival (Scholl *et al*, 1994), and *c-fms* expression confers an increased risk for local relapse (Maher *et al*, 1998). In a large breast cancer tissue array, *c-fms* (Kluger *et al*, 2004) is strongly associated with lymph node metastasis, and poor survival. This strong correlation with prognosis suggests an etiologic role for *c-fms*/CSF-1 in tumor invasion and metastasis.

Tumor-associated macrophages bearing CSF-1 promote progression of breast cancer (Pollard 2004). In mice bearing human breast cancer xenografts, targeting mouse (host) *c-fms* with siRNA, or CSF-1 with antisense, siRNA or antibody suppressed primary tumor growth by 40-50% (Aharinejad *et al*, 2004; Paulus *et al*, 2006), and improved their survival (Aharinejad *et al*, 2004). Hence, paracrine signaling by macrophages bearing CSF-1 also plays a critical role in breast cancer progression. Transgenic models suggest that the absence of CSF-1 results in delay of tumor invasion and metastasis, while targeting CSF-1 to mammary epithelium in these models enables macrophage infiltration and invasive breast cancer to develop and metastasize (Lin *et al*, 2001).

We have reported that glucocorticoids (GC) up-regulate *c-fms* expression both in breast cancer cells (Kacinski *et al*, 1991; Flick *et al*, 2002; Sapi *et al*, 1995), and in primary organ cultures of breast cancer specimens (Kacinski *et al*, 2001). In a study of 329 breast cancer patients, 52% of the breast cancer tissues had functional glucocorticoid receptor (GR) (Allegra *et al*, 1979). This allows for breast cancer responsiveness to circulating, endogenous GCs.

In the *in vivo* environment, with endogenous GCs, we observed extensive metastatic spread by breast cancer cells over-expressing *c-fms*, compared to controls (Toy *et al*, 2005). Parenchymal invasion was demonstrated only by the *c-fms* overexpressing cells. Interrupting the autocrine loop between *c-fms* and CSF-1 inhibits GC-stimulated invasiveness, motility, and adhesiveness *in vitro* of breast cancer cells (Toy *et al*, 2010). This mechanism of increasing *c-fms* by GC becomes aberrantly up-regulated in invasive, metastatic breast cancer.

1.2. Regulation of *c-fms* expression

Regulation of *c-fms* expression is a complex process. Both transcriptional and post-transcriptional regulations are involved to maintain a proper level of *c-fms* expression. This chapter summarizes the research over the last 20 years concerning post-transcriptional regulation of *c-fms* and its expression in breast cancer.

1.3. Stability of *c-fms* transcripts in breast cancer cells

c-fms expression is high in metastatic breast cancer cells, but not detectable in the normal breast cells and non-invasive precursors of breast neoplasms (Kacinski *et al*, 1988, 1990). Unusually long half-life of *c-fms* mRNA partially contributes high expression in metastatic breast cancer cells (Chambers *et al*, 1994, Woo et al, 2011). GCs increase the *c-fms* mRNA half-life from 9.6 h to 18.9 h in BT20 breast cancer cells (Woo et al, 2011). In highly invasive MDA-MB-231 breast cancer cells, *c-fms* mRNA half-life increases up to 27 h in response to GC treatment (Figure 1).

1.4. Post-transcriptional regulation of *c-fms* expression by 3′UTR

mRNA 3′UTR contains *cis*-acting regulatory sequences which are involved in regulation of mRNA stability and polyadenylation (Mignone *et al*, 2003; Bashirullah *et al*, 2001), mRNA degradation (Bevilacqua *et al*, 2003), translation, and subcellular localization of mRNAs (Loya *et al*, 2008; Jansen, 2001). Mutations in 3′UTR could result in diseases and are proposed as 'a molecular hotspot for pathology (Chen *et al*, 2006; Conne *et al*, 2000). Post-transcriptional regulation exerted by 3′UTR is considered an important counterpart to transcriptional regulation for maintaining the proper level of gene products in the cell.

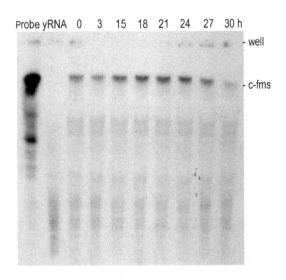

Probe – free probe, yRNA – yeast RNA as negative control, Total RNA was isolated after dexamethasone treatment at the indicated time.

Figure 1. RNase protection analysis of *c-fms* mRNA in MDA-MB-231 cells treated by 400 nM dexamethasone.

Human *c-fms* mRNA 3′UTR encodes 774 nt and contains unique regions including a non-AU-rich-69 nt sequence (3499-3567) which we have described and characterized (Woo *et al*, 2009, 2011), and also several putative target sequences for miRNA binding (Figure 2). The 69 nt sequence contains 3 islets of pyrimidine-rich sequences (CUUU). Mutations in these pyrimidine-rich sequences in 69 nt disrupted vigilin and HuR binding (Woo *et al*, 2009, 2011).

In metazoans, the 69 nt sequence within the 3′-UTR of *c-fms* mRNA is partially conserved between human, mouse, and rat (Figure 2). This region does not contain conventional AU-rich elements (ARE) (Woo *et al*, 2009). Overall, the 69 nt sequence is slightly pyrimidine-rich (>57-61%) and we proposed that primary sequence as well as loop structure may be important for protein binding (Woo *et al*, 2011; Kanamori *et al*, 1998). Indeed, this 69 nt region is predicted to form a stable loop structure (Figure 3).

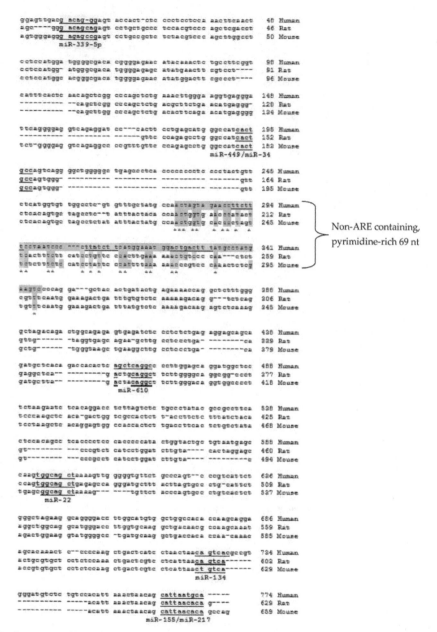

The 69 nt sequence (3499-3567) is partially conserved in human, rat, and mouse.

Figure 2. Alignment of *c-fms* mRNA 3'UTRs of human, rat, and mouse. Six regions are predicted as targets by eight miRNAs.

Human (ΔG = -9.8)   Mouse (ΔG = -2.7)   Rat (ΔG = -4.1)

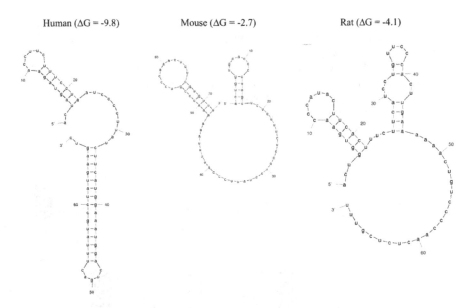

Figure 3. RNA loops of 69 nt are predicted by mfold (http://mfold.rna.albany.edu/?q=mfold).

1.5. microRNAs for *c-fms* mRNA regulation

MicroRNAs (miRNAs) are 21-23 nucleotide single-stranded RNAs, that in general down-regulate translation and enhance mRNA degradation (Huntzinger and Izaurralde, 2011; Braun *et al*, 2011). As a consequence, miRNAs are involved in the regulation of several biological functions (differentiation, hematopoiesis, tumorigenesis, apoptosis, development, proliferation, and growth) (Kim, 2005). They are predicted to regulate more than 60% of human mRNA (Friedman *et al*, 2009). It has been found that mRNAs with long 3'UTRs are more susceptible to miRNA regulation than those with short 3'UTRs as the latter lack the number of binding sites necessary for multiple miRNA binding and regulation (Stark *et al*, 2005).

Bioinformatics analysis predicted eight miRNAs (miR-339-5p, miR-449, miR-34, miR-610, miR-22, miR-134, miR-155, and miR-217) targeting six regions in *c-fms* mRNA 3'UTR (Figure 2). These six target regions are also highly conserved in human, mouse and rat. Among those, two miRNAs (miR-610 and miR-155) were selected by us for further analysis. *C-fms* mRNA level is higher in BT20 epithelial breast cancer cells than in Hey epithelial ovarian cancer cells (Figure 4). In contrast, miR-610 and miR-155 RNA levels show opposite expression patterns with their RNA levels lower in BT20 than in Hey cells. Using a luciferase RNA-fused *c-fms* mRNA 3'UTR reporter system, introduction of miR-610 inhibitors in BT20 cells increased luciferase RNA level by 5.5-fold and luciferase activity by 1.3-fold. The down-regulation of mir-610 has more effects on luciferase RNA levels than translational repression. Some reports describe miRNA effects to be mainly on translational repression, while others describe an effect primarily on mRNA decay. Guo *et al* (2010) reported that the predominant effect of mammalian miRNAs is on mRNA decay which results reduced translation. In contrast, in zebrafish, miR-430 reduced translation initiation prior to inducing mRNA decay (Bazzini *et al*, 2012). Djuranovic *et al* (2012) reported miRNA-mediated translational repression is followed by mRNA deadenylation. Recently, the concept of mRNA destabilization by miRNAs gained support by genome-wide observation studies (Huntzinger and Izaurralde, 2011).

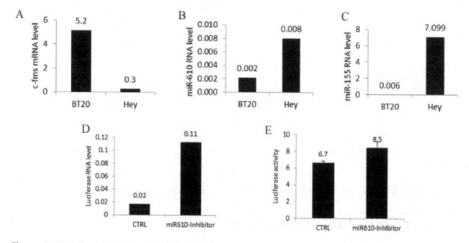

Figure 4. (A) *c-fms* mRNA level is higher in BT20 than in Hey cells. (B) miR-610 RNA level is higher in Hey than in BT20 cells. (C) miR-155 RNA level is higher in Hey than BT20 cells. (D) Using a luciferase RNA-fused *c-fms* mRNA 3′UTR reporter system, introduction of miR-610 inhibitor increased luciferase RNA level by 5.5-fold and (E) luciferase activity by 1.3-fold in BT20 cells.

1.6. RNA-binding proteins for *c-fms* mRNA metabolism and translation

The first evidence supporting post-transcriptional regulation of *c-fms* mRNA by RNA-binding proteins was reported in human monocytes (HL-60 cells) (Weber *et al*, 1989). In their study, TPA (12-O-tetradecanoylphorbol-13-acetate)-induced monocytic differentiation did not change *c-fms* transcription, but increased *c-fms* mRNA level. In addition, treatment of protein synthesis inhibitor cycloheximide decreased half-life of *c-fms* mRNA in TPA-induced HL-60 cells. From this observation, they proposed that a labile protein(s) is involved in stabilization of *c-fms* mRNA.

Chambers *et al*. (1993) reported the existence of mRNA regulatory proteins involved in *c-fms* mRNA destabilization in dexamethasone (Dex) or cyclosporin A (CsA) treated HL-60 cells. Dex or CsA blocked TPA-induced monocytic differentiation as well as TPA-induced adherence and further differentiated morphology. In TPA-induced HL-60 cells, *c-fms* mRNA half life was decreased after the addition of Dex or CsA. The effects of cycloheximide of *c-fms* mRNA decay in this setting suggested the existence of labile destabilizing protein(s).

Furthermore, in breast carcinoma cells (BT20 and SKBR3), Dex-treatment at later time points increased *c-fms* mRNA level without affecting *c-fms* transcription. Addition of protein synthesis inhibitors prevented Dex-induced increase of *c-fms* mRNA level suggesting the presence of Dex-inducible stabilizing protein(s) in breast carcinoma cells (Chambers *et al*, 1994).

RNA-binding proteins: About 1,500 RNA-binding proteins (RBPs) have been identified, which bind to mRNA and modulate mRNA stability and translation. mRNA primary sequences as well as loop structures are known to facilitate regulatory protein binding for post-transcriptional regulation.

HuR – HuR, one of the most extensively studied RBPs, encoded by ELAVL1 (embryonic lethal, abnormal vision, *Drosophila*-like 1) binds *cis*-acting AU-rich elements (AREs) (Barreau *et al*, 2005) and also non-ARE-containing sequences including pyrimidine-rich sequences (Woo *et al*, 2009) in target mRNAs. HuR stabilizes and increases half-life of target mRNAs and therefore enhances their translation (Srikantan and Gorospe, 2011). Our study indicates that HuR binds *c-fms* mRNA 3′UTR and enhances mRNA stability and translation (Woo *et al*, 2009).

In human breast-cancer tissues, HuR is expressed mostly in nucleus (>90%), but expression in cytoplasm is also found. High nuclear expression of HuR is a poor prognostic factor both in breast and ovarian cancer (Woo *et al*, 2009; Yi *et al*, 2009).

Vigilin – Vigilin, a high-density lipoprotein-binding protein, contains 15 K-homology (KH) domains (Goolsby and Shapiro, 2003). The KH domain protein family interacts with ARE-containing mRNAs and enhances mRNA degradation and consequently down-regulates

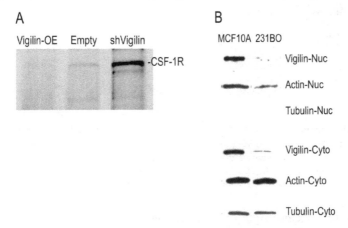

Figure 5. (A) Metabolic labeling and immunoprecipitation of CSF-1R. (B) Immunoblot of Vigilin in both nuclear (Nuc) and cytoplasmic (Cyto) fractions of MCF10A and MDA-MB-231BO cells. Absence of tubulin in nuclear fraction and presence of tubulin in cytoplasmic fraction indicate no cross-contamination in both fractions.

translation (Gherzi *et al*, 2004). In contrast, vigilin interacts largely with unstructured pyrimidine-rich sequences in mRNA 3'UTR (Kanamori *et al*, 1998; Woo *et al*, 2011). We found that vigilin decreases *c-fms* mRNA half-life and down-regulates translation. Ectopic expression of vigilin in breast cancer cells showed that the effects of down-regulation is more pronounced on *c-fms* protein level than on the mRNA level (Woo *et al*, 2011). Metabolic labeling and immunoprecipitation of *c-fms* protein showed that vigilin overexpression down-regulated *c-fms* protein level in BT20 cells (Figure 5A). In contrast, suppression of vigilin by shRNA up-regulated *c-fms* protein level.

Furthermore, immunoblot analysis showed that vigilin expression was lower in metastatic breast cancer MDA-MB-231BO cells than in non-tumorigenic epithelial breast MCF10A cells (Figure 5B). This indicates that a possible suppressive role of vigilin in invasive characters of breast cancer cells.

Both *in vitro* and *in vivo* studies indicate that vigilin and HuR competitively bind to the pyrimidine-rich 69 nt sequence of *c-fms* mRNA 3'UTR (Figure 4, Woo *et al*, 2009, 2011). *In vitro* competition assay showed that affinity of vigilin to the 69 nt sequence is at least 3-fold higher than that of HuR (Figure 6).

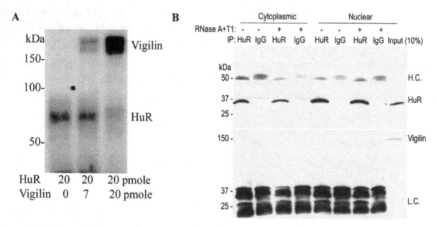

Figure 6. (A) Competition assay between vigilin and HuR by UV crosslink. (B) Co-immunoprecipitation assay. Vigilin and HuR do not present in the same mRNP complexes. IP assays were carried out using cellular lysates from MDA-MB-231 cells in either RNase-free or RNase-treated conditions using anti-human HuR mAb, or IgG. The presence of HuR in the IP materials was monitored by immunoblot. H.C. – heavy chain of IgG. L.C. – Light chain of IgG.

1.7. Effects of HuR and vigilin on invasiveness of breast cancer cells

Increased *c-fms*/CSF-1 levels correlate with the invasive breast cancer phenotype, and with prognosis (Toy, 2005; Toy *et al*, 2010; Sapi, 2004; Kluger *et al*, 2004; Scholl *et al*, 1994, 1993; Maher *et al*, 1998). We studied the ability of BT20 breast cancer cells to invade through a human derived simple matrix *in vitro*. The invasion of BT20 cells was significantly inhibited by the over-expression of vigilin, resulting in a 48% decrease compared to control (Figure 7). In contrast, over-expression of HuR increased invasiveness by 34%. Our findings suggest that vigilin can negatively impact, through suppression of *c-fms* expression, breast cancer cell invasiveness. In contrast, HuR enhances breast cancer cell invasiveness.

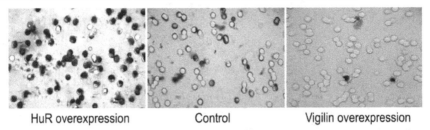

HuR overexpression   Control   Vigilin overexpression

Figure 7. Vigilin and HuR regulate *in vitro* invasiveness of BT20 breast cancer cells. This findings correlate with relative *c-fms* expression.

1.8. Post-translational modification: dimerization and tyrosine-phosphorylation of CSF-1R activation of PIP3/Akt signal transduction pathway

Activation of CSF-1R, product of the *c-fms* gene, requires ligand-induced non-covalent dimerization and phosphorylation of tyrosine residues in CSF-1R (Xiong *et al*, 2011; Li and Stanley, 1991). Here, we focus on one of the major signaling transduction pathways which result from CSF-1R activation. Phosphorylated CSF-1R interacts with PI3K (Phosphatidylinositol 3-kinases) (Shurtleff *et al*, 1990). In turn, PI3K converts PIP2 (Phosphatidylinositol-3,4-bisphosphate) to PIP3 (Phosphatidylinositol-3,4,5-tisphosphate). PIP3 interacts with Akt (protein kinase B, PBK), and activates downstream components in the PIP3/Akt signaling pathway. As a result, several physiological consequences are regulated including cell proliferation, apoptosis, and growth. An activated PIP3/Akt pathway is a common event in human cancer. (Arcaro and Guerreiro, 2007).

In breast cancer cells, multiple components are known to activate phosphorylation of CSF-1R. Endogenous cytokine CSF-1, functioning as an autocrine signal, can bind to the extracellular domain of CSF-1R and activate the cytoplasmic kinase domain leading to autophosphorylation of tyrosine-residues in CSF-1R. There is evidence to suggest that endogenous CSF-1 can also bind CSF-1R without interaction on the membrane surface. Exogenous CSF-1, from other sources such as macrophages, osteoclasts, or fibroblasts, can function in a paracrine manner to activate CSF-1R on the membrane surface. Consequently, phosphorylation of tyrosine residues in CSF-1R activates cell proliferation and invasive potential (Yu *et al*, 2012; Sapi *et al*, 1996). Our study indicates glucocorticoids (dexamethasone) and starvation also activate CSF-1R auto-phosphorylation (Figure 8).

CSF-1R is localized both in the cytoplasm, plasma membrane, and nuclear envelope (Zwaenepoel *et al*, 2012). CSF-1R in the nuclear envelope becomes phosphorylated in response to CSF-1. Phosphorylated CSF-1R in the nuclear envelope triggers the phosphorylation of Akt and p27 inside the nucleus.

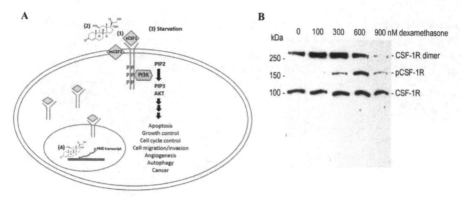

Figure 8. (A) Signal transduction through pCSF-1R/PI3K regulates cell growth and angiogenesis. Both autocrine and paracrine signals (sCSF-1, glucocorticoids, and starvation) trigger dimerization and autophosphorylation of CSF-1R, which interacts with PI3K. The PI3K generates PIP3, which binds to Akt. Activation of PIP3/Akt activates downstream components and regulates growth, apoptosis and cell cycle. (B) Dexamethasone induces autophosphorylation of CSF-1R in starved MDA-MB-231 cells.

2. Discussion

Post-transcriptional and translational regulation of *c-fms* expression by vigilin and HuR in breast cancer cells: mRNA translation and decay are complex multi-staged processes. Mature mRNAs either enter translation or degradation pathways depending on the developmental stages of the cell. We have reported vigilin and HuR, both nuclear-cytoplasmic shuttling RNA-binding proteins, to be involved in post-transcriptional as well as translational regulation of *c-fms* mRNA (Woo *et al*, 2009, 2011). Vigilin binds the pyrimidine-rich 69 nt sequence in the *c-fms* mRNA 3′UTR, to which HuR also binds. Both *in vitro* and *in cell* studies indicate that they compete for the same 69 nt sequence in the *c-fms* mRNA 3′UTR and that dynamic changes in the ratio of vigilin to HuR can influence their ability to associate with the *c-fms* mRNA and post-transcriptionally regulate cellular *c-fms* levels. While vigilin down-regulates *c-fms* translation as well as mRNA stability, HuR, in contrast, has opposite effect on *c-fms* levels; i.e., HuR up-regulates *c-fms* mRNA stability resulting increased *c-fms* protein levels. In our previous study, the polysome profile indicates vigilin is associated with free mRNPs and low MW monosomes. In contrast, HuR was detected with high MW polysomes (Woo *et al*, 2011). Vigilin also represses translation of reporter RNA (luciferase RNA fused with *c-fms* mRNA 3′UTR sequence) in the rabbit reticulocyte lysate cell-free translation system (Woo *et al*, 2011).

Translation can be divided in three phases; initiation, elongation, and termination. Translation initiation is a complicated process for which a large number of eukaryotic initiation factors (eIFs) have been identified (Sonnenberg and Hinnebusch, 2009). Translation initiation starts with the assembly of a 48S quaternary initiation complex comprised of the 40S ribosomal subunit, eIFs, tRNAMet, and m7G cap of the mRNA. In general, this 48S initiation complex scans and base pairs with the AUG initiation codon in

5′UTR of mRNA. This results in formation of the 80S ribosome and is continued in the elongation step of peptide synthesis.

In a 'closed-loop' mRNP model for cap-dependent translational regulation, PABPs bind both to the poly A+ tail at the 3′UTR and eIF4G of the translation initiation complex at the 5′-cap (Huntzinger and Izaurralde, 2011). This mRNA circularization attracts ribosomes to form a translation initiation complex. Subsequently, after translation termination, joining of the 5′- and 3′-ends of the mRNA facilitates the transfer of ribosomal subunits from the 3′ to the 5′-end.

Our results have demonstrated presence of vigilin in free mRNP fractions in human BT20 breast cancer cells. While vigilin association with free mRNPs may prevent 'closed-loop' formation and consequently inhibit *c-fms* protein translation, it was also found to associate with tRNAs and elongation factors (Kruse *et al*, 2003; Vollbrandt *et al*, 2004). Binding of vigilin with these components may deplete the available tRNAs and elongation factors for translation elongation. We propose a model that the impaired translation resulting from vigilin binding may expose both 5′- and 3′-ends of the mRNA through reduced circularization and increase its rate of degradation (Figure 9). In contrast, we propose that HuR binding to *c-fms* mRNA 3′UTR may enhance 'closed-loop' formation which increases the *c-fms* mRNA stability and also translation initiation efficiency. Immunoblot analysis indicates that vigilin is, in general, less expressed in breast cancer cells than in non-tumorigenic breast cells (Woo *et al*, 2011). This indicates that down-regulation of vigilin may be partly responsible for increased *c-fms* level in breast cancer cells. In summary, RNA binding proteins, such as vigilin and HuR are critical regulators for determining the fate of proto-oncogene *c-fms* mRNA, either to be translated or decayed.

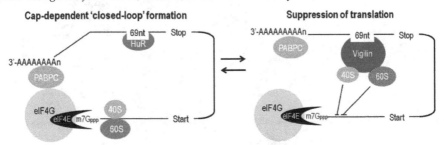

Figure 9. Competition between HuR and vigilin for binding 69 nt of *c-fms* mRNA 3′UTR regulates translational machinery formation. Binding of HuR to 69 nt may induce 'closed-loop' formation. In contrast, binding of vigilin to 69 nt could prevent 'closed-loop' formation.

Future research in post-transcriptional and translational regulation of *c-fms* in breast cancer: Translational inhibition and mRNA degradation are coordinated processes in which translation initiation is inhibited and translation factors (eIFs) are exchanged with repression/degradation complex (hDcp1/2, Hedls) (Fenger *et al*, 2005), resulting in mRNA degradation by exonucleases (Xrn1 and exosomes) (Balagopal and Parker, 2009). In general, 3′-deadenylation leads to 5′-decapping followed by exonucleolytic digestion at either ends of mammalian poly-A⁺-mRNAs (Franks and Lykke-Anderson, 2008; Zheng *et al*, 2008). In human cells, deadenylation is initiated by deadenylase complex (Pan2/3, Caf1, and Ccr4) (Zheng *et al*, 2008). Deadenylated oligo(A) mRNPs are further processed by decapping complex (including Xrn1 for 5'-to-3' decay) or exosomes (for 3'-to-5' decay). In yeast, decapping activators (Dhh1, Pat1, Lsm1-7, Edc1-3, Scd6) were identified which enhance decapping (Nissan *et al*, 2010). Mutated or excess nontranslating mRNAs are stored and degraded in processing bodies (P-bodies, GW-bodies, or Dcp-bodies) and/or stress granules (SGs). During inhibition of translation initiation, elevated numbers of P-bodies and SGs are observed (Shyu *et al*, 2008). Nontranslating mRNPs accumulate both in P-bodies and SGs. Decapping complex (hDcp1/2, Hedls) and mRNA decay fragments are found in P-bodies suggesting presence of 5'-to-3' exonuclease activities (Xrn1). Deadenylation complex (Pan2/3, Caf1, Ccr4) is also present in mouse P-bodies. On the other hand, translation initiation components (eIFs) and RNA-binding proteins (Ataxin-2, Pab1, TIA-R, TIA-1) are found in SGs (Buchan and Parker, 2009). Another very important aspect of mRNA stability is mRNA binding proteins. They can stimulate decapping and degradation processes. Over-expression of cold-inducible RNA-binding protein (CIRP), which represses translation, induces SGs (De Leeuw *et al*, 2007). In contrast, HuR was shown to release translational repression by helping human mRNA associated with P-bodies to re-enter polysomes (Bhattacharyya *et al*, 2006). In mammalian cells, P-bodies and SGs often dock together during translation inhibition. Since vigilin was shown to repress *c-fms* translation, it is crucial to understand mechanisms of transitions of *c-fms* mRNPs between P-bodies, SGs and

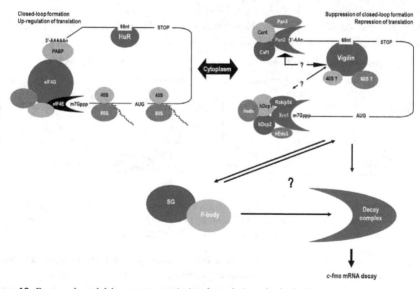

Figure 10. Proposed model for post-transcriptional regulation of *c-fms* by HuR and vigilin. HuR enhances closed-loop formation and increases *c-fms* mRNA stability and translation. In contrast, vigilin prevent closed-loop formation and attracts mRNA degradation complex and down-regulates translation. SG – stress granule

polysomes. A model for these mechanisms is proposed in Figure 10. Elucidating the molecular mechanisms of these exchanges from one state to another is critical to the understanding of regulation of *c-fms* protein levels in breast cancer.

3. Conclusion

In the design of clinical therapeutics, suppression of pathogenic gene expression requires high specificity to prevent off-target toxicity. In order to achieve this, detailed regulatory mechanisms of target gene expression should be elucidated. Understanding the regulatory mechanisms and specific proteins through which vigilin effects translational down-regulation of proto-oncogene *c-fms* in breast cancer can result in more accurate control of its expression.

Based on information available from the last 20 years of research and our recent data, it is now possible to elucidate vigilin's role in translational down-regulation of *c-fms* mRNA in breast cancer. Information obtained from this research will support a model on the manner in which interaction between a specific mRNA (*c-fms*) and proteins (vigilin and HuR) regulates *c-fms* at a translational level. These findings will bring us one step closer to development of a targeted therapy based on these mechanisms.

4. Methods

4.1. Cell culture

A human breast carcinoma cell line BT20 was maintained in MEM (Sigma) supplemented with 0.1 mM non-essential amino acids, 2 mM L-glutamine, 1 mM sodium pyruvate, 1.5 g/L sodium bicarbonate, and 10% fetal bovine serum (Invitrogen) in 5% CO_2 at 37°C. A human breast carcinoma cell line MDA-MB-231 was cultured in DMEM (Sigma) supplemented with 10% fetal bovine serum. For studies using glucocorticoids, cells were grown in starvation medium with 100 nM Dex (Sigma-Aldrich) for 72 h and collected for immunoblot analysis. A human ovarian cancer cell line Hey was grown in DMEM/F12 (Sigma) supplemented with 10% fetal bovine serum.

4.2. Total RNA isolation for semi-quantitative real-time RT-PCR analysis

Cells were grown in 6-well plate for 2-3 days before harvesting. Total RNA was extracted with 500 ul Trizol (Invitrogen) per well. After Trizol extraction, 150 ul of supernatant was carefully removed to avoid genomic DNA contamination. Supernatant was re-extracted by equal volume of chloroform and 100 ul of supernatant was carefully removed and ethanol precipitated for cDNA synthesis.

4.3. Semi-quantitative real-time RT-PCR analysis for *c-fms* mRNAs

Total RNA was oligo-dT$_{18}$ primed by M-MuLV reverse transcriptase (New England Biolab). For PCR analysis, reverse transcriptase reaction was diluted by 10-fold and 2 ul was used for

20 ul PCR reaction. GAPDH mRNA was amplified in PCR reaction as internal loading control.

c-fms PCR primers (forward primer = 5'-GGAGTTGACGACAGGGAGTACCAC-3', reverse primer = 5'- ACGAGGCCAACACCATGAGAACAG-3').

GAPDH PCR primers (forward primer = 5'-CGGGAAACTGTGGCGTGATGGC-3', reverse primer = 5'-AGGAGACCACCTGGTGCTCAGTG-3').

c-fms mRNA expression level was calculated with the ΔΔCᴛ method (Schmittgen and Livak, 2008).

4.4. Stem-loop real-time RT-PCR analysis for miR-610 and miR-155 quantification

miRNA expression was determined by the stem-loop qRT-PCR analysis to increase the specificity of miRNA amplification (Chen *et al*, 2005). cDNAs for miR-610, miR-155, and tRNAGlu specific were synthesized using sequence specific stem-loop forming primers. After 10-fold dilution of reverse transcriptase reaction, 2 ul was used for 20 ul real-time PCR. tRNAGlu was used as internal loading control.

miR-610 reverse transcription primer = 5'-gtcgtatccagtgcagggtccgaggtattcgcact ggatacgactcccag-3')

miR-610 PCR primers (forward primer = 5'- GGCGCTGAGCTAAATGTGTGC-3', reverse primer = 5'- GTGCAGGGTCCGAGGT-3')

miR-155 reverse transcription primer = 5'- gtcgtatccagtgcagggtccgaggtattcgcact ggatacgacacccct-3'

miR-155 PCR primers (forward primer = 5'- GGCGCTTAATGCTAATCGTGATAG-3', reverse primer = 5'- GTGCAGGGTCCGAGGT-3')

tRNAGlu reverse transcription primer = 5'- GTCGTATCCAGTGCAGGGTCCGAGGTATTCGCACT GGATACGAC GGTGAAAG-3'

tRNAGlu PCR primers (forward primer = 5'- CTGGTTAGTACTTGGACGGGAGAC -3', reverse primer = 5'- gtgcagggtccgaggt -3')

4.5. Analysis of *c-fms* mRNA Half Life

The *c-fms* mRNA half-life was determined by RNase protection assay (RPA) (Bordonaro *et al*, 1994). Radioactive-labeled antisense RNA probes of *c-fms* mRNA was generated by *in vitro* transcription. *c-fms* cDNA (237nt, 1789-2025) with 67nt random sequence and 23nt T7 promoter at 3'-end was generated by PCR and used as a templete for *in vitro* transcription. Probes with specific activity of $1x10^5$ cpm were hybridized with 10 μg of total RNA in hybridization buffer (80% deionized formamide, 40 mM PIPES pH6.4, 400 mM NaCl, and 1 mM EDTA) at 42°C overnight. Next morning, unbound RNA was digested by RNase A and

T1 at 37°C for 1 h. After proteinase K treatment at 37°C for 30 min, samples were extracted by phenol-chloroform and precipitated in ethanol. Samples were analyzed on a 5% acrylamide/8M urea gel and exposed on X-ray film.

4.6. Metabolic labeling and immunoprecipitation of *c-fms* proteins

The BT20 cultures at 75-80% confluence were washed with PBS and incubated in labeling medium (Met,Cys-free RPMI1640 (Sigma R-7513), 5% dialyzed FCS, 500ug/ml Glutamine) for 40 min to deplete endogenous methionine and cysteine in cell. For metabolic labeling, 5 ml labeling medium and 50 ul (500 uCi) of 35S-Methionine/35S-Cysteine per T75 flask was added and incubated for 30-40 min. After brief chase in chase medium (labeling medium with 500μg/ml Cysteine-HCl and 100μg/ml Methionine), cells were harvested and lysed in IP buffer (1% Triton x-100, 0.05% NP-40 in TBS, protease inhibitors). For immunoprecipitation of c-fms proteins, 5 ug of *c-fms* monoclonal antibody and 50 μl of Protein A/G-agarose (50% slurrry) (Santa Cruz) were added to cell lysates and incubated overnight at 4°C. Next morning, agarose beads was washed extensively with IP buffer and protein was eluted by SDS sample buffer. Labeled protein was analyzed in 10% SDS-PAGE.

4.7. Gain-of-function and loss-of-function assay

Plasmids encoding a control shRNA or shRNA directed against vigilin were purchased from Origene. The shRNAs correspond to coding region nucleotides 614–642 (5'-AAGCTCG GAAGGACATTGTTGCTAGACTG-3') and 829–863 (5'-CATGAAGTCTTACTCATCTCTG CCGAGCAGGACAA-3'), respectively, of human vigilin (GenBank BC001179). An shRNA containing a non-specific 29nt GFP sequence (TR30003, Origene) was used as a transfection control (Empty). For RNAi, 5 ×106 cells were transfected with 10 μg shRNA plasmid using Fugene HD (Roche) according to the manufacturer's instructions. Transfected cells were maintained in culture medium for 3-4 days to permit knockdown before assays.

For vigilin overexpression, pTetCMV-Fo(AS)-vigilin (Cunningham et al, 2000) was transfected using Fugene HD (Roche). The BT20 cells at 75-80% confluence in 6-well plates were transfected with 5 μg of plasmids. The overexpression effects were monitored for 3-4 days by qRT-PCR and western blot analyses.

4.8. UV crosslinking and label transfer with *c-fms* mRNA 3'UTR

UV cross-linking of HuR and vigilin was performed as described previously (Urlaub *et al*, 2000) with modifications. RNAs of *c-fms* 3'UTR labeled with 32P-UTP were incubated with recombinant HuR or recombinant vigilin proteins. The 15 μl reaction mixture contained 5 mM HEPESpH7.6, 1.25 mM MgCl2, 3.8% glycerol, 0.02 mM DTT, 1 mM EDTA, 25 mM KCl, 50 ng yeast tRNA, 50 ng heparin, 1 mM ATP, and 32P-labeled RNA probe (50,000 cpm). After incubation at 30°C for 20 min, reaction mixture in a 96-well polystyrene plate on ice was illuminated at 254 nm, 125 mJoule for 120 seconds using a GS Gene Linker UV Chamber (Bio-Rad). After crosslink, excess RNA was digested by RNase A for 30 min at 37°C. Crosslinked protein was fractionated in 10% SDS-PAGE.

4.9. Invasion assay

The Membrane Invasion Culture System (MICS chamber) was used to quantitate, the degree of invasion of MDA-MB-231 transiently transfected vigilin or HuR overexpressing clones. Breast cancer cells were cultured in the presence of 100 nM Dex and remained under starved conditions for transfection duration prior to the invasion assays. Parent or transfected cells, 1×10^5 per well in a 6-well plate, were seeded onto 10-μm pore filters coated with a human defined matrix containing 50 μg/ml human laminin, 50 μg/ml human collagen IV, and 2 mg/ml gelatin in 10 mM acetic acid.

Author details

Ho-Hyung Woo and Setsuko K. Chambers
Arizona Cancer Center, University of Arizona, Tucson, AZ, USA

Acknowledgement

This work was supported by Department of Defense grant DAMD 17-02-1-0633 (to S.K.C), by Arizona Biomedical Research Commission grant 07-061 (to S.K.C.), and the Rodel Foundation (to S.K.C.).

5. References

Aharinejad, S., Paulus, P., Sioud, M., Hofmann, M., Zins, K., Schafer, R., Stanley, E.R., Abraham, D. (2004). Colony-stimulating factor-1 blockade by antisense oligonucleotides and small interfering RNAs suppresses growth of human mammary tumor xenografts in mice. *Cancer Res.* 64: 5378-5384.

Allegra, J.C., Lippman, M.E., Thompson, E.B., Simon, R., Barlock, A., Green, L., Huff , K.K., Do, H.M. & Aitken, S.C. (1979). Distribution, frequency, and quantitative analysis of estrogen, progesterone, androgen, and glucocorticoids receptors in human breast cancer. *Cancer Res.* 39: 1447-1454.

Arcaro, A. & Guerreiro, A.S. (2007). The Phosphoinositide 3-kinase pathway in human cancer: genetic alterations and therapeutic implications. *Current Genomics* 8: 271-306.

Balagopal, V. & Parker R. (2009). Polysomes, P bodies and stress granules: states and fates of eukaryotic mRNAs. *Curr. Op. Cell Biol.* 21: 403-408.

Barreau, C., Paillard, L. & Osborne, B. (2005). AU-rich elements and associated factors: are there unifying principles? *Nucleic Acids Res.* 33: 7138-7150.

Bashirullah, A, Cooperstock, R.L. & Lipshitz, H.D. (2001). Spatial and temporal control of RNA stability. *PNAS* 98: 7025–7028.

Bazzini, A., Lee, M.T. & Giraldez A.J. (2012). Ribosome profiling shows that miR-430 reduces translation before causing mRNA decay in Zebrafish. *Science* 336: 233-237.

Bevilacqua, A., Cerian, M.C. Capaccioli, S. & Nicolin, A. (2003). Post-transcriptional regulation of gene expression by degradation of messenger RNAs. *J. Cell. Physiol.* 195: 356-372.

Bhattacharyya, S.N., Habermacher, R., Martine, U., Closs, E.I. & Filipowicz, W. (2006). Relief of microRNA-mediated translational repression in human cells subjected to stress. *Cell* 125: 1111-1124.

Bordonaro, M., F. Saccomanno, C.F., L. Nordstrom, J.L. (1994) An improved T1/A ribonuclease protection assay, BioTechniques 16, 428-430.

Buchan, J.R. & Parker R. (2009) Eukaryotic stress granules: the ins and outs of translation. *Mol. Cell* 36: 932-941.

Chambers, S.K. (2009). Role of CSF-1 in progression of epithelial ovarian cancer. *Future Oncol.* 5: 1429-1440.

Chambers, S.K., Kacinski, B.M., Ivins, C.M. & Carcangiu, M.L. (1997). Overexpression of epithelial CSF-1 and CSF-1 receptor: a poor prognostic factor in epithelial ovarian cancer; contrasted to a protective effect of stromal CSF-1. *Clin. Cancer Res.* 3: 999-1007.

Chambers, S.K., Gilmore-Hebert, M., Wang, Y., Rodov, S., Benz, E.J. Jr, & Kacinski, B.M. (1993). Posttranscriptional regulation of colony-stimulating factor-1 (CSF-1) and CSF-1 receptor gene expression during inhibition of phorbol-ester-induced monocytic differentiation by dexamethasone and cyclosporin A: potential involvement of a destabilizing protein. *Exp Hematol.* 21: 1328-1334.

Chambers, S.K., Wang, Y., Gilmore-Hebert, M., & Kacinski, M. (1994). Post-transcriptional regulation of *c-fms* proto-oncogene expression by dexamethasone and of CSF-1 in human breast carcinomas in vitro. *Steroids* 59: 514-522.

Chen, C., Ridzon, D.A., Broomer, AJ, *et al.* (2005). Real-time quantification of microRNAs by stem-loop RT-PCR. *Nucleic Acids Res* 33: e179.

Chen J-M, Fe´rec. & Cooper D.N. (2006). A systematic analysis of disease-associated variants in the 3′ regulatory regions of human protein-coding genes II: the importance of mRNA secondary structure in assessing the functionality of 3′ UTR variants. *Hum Genet* 120: 301–333.

Conne, B., Stutz, A. & Vassalli J.-D. (2000). The 3′ untranslated region of messenger RNA: A molecular 'hotspot' for pathology? *Nature Med* 6: 637-641.

Cunningham, K. S., Dodson, R.E., Nagel, M.A., Shapiro, D.J. & Schoenberg D.R. (2000). Vigilin binding selectively inhibits cleavage of the vitellogenin mRNA 3′-untranslated region by the mRNA endonucleases polysomal ribonuclease 1. *PNAS* 97: 12498-12502.

Dai, X-M., Ryan, G.R., Hapel, A.J., Dominguez, M.G., Russell, R.G., Kapp, S., Sylvestre, V. & Stanley, E.R. (2002). Targeted disruption of the mouse colony-stimulating factor 1 receptor gene results in osteopetrosis, mononuclear phagocyte deficiency, increased primitive progenitor cell frequencies, and reproductive defects. *Blood* 99: 111-120.

De Leeuw, F., Zhang, T., Wauquier, C., Huez, G., Kruys, V. & Gueydan, C. (2007). The cold-inducible RNA-binding protein migrates from the nucleus to cytoplasmic stress granules by a methylation-dependent mechanism and acts as a translational repressor. *Exp. Cell Res*. 313: 4130-4144.

Djuranovic, S., Nahvi, A., & Green R. (2012). miRNA-mediated gene silencing by translational repression followed by mRNA deadenylation and decay. *Science* 336: 237-240.

Fenger, M., Fillman, C., Norrild, B. & Lykke-Anderson, J. (2005). Multiple processing body factors and the ARE binding protein TTP activate mRNA decapping. *Mol. Cell* 20: 905-915.

Filderman, A.E., Bruckner, A., Kacinski, B.M., Deng, N. & Remold, H.G. (1992). Macrophage colony-stimulating factor (CSF-1) enhances invasiveness in CSF-1 receptor-positive carcinoma cell lines. *Cancer Res*. 52: 3661-3666.

Flick, M.B., Sapi, E., Perrotta, P.L., Maher, M.G., Halaban, R., Carter, D. & Kacinski, B.M. (1997). Recognition of activated CSF-1 receptor in breast carcinomas by a tyrosine 723 phosphospecific antibody. *Oncogene* 14: 2553-2561.

Flick, M.B., Sapi, E. & Kacinski, B.M. (2002). Hormonal regulation of the c-fms proto-oncogene in breast cancer cells is mediated by a composite glucocorticoid response element. *J Cell Biochem*. 85: 10-23.

Franks, T.M. & Lykke-Anderson J. (2008). The control of mRNA decapping and P-body formation. *Mol. Cell* 32: 605-615.

Friedman, R.C., Farh, K.K., Burge, C.B. & Bartel, D.P. (2009). Most mammalian mRNAs are conserved targets of microRNAs. *Genome Res*. 19: 92-105.

Gherzi, R., K. Y. Lee, P. Briata, D. Wegmüller, C. Moroni, M. Karin. & Chen C.Y. (2004). A KH domain RNA binding protein, KSRP, promotes ARE-directed mRNA turnover by recruiting the degradation machinery. *Mol. Cell* 14: 571-583.

Goolsby, K.M., Shapiro, D.J. (2003). RNAi-mediated depletion of the 15 KH domain protein, vigilin, induces death of dividing and non-dividing human cells but does not initially inhibit protein synthesis. *Nucleic Acids Res*. 31: 5644–5653.

Guo, H, Ingolia NT, Weissman JS, Bartel D.P. (2010). Mammalian microRNAs predominantly act to decrease target mRNA levels. *Nature* 466: 835-840.

Huntzinger, E, Izaurralde E. (2011). Gene silencing by microRNAs: contributions of translational repression and mRNA decay. *Nature Reviews: Genetics* 12: 99-110.

Ide, H., Seligson, D.B., Memarzadeh, S., Xin, L., Horvath, S., Dubey, P., Flick, M.B., Kacinski, B.M., Palotie, A., Witte, O.N. (2002). Expression of colony-stimulating factor 1 receptor during prostate development and prostate cancer progression. *PNAS*. 99: 14404-14409.

Jansen, R.-P. (2001). mRNA localization: message on the move. *Nature Reviews* 2: 247-256.

Kacinski, B.M., Flick, M.B. & Sapi, E. (2001). RU-486 can abolish glucocorticoid-induced increases in CSF-1 receptor expression in primary human breast carcinoma specimens. *J Soc Gynecol Investig*. 8: 114-116.

Kacinski, B.M., Carter, D., Mittal, K., Kohorn, E.I., Bloodgood, R.S., Donahue, J., Donofrio, L., Edwards, R., Schwartz, P.E., Chambers, J.T. & Chambers, S.K. (1988). High level expression of fms proto-oncogene mRNA is observed in clinically aggressive human endometrial adenocarcinomas. *Int. J. Radiat. Oncol. Biol. Phys.* 15: 823-829.

Kacinski, B.M., Carter, D., Mittal, K., Yee, L.D., Scata, K.A., Donofrio, L., Chambers, S.K., Wang, K., Yang-Feng, T., Rohrschneider, L.R. & Rothwell, V.M. (1990). Ovarian adenocarcinomas express *fms*-complementary transcripts and *fms* antigen, often with coexpression of CSF-1. *Am. J. Pathol.* 137: 135-147.

Kacinski, B.M., Scata, K.A., Carter, D., Yee, L.D., Sapi, E., King, B.L., Chambers, S.K., Jones, M.A., Pirro, M.H., Stanley, E.R. & Rohrschneider, L.R. (1991). FMS (CSF-1 receptor) and CSF-1 transcripts and protein are expressed by human breast carcinomas in vivo and in vitro. *Oncogene* 6: 941-952.

Kanamori, H., Dodson, R.E. & Shapiro, D.J. (1998). *In vitro* genetic analysis of the RNA binding site of vigilin, a multi-KH-domain protein. *Mol. Cell. Biol.* 18, 3991–4003

Kim, V.N. (2005). MicroRNA biogenesis: coordinated cropping and dicing. *Nat Rev Mol Cell Biol.* 6: 376-385.

Kluger, H. M., Dolled-Filhart, M.D., Rodov, S., Kacinski, B.M., Camp, R.L. & Rimm, D.L. (2004). Macrophage colony-stimulating factor-1 receptor expression is associated with poor outcome in breast cancer by large cohort tissue microarray analysis. *Clin. Cancer Res.* 10: 173-177.

Kruse, C., Willkomm, D., Gebken, J., Schuh, A., Stossberg, H., Vollbrandt, T., & Müller, P.K. (2003). The multi-KH protein vigilin associates with free and membrane-bound ribosomes. *Cell Mol. Life Sci.* 60: 2219-2227.

Li, W. & Stanley, E.R. (1991). Role of dimerization and modification of the CSF-1 receptor in its activation and internalization during the CSF-1 response. *The EMBO J.* 10: 277-288.

Lin, E.Y., Nguyen, A.V., Russell, R.G., Pollard, J.W. (2001). Colony-stimulating factor 1 promotes progression of mammary tumors to malignancy. *J Exp Med.* 193: 727-739.

Loya, A., Pnueli, L., Yosefzon, Y., Wexler, Y., Ziv-Ukelson, M. & Arava, Y. (2008). The 39-UTR mediates the cellular localization of an mRNA encoding a short plasma membrane protein. *RNA* 14:1352–1365.

Maher, M.G., Sapi, E., Turner, B., Gumbs, A., Perrotta, P.L., Carter, D., Kacinski, B.M. & Haffty B.G. (1998). Prognostic significance of colony-stimulating factor receptor expression in Ipsilateral breast cancer recurrence. *Clin. Cancer Res.* 4: 1851-1856.

Mignone, F., Gissi, C., Liuni, S. & Pesole, G. (2003). Untranslated regions of mRNAs. *Genome Biology* 3: 0004.1–0004.10.

Moncini, S., Bevilacqua, A., Venturin, M., Fallini, C., Ratti, A., Nicolin, A. & Riva, P. (2007). The 3' untranslated region of human cyclin-dependent kinase 5 regulatory subunit 1 contains regulatory elements affecting transcript stability. *BMC Molecular Biology* 8: 111.

Nissan, T., Rajyaguru, P., She, M., Song, H. & Parker, R. (2010). Decapping activators in *Saccharomyces cerevisiae* act by multiple mechanisms. *Mol. Cell* 39: 773-783.

Paulus, P., Stanley, E.R., Schafer, R., Abraham, D., Aharinejad, S. (2006). Colony-Stimulating Factor-1 Antibody Reverses Chemoresistance in Human MCF-7 Breast Cancer Xenografts. *Cancer Res.* 66: 4349-4356.

Pollard, J.W., Stanley, E.R., Paul, M.W. (1996). Pleiotropic roles for CSF-1 in development defined by the mouse mutation osteopetrotic. *Adv. Dev. Biochem.* 4: 153-193.

Pollard, J.W. (2004). Tumour-educated macrophages promote tumour progression and metastasis. *Nat. Rev. Cancer* 4: 71-78.

Price, F.V., Chambers, S.K., Chambers, J.T., Carcangiu, M.L., Schwartz, P.E., Kohorn, E.I., Stanley, E.R., Kacinski, B.M. (1993). CSF-1 concentration in primary ascites of ovarian cancer is a significant predictor of survival. *Am J Obstet Gynecol.* 168: 520-527.

Rettenmier, C.W., Sacca, R., Furman, W.L., Roussel, M.F., Holt, J.T., Nienhuis, A.W., Stanley, E.R. & Sherr, C.J. (1989). Expression of the human c-fms proto-oncogene product (colony-stimulating factor-1 receptor) on peripheral blood mononuclear cells and choriocarcinoma cell lines. *J Clin Invest.* 77: 1740-1746.

Roberts, W.M., Shapiro, L.H., Ashmun, R.A. & Look, A.T. (1992). Transcription of the human colony-stimulating factor-1 receptor gene is regulated by separate tissue-specific promoters. *Blood* 79: 586-593.

Sapi, E., Flick, M.B., Rodov, S., Gilmore-Hebert, M., Kelley, M., Rockwell, S. & Kacinski, B.M. (1996). Independent regulation of invasion and anchorage-independent growth by different autophosphorylation sites of the macrophage colony-stimulating factor 1 receptor. *Cancer Res.* 56: 5704-5712.

Sapi, E., Flick, M.B., Gilmore-Hebert M., Rodov, S. & Kacinski, B.M. (1995). Transcriptional regulation of the *c-fms* (CSF-1R) proto-oncogene in human breast carcinoma cells by glucocorticoids. *Oncogene* 10: 529-42.

Sapi, E. (2004). The role of CSF-1 in normal physiology of mammary gland and breast cancer: an update. *Exp Biol Med* 229(1): 1-11.

Schmittgen, T.D. & Livak, K.J. (2008). Analyzing real-time PCR data by the comparative CT method. *Nature Protocol* 3: 1101-1108.

Scholl, S.M., Mosseri, V., Tang, R., Beuvon, F., Palud, C., Lidereau, R. & Pouillart, P. (1993). Expression of colony-stimulating factor-1 and its receptor (the protein product of c-fms) in invasive breast tumor cells. Induction of urokinase production via this pathway? *Ann N Y Acad Sci.* 698: 131-135.

Scholl, S.M., Pallud, C., Beuvon, F., Hacene, K., Stanley, E.R., Rohrschneider, L., Tang, R., Pouillart, P. & Lidereau, R. (1994). Anti-colony-stimulating factor-1 antibody staining in primary breast adenocarcinomas correlates with marked inflammatory cell infiltrates and prognosis. *J Natl Cancer Inst.* 86: 120-126.

Shurtleff, S.A., Downing, JR., Rock, C.O., Hawkins, S.A., Roussel, M.F. & Sherr, C.J. (1990). Structural features of the colony-stimulating factor receptor that affect its association with phosphatidylinositol 3-kinase. *The EMBO J.* 9: 2415 – 2421.

Shyu, A.B., Wilkinson, M.F. & van Hoof, A. (2008). Messenger RNA regulation: to translate or to degrade. *EMBO J.* 27: 471-481.

Sonenberg N. & Hinnebusch A.G. (2009). Regulation of translation initiation in eukaryotes: mechanisms and biological targets. *Cell* 136: 731-745.

Srikantan, S. & Gorospe, M. (2011) Unclipsing HuR nuclear function. *Mol. Cell.* 43: 319-321.

Stark, A., Brennecke, J., Bushati, N., Russell, R.B. & Cohen, S.M. (2005). Animal MicroRNAs confer robustness to gene expression and have a significant impact on 3'UTR evolution. *Cell* 123: 1133-1146.

Tang, R., Kacinski, B., Validire, P., Beuvon, F., Sastre, X., Benoit, P., de la Rochefordiere, A., Mosseri, V., Pouillart, P., Scholl, S. (1990). Oncogene amplification correlates with dense lymphocyte infiltration in human breast cancers: a role for hematopoietic growth factor release by tumor cells? *J. Cell Biochem.* 44: 189-198.

Toy, E.P., Bonafe, N., Savlu, A., Zeiss, C., Zheng, W., Flick, M., Chambers, S.K. (2005). Correlation of tumor phenotype with c-fms proto-oncogene expression in an in vivo intraperitoneal model for experimental human breast cancer metastasis. *Clin. Exp. Metastasis.* 22: 1-9.

Toy, E.P., Lamb, L., Azodi, M., Roy, W.J, Woo, H.H. & Chambers, S.K. (2010). Inhibition of the *c-fms* proto-oncogene autocrine loop and tumor phenotype in glucocorticoid stimulated human breast carcinoma cells. *Breast Cancer Res. Treat* 129: 411-419.

Urlaub, H., Hartmuth, K., Kostka, S., Grelle, G.M. & Luhrmann, R. (2000). A general approach for identification of RNA-protein cross-linking sites within native human spliceosomal small nuclear ribonucleoproteins (snRNPs). Analysis of RNA-protein contacts in native U1 and U4/U6.U5 snRNPs. *J Biol Chem.* 275: 41458-41468.

Vollbrandt, T., Willkomm, D., Stossberg, H., Kruse, C. (2004). Vigilin is co-localized with 80S ribosomes and binds to the ribosomal complex through its C-terminal domain. *Int. J. Biochem. Cell Biol.* 36: 1306-1318.

Weber, B., Horiguchi, J., Luebbers, R., Sherman, M., & Kufe, D. (1989). Posttranscriptional stabilization of *c-fms* mRNA by a labile protein during human monocytic differentiation. *Mol. Cell Biol.* 9: 769-775.

Woo, H.H., Zhou, Y., Yi, X., David, C.L., Zheng, W., Gilmore-Hebert, M., Klugger, H.M., Ulukus, E.C., Baker, T., Stoffer, J.B. & Chambers, S.K. (2009). Regulation of non-AU-rich element containing *c-fms* proto-oncogene expression by HuR in breast cancer. *Oncogene* 28: 1176-1186.

Woo, H.H., Yi, X., Lamb, T., Menzl, I., Baker, T., Shapiro, D.J. & Chambers, S.K. (2011). Posttranscriptional suppression of proto-oncogene *c-fms* expression by vigilin in breast cancer. *Mol. Cell. Biol.* 31: 215-225.

Xiong, Y., Song, D., Cai, Y., Yu, W., Yeung, Y.-G. & Stanley, E.R. (2011). A CSF-1 Receptor Phosphotyrosine 559 Signaling Pathway regulates Receptor ubiquitination and tyrosine phosphorylation. *JBC.* 286: 952–960.

Yu, W., Chen, J., Xiong, Y., Pixley, F.J., Yeung, Y.-G. & Stanley, E.R. (2012).Macrophage proliferation is regulated through CSF-1 receptor tyrosines 544, 559 and 807. *JBC.* M112.355610.

Yi, X., Zhou, Y., Zheng, W. & Chambers, S. (2009). HuR expression in the nucleus correlates with high histological grade and poor disease-free survival in ovarian cancer. *Australian and New Zealand J Obstetrics and Gynaecology* 49: 93-98.

Zwaenepoel, O., Tzenaki, N., Vergetaki, A., Makrigiannakis, A., Vanhaesebroeck, B. & Papakonstanti, E.A. (2012). Functional CSF-1 receptors are located at the nuclear envelope and activated via the p110δ isoform of PI 3-kinase. *The FASEB J*. 26: 691-706.

Zheng, D., Ezzeddine, N., Chen, C.Y., Zhu, W., He, X. & Shyu, A.B. (2008). Deadenylation is prerequisite for P-body formation and mRNA decay in mammalian cells. *JCB*. 182: 89-101.

microRNA: New Players in Metastatic Process

Tiziana Triulzi, Marilena V. Iorio, Elda Tagliabue and Patrizia Casalini

Additional information is available at the end of the chapter

1. Introduction

In the last years new players have been revealed in cancer biology: microRNA (miRNAs or miRs) a class of small non coding RNAs (19-22 nts) able to regulate gene expression at post-transcriptional level, binding through partial sequence homology mainly the 3' UTR of target mRNAs, and causing block of translation and/or mRNA degradation.

miRNAs are generated by an endogenous transcript, they represent approximately 1% of the genome of different species, and each of them has hundreds of different conserved or non conserved targets: it has been estimated that about 30% of the genes are regulated by at least one miRNA. miRNA genes, expressed in several organisms, including *Homo Sapiens*, are highly conserved across different species [1].

This discovery resulted in a pattern shift in our understanding of gene regulation because miRNAs are now known to repress thousands of target genes and coordinate normal processes, including cellular proliferation, differentiation and apoptosis. They are highly specific for tissue and developmental stage, and play crucial functions in the regulation of important processes, such as development, and stress response. In the last few years, miRNAs have indeed taken their place in the complex circuitry of cell biology, revealing a key role as regulators of gene expression.

In 2002, Croce and colleagues first demonstrated that a miRNA cluster was frequently deleted or downregulated in chronic lymphocytic leukemia. This discovery suggested that non-coding genes were contributing to the development of cancer, and paved the way for a closer investigation of miRNA loss or amplification in tumors.

miRNAs expression profiling has indeed provided evidence of the association of these tiny molecules with tumor development, progression and response to therapy, suggesting their possible use as diagnostic, prognostic and predictive biomarkers. It has been demonstrated that miRNAs can act either as oncogenes or tumor suppressors, and more recently it has been demonstrated that a miRNAs can exploit both functions according to the cellular context of their target genes. Another important issue concerns the role of miRNAs in regulating the interaction between cancer cells and the microenvironment with respect to neo-angiogenesis or tissue invasion and metastasis.

Outgrowths of disseminated metastases remain the primary cause of mortality in cancer patients, but the molecular and cellular mechanisms regulating metastatic spread remain largely unknown. Metastatic processes involve multiple steps, including detachment from primary tumors, crossing the basement membrane barriers and extracellular matrix, intravasation into the circulation, survival within the vasculature, extravasation into distant tissues, and finally, establishment of secondary tumors [2] . These processes rely on coordinated spatio-temporal expression of various genes and finely regulated protein products, which govern the ability of tumor cells to successfully complete the intricate task, and the pivotal role of miRNAs in metastasis has emerged only recently.

2. miRNAs biogenesis and mechanism of action

miRNAs are generated by endonucleolytic cleavage of hairpin precursor transcripts by Dicer ribonuclease (RNase) III–like proteins and can direct the cleavage of target transcripts by Argonaute RNAse H–like proteins in a sequence-specific manner. miRNAs can also inhibit translation of target mRNAs.

miRNAs are transcribed for the most part by RNA Polimerase II as long primary transcripts characterized by hairpin structures (pri-microRNAs), and part of them are transcribed as distinct transcriptional units. 50% of known miRNA genes are located nearby other microRNAs, supporting the hypothesis that clustered miRNAs, representing miRNA families which are commonly related in sequence and function, can be transcribed from their own promoters as polycistronic pri-microRNAs.

According to their genomic localization, microRNAs can be classified in:

a) exonic microRNAs located in non coding transcripts, b) intronic microRNAs located in non coding transcripts and microRNA located in protein-coding trancripts, c) mixed miRNA genes that can be assigned to one of the above groups depending on the given splicing pattern. Exonic microRNAs are transcribed within the pri-miR (up to 1 kb long) containing both the 5'-cap and the 3'-poly-A tail. The miRNAs localized within introns of protein-encoding or -non-encoding genes have been denominated "miRtrons". miRtrons are regulatory RNAs transcribed within the mRNA of the host gene generating a hairpin structure, recognized and cleaved by the spliceosome machinery without Drosha-mediated cleavage.

The initial step in pri-miRNA processing (Figure 1) is performed in the nucleus by the enzymatic activity of an RNAse III-type protein called Drosha. Drosha is a highly conserved 160 kDa protein containing two RNAse III domains and one double-strand RNA-binding domain. Drosha forms a huge complex, 500 kDa in *D. melanogaster* and 650 kDA in *H. sapiens*, known as Microprocessor complex, which generates a ~70-nucleotides precursor miRNA (pre-miRNA) and contains the co-factor Di George syndrome critical region 8 (DGCR8), also known as Pasha in *D. melanogaster* and *C. elegans*.

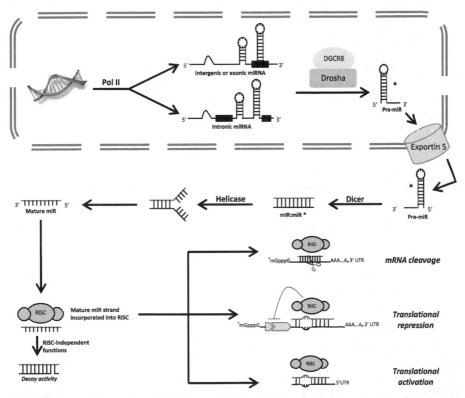

Figure 1. An overview of microRNAs biogenesis and mechanism of action.

The originated precursor molecules are then actively exported by a Ran-GTP and Exportin 5-mediated mechanism to the cytoplasm, where the second step of pre-miRNA processing (dicing) is mediated by the RNAse III Dicer (~200 kDa), which acts in complex with the transactivating response RNA-binding protein (TRBP), or PACT (also known as PRKRA), and Argonaute (AGO1-4), generating a dsRNA of approximately 22 nucleotides, named miR:miR*. This dsRNA includes the mature miRNA guide, and the complementary passenger strand, the miRNA* (star miRNA) (many publications refer to the two strand pair as miR-3p/miR-5p, referring to the direction of the functional miRNA). Whereas one of the two strands is selected as guide strand according to thermodynamic properties, the complementary one is usually subjected to degradation. The so called miRNA* was initially thought to be the strand subjected to degradation, instead more recent evidence suggests that it does not simply represent a non-functional bioproduct of miRNA biogenesis, but it can be selected as a functional strand and play significant biological roles [3] .

More in details, guided by the sequence complementarity between the small RNA and the target mRNA, miRNA-RISC-mediated gene inhibition is commonly divided into three processes: (i) site-specific cleavage, (ii) enhanced mRNA degradation and (iii) translational inhibition. The first process, commonly defined as RNA interference (RNAi) and restricted to miRNAs with a perfect or near-perfect match to the target RNA, is a very rare event in mammals, where it is carried out exclusively by Ago2. By contrast, the other two processes are more commonly associated with mismatched miRNA/target sequences, which is the most likely scenario in mammals. The combination of these two processes is commonly defined as a non-cleavage repression, and can be carried out by any of the four mammalian Ago proteins [4] . However, the exact mechanism through which miRNAs can impair translation is still debated.

Moreover, even though it is known that microRNAs mainly recognize complementary sequences in the 3' untraslated regions (UTRs) of their target mRNAs, more recent studies have reported that they can also bind to the 5'UTR or the ORF [5-8] and, even more surprisingly, they can upregulate translation upon growth arrest conditions [9] .

Finally, whereas the 5' end of the microRNA (the so called "seed site") has always been considered the most important for the binding to the mRNA, recently the target sites have been further divided into three main classes, according to grade and localization of the complementarity [10] : the dominant seed site targets (5' seed-only), the 5' dominant canonical seed site targets (5' dominant) and the 3' complementary seed site targets (3' canonical).

Considering the different rules regulating the interaction between a microRNA and its target mRNA, it is not surprising that each miRNA has the potential to target a large number of genes [11-14]. Conversely, an estimated 60% of the mRNAs have one or more evolutionarily conserved sequences that are predicted to interact with miRNAs. Bioinformatical analysis predicts that the 3' UTR of a single gene is frequently targeted by several different miRNAs [11] . Many of these predictions have been validated experimentally, suggesting that miRNAs might cooperate to regulate gene expression (a list of computational tools for miRNA target prediction is reported in Table 1).

name	website
miRNA map	http://mirnamap.mbc.nctu.edu.tw/
miRBASE	http://mirbase.org/
microRNA	http://www.microrna.org/microrna/home.do
coGemiR	http://www.cogemir.tigem.it/
miRGEN	http://www.diana.pcbi.upenn.edu/miRGen.html
deepBase	http://www.deepbase.sysu.edu.cn

Table 1. miRNA databases.

To complicate the already intricate scenario, it has been recently reported that miRNAs can bind to ribonucleoproteins in a seed sequence and a RISC-independent manner and then interfere with their RNA binding functions (decoy activity) [15] . Three studies have reported that miRNAs can also regulate gene expression at the transcriptional level by direct binding to the DNA [16-18].

Overall, these data show the complexity and widespread regulation of gene expression by miRNAs that should be taken into consideration when developing miRNA-based therapies.

3. Metastasis

The most deleterious effect of cancer is metastases development, indeed tumor metastasis is the primary cause of death in cancer patients. The ability to metastasize is a hallmark of malignant tumors [19] . Metastases represent the end point of a multi-step process that consists of local invasion through surrounding extracellular matrix and stromal cells, intravasation into the blood vessels, survival in the circulation, extravasation, and colonization of distant tissues [20]. Each step in this process represents a physiological barrier that must be overcome by the tumor cell to successfully metastasize. Malignant cells overcome these barriers through the accumulation of genetic and epigenetic changes, including modifications in microRNA expression profiles. Despite great improvement in the knowledge of metastasis biology, the molecular mechanisms which underlie this intricate process are still not completely understood.

Tumor cells can invade surrounding tissues as cohesive multicellular units or as individual cells, and individual cells can invade through the 'amoeboid invasion' or the 'mesenchymal invasion' programs [21] . Amoeboid movement depends mainly from Rho/ROCK expression, and is independent from adhesion and proteolytic degradation of ECM [22,23]. On the contrary, mesenchymal motility depends upon interaction of carcinoma cells with the extracellular matrix through integrin recruitment and upon pericellular ECM proteolysis of the moving cells. Cells that use this program to invade are characterized by an elongated and polarized morphology, achievable with an epithelial to mesenchymal transition (EMT). EMT, first described as typical of embryonic development, generates cells with mesenchymal features phenotypically similar to invading cells. The EMT transcriptional programme has been associated with activation of several key transcriptions factors, including Snail1 and Snail2 (Slug), Twist, ZEB-1-2, etc, which lead to the regulation of a series of proteins causing decrease of E-cadherin for disruption of adherent junctions, increase in N-cadherin and Met proto-oncogene to drive motility, as well as increase in MMPs and urokinase–type plasminogen activator/urokinase–type plasminogen receptor (uPA/uPAR) proteolytic systems to degrade 3D barriers [24,25].

The overexpression of many of these EMT regulators have been shown to correlate with disease relapse and decreased survival in patients with breast, colorectal, and ovarian carcinomas, suggesting that the induction of EMT leads to more aggressive tumors and poorer clinical outcomes.

Once tumor cells have invaded local microenvironment, they should intravasate, survive in the circulation and extravasate at distant sites. To successfully perform these steps, they have to cross the pericyte and endothelial cell barriers that form the walls of microvessels. In order to overcome physical barriers which represent an obstacle to extravasation in tissues with low intrinsic microvessel permeability, primary tumors are capable of secreting factors that perturb these distant microenvironments and induce vascular hyperpermeability. The ability of the cancer cell to develop into a metastatic lesion at distant sites is the most limiting step in cancer metastasis formation. Indeed, the disseminated tumor cells may stay in a quiescent state for long time, probably due to incompatibilities with the foreign microenvironments that surround them [2]. Some have proposed that carcinoma cells can address the problem of an incompatible microenvironment at the metastatic site via the establishment of a "premetastatic niche" [26].

4. miRNAs and metastasis

Remarkably, a regulatory role for miRNAs in metastasis has been recognized, and the term "metastamir" has been coined by Welch and colleagues to refer to those regulatory miRNAs not just involved in tumorigenesis, but specific in the promotion or suppression of various steps of metastasis [27]. To date, microRNAs have mostly been found to influence the initial stages of metastasis, affecting cell migration and invasion (Figure 2). Although a particular miRNA that specifically regulates cancer cell intravasation and extravasation has not yet been identified, it is still believed that these steps may also be regulated by miRNAs.

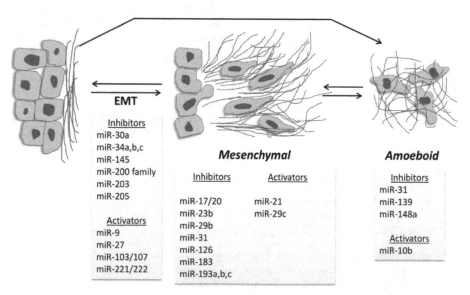

Figure 2. microRNAs implicated in the regulation of EMT and cell migration.

Several miRNAs have been found to regulate the EMT process, and the most well-known among them is the miR-200 family, which includes miR-200a, miR-200b, miR-200c, miR-141 and miR-429.

miR-200 family is recognized as a master regulator of the epithelial phenotype by post transcriptionally suppression of the expression of the ZEB1 and ZEB2 EMT-inducing transcription factors in breast [28] and gastric cancer [29]. Acting in the opposite direction, ZEB1 and ZEB2, which promote not only tumor cell dissemination, but also the tumor-initiating capacity, has been shown to transcriptionally repress miR-200 family members, thereby establishing a double negative feedback loop that causes the reinforcement of cells in either the mesenchymal or epithelial state [25]. This miR family, as others able to control epithelial–mesenchymal plasticity, is likely to also affect events at metastatic sites. Recently, the putative DNA methylation-associated inactivation of various miR-200 members has been described in cancer. miR-200 epigenetic silencing resulted to be not a static and fixed process, instead there can be a shift to hypermethylated or unmethylated 5'-CpG island status corresponding to the EMT and mesenchymal-epithelial-transition (MET) phenotypes, respectively. In fact, careful laser microdissection in human colon revealed that in normal colon mucosa crypts (epithelia) and stroma (mesenchyma) 5'-CpG island status are unmethylated and methylated at these loci, respectively, and that the colorectal tumors undergo selective miR-200 hypermethylation of their epithelial component. These findings indicate that the epigenetic silencing plasticity of the miR-200 family contributes to the evolving and adapting phenotypes of human tumors [30].

Unexpectedly, it was reported that overexpression of miR-200 enhances macroscopic metastases in mouse breast cancer models. These findings were surprising but provide yet another example of the opposing activities of some miRNAs [31]. miR-200 levels are indirectly downregulated by miR-103/107 that target Dicer, a key component of the miRNA processing machinery. Accordingly, miR-103/107 are associated with metastasis and poor outcome in human breast cancer [32].

The transcription factor ZEB1 can also repress the expression of stemness-inhibiting miR-203 [33]. Recently, miR-203 was reported as a metastasis suppressor miRNA, targeting Slug [34] and Snail1 [35] and is often silenced in different malignancies including hepatocellular carcinoma, prostate cancer, oral cancer, breast cancer and hematopoietic malignancy. Snail1 and Slug play a key role during the early step of EMT, activating expression of ZEB factors in a context-dependent manner. Functionally, ectopic expression of miR-203 in BT549 and MDA-MB-231 breast cancer cell lines caused cell cycle arrest and apoptosis and inhibited cell invasion and migration *in vitro*. Thus the miR-203 and miR-200 feedback loops control cell plasticity in epithelial homeostasis. Snail1 is also regulated by miR-30a in non-small cell lung cancer (NSCLC), where it is dowmodulated [36].

Opposite to miR-200 family, miR-221/222 family promotes a poorly differentiated mesenchymal-like phenotype in breast cancer, and is highly expressed in triple negative breast cancers that basally expressed EMT markers. Increasing miR-221 or miR-222 can affect various characteristics associated with EMT, including increased invasive capacity,

[37,38], and anoikis resistance [39]. Forced expression of miR-221/222 in luminal breast cancer cells causes a decrease in E-cadherin and an increase in the mesenchymal marker vimentin [40]. Luminal cells expressing miR-221/222 gained a more mesenchymal morphology and had increased migratory and invasive capacity [41]. Furthermore, miR-221 and miR-222 can regulate angiogenesis, repressing the proliferative and angiogenic properties of c-Kit in endothelial cells [42]. In addition other miRNAs can manage EMT, such as the ZEB1- and ZEB2-suppressing miR-205 [28], which has also been shown to exert an oncosuppressive activity in breast cancer [43,44] prostate cancer [45] and melanoma [46]; and miR-27, which promotes EMT in gastric cancer cell directly targeting APC gene and activating the Wnt pathway [47].

Recently, the inhibition of EMT by p53 has been described as a new mode of tumor suppression which presumably prevents metastasis. p53 activation down-regulates Snail via induction of the miR-34a/b/c genes, which directly target Snail transcription factor. Ectopic miR-34a expression caused down-regulation of Slug and ZEB1, as well as the stemness factors BMI1, CD44, CD133, OLFM4 and c-MYC, thus provoking MET. Conversely, the transcription factors Snail and ZEB1 repress miR-34a and miR-34b/c expression [48]. Recently it has been described that miR-34 suppress also c-MET in hepatocellular carcinoma [49] and in osteosarcoma cells [50].

EMT is characterized by cadherin switching (from E-cadherin to N-cadherin), that correlates with a profound change in cell phenotype and behavior. miR-9, identified as a new "metastomiR" and activated by MYC and MYCN, directly targets CDH1, the E-cadherin-encoding messenger RNA, leading to increased cell motility and invasiveness, activation of β-catenin signaling and upregulation of VEGF. Moreover, overexpression of miR-9 in non-metastatic breast tumor cells enables these cells to form pulmonary micrometastases in mice, and in colorectal cancer cells it promotes cell motility [51]. Conversely, inhibition of miR-9 in highly malignant cells impairs metastasis formation [52].

N-cadherin (CDH2) was proved to be a direct target of miR-145 by Gao P and coworkers [53]. miR-145, suppressing N-cadherin protein translation and indirectly downregulating also its downstream effector matrix metallopeptidase 9 (MMP9), suppresses metastases. It has been reported that miR-145 exerts its anti metastatic role by directly targeting also the metastatic gene *mucin 1* [54] in breast cancer and VEGF in osteosarcoma cells [55]. Moreover, suppression of Mucin1 by miR-145 causes a reduction of β-catenin as well as the oncogenic Cadherin 11 [54]. Accordingly miR-145, acting as a metastasis suppressor, is stepwise downregulated in normal gastric mucosa, primary gastric cancers and their secondary metastases [53] , and in osteosarcoma in comparison to normal tissues [55].

Several miRNAs such as miR-34a [56], miR-373 and miR-520c [57] and mir-328 [58] have been reported to regulate the cell-surface glycoprotein encoding gene CD44 (cell surface receptor for hyaluronan). Cell lines with high CD44+/CD24– cell numbers are basal/mesenchymal or myoepithelial types and are more invasive than other cell lines [59]. miR-520/373 has been also reported to directly target TGFBR2 and to induce the suppression of Smad-dependent expression of the metastasis-promoting genes parathyroid hormone-related protein, plasminogen activator inhibitor-1 and angiopoietin-like 4, thus impairing tumor cell invasion, *in vitro* and *in vivo*. Remarkably, decreased expression of miR-520c correlated with lymph node metastasis specifically in ER negative breast tumors [60].

Recently Han M and coworkers [61] demonstrated that miR-21 regulates epithelial-mesenchymal transition phenotype and hypoxia-inducible factor-1α (HIF-1α) expression in sphere forming breast cancer stem cells (CSC). Indeed inhibition of miR-21 by antagomir led to reversal of EMT, down-expression of HIF-1α, as well as suppression of invasion and migration, which indicates a key role of miR-21 in regulating CSC-associated features.

EMT is a profound change in cell phenotype that causes immotile epithelial cells to acquire traits such as motility, invasiveness, anoikis and the ability to adapt to environmental changes to continue to invade successfully. Mesenchymal motility program is characterised by elongated and polarized cell morphology and depends upon ECM proteolysis of the moving cells and from integrin interaction with the extracellular matrix.

Urokinase, a serin protease, activating plasmin triggers a proteolysis cascade that, depending on the physiological environment, participates in extracellular matrix degradation. miR-193a/b overexpression in MDA-MB-231 and MDA-MB-435 breast carcinoma cells significantly reduced its direct target uPA protein amounts and inhibited cell invasion [62]. In an immunodeficient mouse model, miR-193b significantly inhibited the growth and dissemination of xenografted tumors [63]. The expression of miR-193b is downregulated in metastatic breast cancer, and this microRNA is in turn able to upregulate uPA expression and to contribute to the progression of breast cancer. Recently, miR-23b was reported to directly target uPA and c-MET and to decrease migration and proliferation of human hepatocellular carcinoma cells [64]. Plasminogen activation can be regulated also indirectly by mir-17/20 expression, which is usually downregulated in highly invasive breast cancer cell lines and node-positive breast cancer specimens [65]. microRNA17/20 directly repressed IL-8 by targeting its 3' UTR, and inhibited cytokeratin 8 via the cell cycle control protein cyclin D1, a secreted plasminogen activator. Indeed cell-conditioned medium from microRNA17/20-overexpressing non invasive breast cancer cell MCF7 was sufficient to inhibit MDA-MB-231 cell migration and invasion [65]. The invasion-related urokinase receptor is also indirectly regulated by a miRNA. Indeed, oncogenic miR-21, elevated in different tumor types, included colorectal cancer [66] melanoma and breast cancer [67], post-transcriptionally regulates PDCD4, that can suppress invasion and intravasation, at least in part by inhibiting expression of uPAR gene via the transcription factors Sp1/Sp3. Thus, miR-21 is able to enhance cancer cell intravasation, extravasation and metastasis in addition to cell proliferation.

The restoration in hepatocellular carcinoma cells of miR-122 that exerts some of its action via regulation of ADAM17 caused a dramatic reduction of *in vitro* migration, invasion, *in vivo* tumorigenesis, angiogenesis, and local invasion in the liver of nude mice [68]. Under the transcriptional control of HNF1A, HNF3A and HNF3B, miR-122 is specifically repressed in a subset of primary tumors that are characterized by poor prognosis [69].

ADAM9 is directly target by miR-126, which expression is reduced in invasive ductal adenocarcinoma (IDA) and pancreatic cancer cell lines. Re-expression of miR-126 and siRNA-based knockdown of ADAM9 in pancreatic cancer cells resulted in reduced cellular migration, invasion, and induction of epithelial marker E-cadherin [70]. It also directly regulates the adaptor protein Crk that binds to several tyrosine-phosphorylated proteins, inhibiting cell growth by inducing cell cycle arrest in G0/G1 phase, migration and invasion *in vitro* as well as tumorigenicity and metastasis *in vivo* in gastric cancer [71].

Matrix metalloproteinase-2 (MMP2), involved in matrix degradation and involved in angiogenesis, is directly regulated by miR-29b, whose down modulation promotes angiogenesis, invasion, and metastasis of hepatocellular carcinomas [72]. MMP2 was confirmed to be a miR-29b target apart from Mcl-1, COL1A1, and COL4A1 also in prostate cancer cells [73].

miR-29c-targeted genes identified in nasopharyngeal carcinomas (NPC) encode extracellular matrix proteins, including multiple collagens and Laminin γ1, that are associated with tumor cell invasiveness in culture and increased metastasis in animal models and multiple human solid tumors as well as fibrillin SPARC [74]. Interestingly, introduction of miR-29c led to a reduced transcription of these genes in cultured cells, and the down-regulation of mir-29c level in NPC human cancer correlated with increase of target mRNAs, which could facilitate rapid matrix generation and renewal during tumor growth and the acquisition of tumor motility.

It was demonstrated that miR-183 targets ezrin, an intermediate between the plasma membrane and the actin cytoskeleton involved, together with radixin, in epithelial cell morphogenesis and adhesion [75], and may play a central role in the regulation of migration and metastasis in breast cancer [76], osteosarcoma [77] and lung cancer [78]. miR-183 is markedly down-regulated in osteosarcoma cells and tissues compared with matching normal bone tissues and its expression levels significantly correlated with lung metastasis as well as with local recurrence of osteosarcoma [77].

miR-223 is overexpressed in metastatic gastric cancer cells and stimulates non metastatic gastric cancer cells to migrate and to invade. Mechanistically, miR-223, induced by the transcription factor Twist, post transcriptionally downregulates EPB41L3 expression, thought to be involved in tethering the F-actin cytoskeleton to membrane proteins. Another functional downstream target of miR-223 is FBXW7, shown to have important roles in regulating the stability of multiple oncoprotein substrates, including Cyclin E, c-MYC, Notch, c-Jun, and Mcl-1. Overexpression of miR-223 is associated with poor metastasis-free survival in primary gastric carcinomas [79], with lymph node metastasis in gastric cancer, and poorer prognosis in oesophageal squamous cell carcinoma patients [80].

Cells can move also through an "amoeboid invasion" program. This motility style is largely independent from cell-ECM contact and from proteolytic degradation of ECM from MMPs. Furthermore, cell-ECM attachments of amoeboid moving cells are not organized in large focal adhesions but are very diffuse, and much weaker cell-ECM attachments are required, indeed, amoeboid movement cannot be blocked by inhibition of integrin function. The amoeboid invasion depends from Rho/ROCK expression, and their expression can be regulated also by miRNAs.

miR-10b, the first miRNA described to be pro-metastatic by Ma and colleagues in 2007 [81], inhibits the translation of mRNA encoding HOXD10, increasing the expression of Rho C, and thus leading to tumor cell invasion and metastasis. Ectopic expression of this miRNA endowed non-aggressive human breast cancer cells with the capacity to become invasive, as well as seed distant micrometastases when implanted as xenografts in immunodeficient mice. miR-10b was down-regulated in most breast cancers in comparison with normal mammary tissues, whereas it was highly expressed in about 50% of breast metastatic tumors. Induced by transcription factor Twist, miR-10b function as a metastasis driver in different types of cancer: i.e pancreatic [82], gastric [83] and colorectal [84] cancers.

RhoA, another member of Ras homolog gene family, was described also as a target for miR-155, a Smad4 regulated miR in breast cancer [85].

Mir-31 is able to inhibit multiple steps in the metastatic process: local invasion, one or more early post-intravasation events (intraluminal viability, extravasation efficiency and/or capacity to initially survive in the lung parenchyma), and metastatic colonization. MiR-31 carries out its anti-metastatic function regulating three genes: Rho A, Integrin $\alpha5$ and Radixin. Via suppression of Rho A, it is able to inhibit *in vitro* invasiveness [86,87]. Notably it also reduces Integrin $\alpha5$, a key effector of the mesenchymal invasion program, causing concomitant inhibition of both single-cell invasion programs. Controlling expression of Radixin, miR-31 causes anoikis-mediated cell death. In agreement with these data, miR-31 expression has been found to be attenuated in human breast [88-90], prostate [91], ovary [92], stomach [93,94] and bladder cancer [95]. Moreover miR-31 levels in primary human breast tumors were inversely associated with distant metastases [86]. Paradoxically, upregulation of miR-31 in human colorectal [96,97], liver [98] and head-and-neck tumors [99,100], as well as squamous cell carcinomas of the tongue [101] has also been observed [102] .

ROCK1 and ROCK2, the downstream targets of Rho A and Rho C, are regulated by miR-148a [103] and by miR-139 [104], respectively, which all behave as anti-metastatic miRNAs. Overexpression of miR-148a in gastric cancer cells [103] as well as in head and neck cancer cells [105], and of miR-139 in hepatocellular carcinoma cells (HCC) [104], suppressed cell migration and invasion *in vitro* and lung metastasis formation *in vivo*. Accordingly, miR-148a expression was suppressed in gastric cancer compared with their corresponding non tumor tissues, and the downregulated miR-148a was significantly associated with tumor node metastasis and miR-139 expression is reduced in metastatic HCC tumors compared with primary tumors.

In addition, others miRNAs with prominent roles in breast cancer metastasis have been reported.

The c-MYC regulated miR-17-92 cluster, which targets the connective tissue growth factor (CTGF) and the anti-angiogenic adhesive glycoprotein Thrombospondin 1 (TSP1) is shown to be elevated in metastatic breast cancer cells compared with nonmetastatic cells. miRNAs belonging to this cluster, attenuating also the TGFβ signaling pathway, indirectly shut down clusterin and angiopoietin-like 4 expressions, thereby stimulating angiogenesis and tumor cell growth [106]. Accordingly, blockade of miR-17 is shown to decrease breast cancer cell invasion/migration *in vitro* and metastasis *in vivo* [107]. Furthermore miR-17 and miR-20a were found to be significantly associated with reduced progression free survival in gastrointestinal cancer patients [108] .

The team led by Joan Massague [109] found that miR-335, miR-126, and miR-206 are metastasis-suppressors. Authors performed array-based miRNA profiling in MDA-MB-231 breast cancer cell derivatives (LM2) highly breast cancer cell derivatives highly metastatic to bone and lung, and found a signature of six genes (miR-335, miR-126, miR-206, miR-122a, miR-199a*, and miR-489) whose expression was highly decreased in metastatic cells. Restoring the expression of miR-335, miR-126 or miR-206 in LM2 cells decreased the lung colonizing activity of these cells by more than fivefold. They found that miR-335 suppresses metastasis and migration by targeting the progenitor cell transcription factor SOX4 and TNC messenger RNAs. Consequently, loss of miR-335 leads to the activation of SRY-box containing SOX4 and TNC, which are responsible for the acquisition of metastatic properties. Notably, knockdown of SOX4 and TNC using RNA interference diminished *in vitro* invasive ability and *in vivo* metastatic potential, evidencing that both genes are key effectors of metastasis [110]. miR-126, has recently been described to suppress metastatic endothelial recruitment, metastatic angiogenesis and metastatic colonization through coordinate targeting of IGFBP2, PITPNC1 and MERTK, novel pro-angiogenic genes and biomarkers of human metastasis through the IGFBP2/IGF1/IGF1R and GAS6/MERTK signaling pathways [111]. In addition, low expression of miR-335 or miR-126 in primary tumors from patients was associated with poor distal metastasis-free survival.

IGF1R was identified as a direct target of miR-493 that has been described as a metastasis inhibitor. Indeed, high levels of miR-493 and miR-493(*), but not pri-miR-493, in primary colon cancer were inversely related to the presence of liver metastasis, and attributed to an increase of miR-493 expression during carcinogenesis [112].

Raf kinase inhibitor protein (RKIP) represses breast tumour cell intravasation and bone metastasis through inhibition of MAPK leading to decreased transcription of LIN28 by Myc. Suppression of LIN28 enables enhanced let-7 processing in breast cancer cells. let-7 appears to play a major role in regulating stemness however elevated let-7 expression inhibits HMGA2, a chromatin remodelling protein that activates pro-invasive and pro-metastatic genes, including Snail. LIN28 depletion and let-7 expression suppress bone metastasis, and LIN28 restores bone metastasis in mice bearing RKIP-expressing breast tumour cells [113].

miR-146a is very similar to miR-146b, which is encoded by a different gene, but differs by only two bases and appears to function redundantly in many systems as mediators of inflammatory signaling, influencing differentiation, proliferation and apoptosis. They are pleiotropic regulators of tumorigenesis, as altered expression of both miR-146a/b have been linked with cancer risk, tumor histogenesis and invasive and metastatic capacity in diverse cancers [114]. In fact Hurst and coworkers [27], showed that breast cancer metastasis suppressor 1 (BRMS1), a protein that regulates expression of multiple genes [115] leading to suppression of metastasis, significantly up-regulates miR-146a and miR-146b in metastatic breast cancer cells. Transduction of miR-146a or miR-146b into MDA-MB-231 inhibited invasion and migration *in vitro*, and suppressed experimental lung metastasis. Bhaumik et al. confirmed that expression of miR-146a/b in MDA-MB-231 cells, impaired invasion and migration capacity by suppressing NF-κB activity [116]. In Table 2 both suppressing and promoting metastasis related miRNAs are summarized.

miRNA	Target
Suppressing miRNAs	
miR-17/20	IL8, Cyclin D1
miR-23b	c-MET, uPA
miR-29b	COL1A1,COL4A1, MMP-2
miR-29c	Laminin γ1, collagens
miR-30a	Snail
miR-31	Integrin α5, Radixin, Rho A
miR-34a	Snail, CD44, c-MET
miR-122	ADAM17
miR-126	ADAM9, Crk, IGFBP2, PTPNC1, MERTK
miR-139	ROCK2
miR-145	Mucin 1, N-cadherin, VEGF
miR-146a,b	NF-κB
miR-148a	ROCK
miR-155	Rho A
miR-183	Ezrin
miR-193a,b	uPA
miR-203	Slug, Snail1
miR-205	ZEB1, ZEB2
miR-335	SOX4, TNC
let-7	HMGA2, RAS
miR-200 family	ZEB1, ZEB2
miR-328	CD44
miR-373/520c	CD44, TGFBR2
miR-493	IGF1R
Promoting miRNAs	
miR-9	E-cadherin
miR-10b	HOXD10
miR-17-92	CTGF, TSP1
miR-21	PDCD4
miR-27	APC
miR-103/107	Dicer
miR-221/222	TRPS1
miR-223	EPB41L3, FBXW7

Table 2. microRNAs and their targets relevant in metastasis.

5. miRNAs as prognostic biomarkers

After early studies indicating the role of microRNA genes in the pathogenesis of human cancer, platforms to assess the global expression of microRNA genes in normal and diseased tissues have been developed. Gene expression profiling has already demonstrated its effectiveness at subtyping various cancers, however miRNA profiles are equally discriminatory and can even be more informative, as changes in their expression can provide insights into the myriad of gene permutations observed in various cancer subtypes: links have indeed been made between misregulated miRNAs and the target genes that are affected, thus unraveling some of the unique gene networks involved [117]. miRNA profiles may identify cancer-specific signatures distinguishing between normal and cancerous tissue [118-121], but they can also discriminate different subtypes of a particular cancer [119,122,123].

To discover microRNAs regulating the critical transition from ductal carcinoma in situ to invasive ductal carcinoma, a key event in breast cancer progression, Volinia et al. [124] performed a microRNA profile on 80 biopsies from invasive ductal carcinoma, 8 from ductal carcinoma in situ, and 6 from normal breast selected from a recently published deep-sequencing dataset [125]. They found that the microRNA profile established for the normal breast to ductal carcinoma in situ transition was largely maintained in the in situ to invasive ductal carcinoma transition. Nevertheless, a nine-microRNA signature that differentiated invasive from in situ carcinoma was identified. Specifically, let-7d, miR-210, and -221 were down-regulated in the in situ and up-regulated in the invasive transition, thus featuring an expression reversal along the cancer progression path. Additionally, they identified microRNAs for overall survival and time to metastasis. Five noncoding genes were associated with both prognostic signatures miR-210, -21, -106b*, -197, and let-7i, with miR-210 the only one also involved in the invasive transition.

Concerning the possibility to use miRNAs as prognostic markers to predict outcome, several groups have successfully addressed this issue [123,126-130] and in particular, concerning involvement of microRNAs in metastatic disease. For example several studies conducted on samples from patient with lung cancer assessed the involvement of metastamiRs: Landi et al [122] analyzed 107 male with early-stage squamous cell lung cancers (SQ) and found 5 miRNAs (miR-25, -34c-5p, -191, let- 7e, miR-34a) whose high expression strongly predicted longer SQ survival [122]. In another study, based on miRNA expression profiling of lung adenocarcinoma and SQ, ten miRNAs (hsa-miR-450b-3p, hsa-miR-29c*, hsa-miR-145*, hsa-miR-148a*, hsa-miR-1, hsa-miR-30d, hsa-miR-187, hsa-miR-218, hsa-miR-708* and hsa-miR-375) associated with brain metastasis were identified including miR-145*, which inhibit cell invasion and metastasis. Two miRNA signatures that are highly predictive of recurrence free survival of 357 stage I NSCLC were also identified, one independent of cancer subtype, the other specific for adenocarcinoma or SQ subtype [131]. From a small cohort of 20 NSCLC patients, Donnem and co-workers [132] in addition to miR differentially expressed between NSCLC tumors and normal control, found 37 miRs up/down regulated in tumors derived from patients with short versus long disease specific survival (DSS) including upregulated miR-31, miR-183, let-7a, miR-193b and downregulated miR-205, miR-378, miR-708 and miR-

29c. A further analysis comparing short versus long DSS patients tumors identified significantly altered angiogenesis-related miRs (miR-21, miR-106a, miR-126, miR-155, miR-182, miR-210 and miR-424) [123], on the basis of a small number of cases, found that the reduced expression of miR-17-5p and -30c in malignant mesothelioma correlated with better survival in patients with the sarcomatoid subtype.

Studies relative to tumors in other body districts have been carried out to determine the involvement of miRs in metastatic disease. Heinzelman et al, analysed miRNA expression of 30 human clear cell renal carcinoma (ccRCC) including 10 non-metastatic tumors, 4 tumors with metastasis after 3 years or later and 4 tumors with primary metastasis. They detected a miRNA signature that distinguishes between metastatic and non-metastatic ccRCC, including miR-451, miR-221, miR-30a, miR-10b and miR-29a. Furthermore, the authors identified a group of 12 miRNAs, such as let-7 family, miR-30c, miR-26a, which are decreased in highly aggressive primary metastatic tumours. They found also correlations between expression levels of specific miRNAs with progression-free survival and overall survival [133].

Veerla et al [95], by miRNA expression analysis of 34 cases of urothelial carcinomas identified 51 miRNAs that discriminated the 3 pathological subtypes Ta, T1 and T2-T3. A score based on the expression levels of the 51 miRNAs, identified muscle invasive tumors with high precision and sensitivity. miRNAs showing high expression in muscle invasive tumors included miR-222 and miR-125b and in Ta tumors miR-10a. Moreover authors identified 2 miRNAs, miR-452 and miR-452*, associated with metastases in the lymph nodes and with a strong prognostic impact on death as endpoint.

353 gastric samples from two independent subsets of patients from Japan were analysed by Ueda et al [119], with the aim to assess the relation between microRNA expression and prognosis of gastric cancer. They found a progression-related signature including miR-125b, miR-199a, and miR-100 as the most important microRNAs involved. Moreover they found that low expression of let-7g and miR-433 and high expression of miR-214 were associated with unfavourable outcome in overall survival independent of clinical covariates, including depth of invasion, lymph-node metastasis, and stage.

6. Conclusion

Although miRs that have been demonstrated to be implicated in the metastatic process might represent a possible therapeutic tool, there have been so far few reported successes in the development of miRNAs for use in therapy. There are two main strategies to target miRNAs expression in cancer. Direct strategies involve the use of oligonucleotides or virus-based constructs to either block the expression of an oncogenic miRNA or to reintroduce a tumor suppressor miRNA lost in cancer. The indirect strategy involves the use of drugs to modulate miRNAs expression by targeting their transcription and their processing. Indeed, even though a number of reports have described the possibility to reintroduce or inhibit microRNAs (reviewed by Iorio and Croce, [134]), there are still many issues that need to be addressed for an effective translation in clinics, as the development of efficient methods of a specific drug delivery, and the accurate prevision of putative unwanted off target effects.

Nevertheless, the results obtained up to date seem quite promising and encouraging, and even though we still have to improve the knowledge in microRNA field to even think of future therapeutic applications, we might be not so far from there.

Author details

Tiziana Triulzi, Elda Tagliabue* and Patrizia Casalini
Molecular Targeting Unit, Department of Experimental Oncology and Molecular Medicine, Fondazione IRCCS , Istituto Nazionale dei Tumori, Milan; Italy

Marilena V. Iorio
Start-Up Unit, Department of Experimental Oncology and Molecular Medicine, Fondazione IRCCS , Istituto Nazionale dei Tumori, Milan; Italy

Acknowledgement

Authors gratefully acknowledge Dr. Viola Regondi for figures preparation.

7. References

[1] Bartel DP. MicroRNAs: genomics, biogenesis, mechanism, and function. Cell 2004 Jan 23;116:281-97.
[2] Chambers AF, Groom AC, MacDonald IC. Dissemination and growth of cancer cells in metastatic sites. Nat Rev Cancer 2002 Aug;2:563-72.
[3] Bhayani MK, Calin GA, Lai SY. Functional relevance of miRNA sequences in human disease. Mutat Res 2012 Mar 1;731(1-2):14-9.
[4] Su H, Trombly MI, Chen J, Wang X. Essential and overlapping functions for mammalian Argonautes in microRNA silencing. Genes Dev 2009 Feb 1;23(3):304-17.
[5] Orom UA, Nielsen FC, Lund AH. MicroRNA-10a binds the 5'UTR of ribosomal protein mRNAs and enhances their translation. Mol Cell 2008 May 23;30(4):460-71.
[6] Lytle JR, Yario TA, Steitz JA. Target mRNAs are repressed as efficiently by microRNA-binding sites in the 5' UTR as in the 3' UTR. Proc Natl Acad Sci U S A 2007 Jun 5;104(23):9667-72.
[7] Moretti F, Thermann R, Hentze MW. Mechanism of translational regulation by miR-2 from sites in the 5' untranslated region or the open reading frame. RNA 2010 Dec;16(12):2493-502.
[8] Qin W, Shi Y, Zhao B, Yao C, Jin L, Ma J, et al. miR-24 regulates apoptosis by targeting the open reading frame (ORF) region of FAF1 in cancer cells. PLoS One 2010 Feb 25;5(2):e9429.
[9] Vasudevan S, Tong Y, Steitz JA. Switching from repression to activation: microRNAs can up-regulate translation. Science 2007 Dec 21;318(5858):1931-4.

---

* Corresponding Author

[10] Brennecke J, Stark A, Russell RB, Cohen SM. Principles of microRNA-target recognition. PLoS Biol 2005 Mar;3(3):e85.

[11] Lewis BP, Burge CB, Bartel DP. Conserved seed pairing, often flanked by adenosines, indicates that thousands of human genes are microRNA targets. Cell 2005 Jan 14;120(1):15-20.

[12] Krek A, Grun D, Poy MN, Wolf R, Rosenberg L, Epstein EJ, et al. Combinatorial microRNA target predictions. Nat Genet 2005 May;37(5):495-500.

[13] Betel D, Wilson M, Gabow A, Marks DS, Sander C. The microRNA.org resource: targets and expression. Nucleic Acids Res 2008 Jan;36(Database issue):D149-D153.

[14] Friedman RC, Farh KK, Burge CB, Bartel DP. Most mammalian mRNAs are conserved targets of microRNAs. Genome Res 2009 Jan;19(1):92-105.

[15] Beitzinger M, Meister G. Preview. MicroRNAs: from decay to decoy. Cell 2010 Mar 5;140(5):612-4.

[16] Khraiwesh B, Arif MA, Seumel GI, Ossowski S, Weigel D, Reski R, et al. Transcriptional control of gene expression by microRNAs. Cell 2010 Jan 8;140(1):111-22.

[17] Gonzalez S, Pisano DG, Serrano M. Mechanistic principles of chromatin remodeling guided by siRNAs and miRNAs. Cell Cycle 2008 Aug 15;7(16):2601-8.

[18] Kim DH, Saetrom P, Snove O, Jr., Rossi JJ. MicroRNA-directed transcriptional gene silencing in mammalian cells. Proc Natl Acad Sci U S A 2008 Oct 21;105(42):16230-5.

[19] Hanahan D, Weinberg RA. The hallmarks of cancer. Cell 2000;100:57-70.

[20] Gupta GP, Massague J. Cancer metastasis: building a framework. Cell 2006 Nov 17;127(4):679-95.

[21] Friedl P, Wolf K. Tumour-cell invasion and migration: diversity and escape mechanisms. Nat Rev Cancer 2003 May;3(5):362-74.

[22] Friedl P, Wolf K. Plasticity of cell migration: a multiscale tuning model. J Cell Biol 2010 Jan 11;188(1):11-9.

[23] Wolf K, Mazo I, Leung H, Engelke K, von Andrian UH, Deryugina EI, et al. Compensation mechanism in tumor cell migration: mesenchymal-amoeboid transition after blocking of pericellular proteolysis. J Cell Biol 2003 Jan;%20;160(2):267-77.

[24] Kalluri R. EMT: when epithelial cells decide to become mesenchymal-like cells. J Clin Invest 2009 Jun;119(6):1417-9.

[25] Thiery JP. Epithelial-mesenchymal transitions in development and pathologies. Curr Opin Cell Biol 2003 Dec;15:740-6.

[26] Psaila B, Lyden D. The metastatic niche: adapting the foreign soil. Nat Rev Cancer 2009 Apr;9(4):285-93.

[27] Hurst DR, Edmonds MD, Welch DR. Metastamir: the field of metastasis-regulatory microRNA is spreading. Cancer Res 2009 Oct 1;69(19):7495-8.

[28] Gregory PA, Bert AG, Paterson EL, Barry SC, Tsykin A, Farshid G, et al. The miR-200 family and miR-205 regulate epithelial to mesenchymal transition by targeting ZEB1 and SIP1. Nat Cell Biol 2008 May;10(5):593-601.

[29] Kurashige J, Kamohara H, Watanabe M, Hiyoshi Y, Iwatsuki M, Tanaka Y, et al. MicroRNA-200b Regulates Cell Proliferation, Invasion, and Migration by Directly Targeting ZEB2 in Gastric Carcinoma. Ann Surg Oncol 2012 Feb 4.

[30] Davalos V, Moutinho C, Villanueva A, Boque R, Silva P, Carneiro F, et al. Dynamic epigenetic regulation of the microRNA-200 family mediates epithelial and mesenchymal transitions in human tumorigenesis. Oncogene 2011 Aug 29;10.

[31] Korpal M, Ell BJ, Buffa FM, Ibrahim T, Blanco MA, Celia-Terrassa T, et al. Direct targeting of Sec23a by miR-200s influences cancer cell secretome and promotes metastatic colonization. Nat Med 2011 Aug 7;17(9):1101-8.

[32] Martello G, Rosato A, Ferrari F, Manfrin A, Cordenonsi M, Dupont S, et al. A MicroRNA targeting dicer for metastasis control. Cell 2010 Jun 25;141:1195-207.

[33] Wellner U, Schubert J, Burk UC, Schmalhofer O, Zhu F, Sonntag A, et al. The EMT-activator ZEB1 promotes tumorigenicity by repressing stemness-inhibiting microRNAs. Nat Cell Biol 2009 Dec;11(12):1487-95.

[34] Zhang Z, Zhang B, Li W, Fu L, Fu L, Zhu Z, et al. Epigenetic Silencing of miR-203 Upregulates SNAI2 and Contributes to the Invasiveness of Malignant Breast Cancer Cells. Genes Cancer 2011 Aug;2(8):782-91.

[35] Moes M, Le BA, Crespo I, Laurini C, Halavatyi A, Vetter G, et al. A Novel Network Integrating a miRNA-203/SNAI1 Feedback Loop which Regulates Epithelial to Mesenchymal Transition. PLoS One 2012;7(4):e35440.

[36] Kumarswamy R, Mudduluru G, Ceppi P, Muppala S, Kozlowski M, Niklinski J, et al. MicroRNA-30a inhibits epithelial-to-mesenchymal transition by targeting Snail and is downregulated in non-small cell lung cancer. Int J Cancer 2012 May 1;130(9):2044-53.

[37] Zheng C, Yinghao S, Li J. MiR-221 expression affects invasion potential of human prostate carcinoma cell lines by targeting DVL2. Med Oncol 2011 Apr 13.

[38] Guttilla IK, Phoenix KN, Hong X, Tirnauer JS, Claffey KP, White BA. Prolonged mammosphere culture of MCF-7 cells induces an EMT and repression of the estrogen receptor by microRNAs. Breast Cancer Res Treat 2012 Feb;132(1):75-85.

[39] Gramantieri L, Fornari F, Ferracin M, Veronese A, Sabbioni S, Calin GA, et al. MicroRNA-221 targets Bmf in hepatocellular carcinoma and correlates with tumor multifocality. Clin Cancer Res 2009 Aug 15;15(16):5073-81.

[40] Stinson S, Lackner MR, Adai AT, Yu N, Kim HJ, O'Brien C, et al. TRPS1 targeting by miR-221/222 promotes the epithelial-to-mesenchymal transition in breast cancer. Sci Signal 2011 Jun 14;4(177):ra41.

[41] Howe EN, Cochrane DR, Richer JK. The miR-200 and miR-221/222 microRNA Families: Opposing Effects on Epithelial Identity. J Mammary Gland Biol Neoplasia 2012 Mar;17(1):65-77.

[42] Poliseno L, Tuccoli A, Mariani L, Evangelista M, Citti L, Woods K, et al. MicroRNAs modulate the angiogenic properties of HUVECs. Blood 2006 Nov 1;108(9):3068-71.

[43] Iorio MV, Casalini P, Piovan C, Di Leva G, Merlo A, Triulzi T, et al. microRNA-205 regulates HER3 in human breast cancer. Cancer Res 2009 Mar 15;69:2195-200.

[44] Piovan C, Palmieri D, Di Leva G, Braccioli L, Casalini P, Tortoreto M, et al. Oncosuppressive role of p53-induced miR-205 in triple negative breast cancer. Mol Oncol 2012;In press.

[45] Gandellini P, Folini M, Longoni N, Pennati M, Binda M, Colecchia M, et al. miR-205 Exerts tumor-suppressive functions in human prostate through down-regulation of protein kinase Cepsilon. Cancer Res 2009 Mar 15;69:2287-95.

[46] Dar AA, Majid S, de SD, Nosrati M, Bezrookove V, Kashani-Sabet M. miRNA-205 suppresses melanoma cell proliferation and induces senescence via regulation of E2F1 protein. J Biol Chem 2011 May 13;286(19):16606-14.

[47] Zhang Z, Liu S, Shi R, Zhao G. miR-27 promotes human gastric cancer cell metastasis by inducing epithelial-to-mesenchymal transition. Cancer Genet 2011 Sep;204(9):486-91.

[48] Siemens H, Jackstadt R, Hunten S, Kaller M, Menssen A, Gotz U, et al. miR-34 and SNAIL form a double-negative feedback loop to regulate epithelial-mesenchymal transitions. Cell Cycle 2011 Dec 15;10(24):4256-71.

[49] Li N, Fu H, Tie Y, Hu Z, Kong W, Wu Y, et al. miR-34a inhibits migration and invasion by down-regulation of c-Met expression in human hepatocellular carcinoma cells. Cancer Lett 2009 Mar 8;275:44-53.

[50] Yan K, Gao J, Yang T, Ma Q, Qiu X, Fan Q, et al. MicroRNA-34a Inhibits the Proliferation and Metastasis of Osteosarcoma Cells Both In Vitro and In Vivo. PLoS One 2012;7(3):e33778.

[51] Zhu L, Chen H, Zhou D, Li D, Bai R, Zheng S, et al. MicroRNA-9 up-regulation is involved in colorectal cancer metastasis via promoting cell motility. Med Oncol 2011 May 12.

[52] Ma L, Reinhardt F, Pan E, Soutschek J, Bhat B, Marcusson EG, et al. Therapeutic silencing of miR-10b inhibits metastasis in a mouse mammary tumor model. Nat Biotechnol 2010 Apr;28:341-7.

[53] Gao P, Xing AY, Zhou GY, Zhang TG, Zhang JP, Gao C, et al. The molecular mechanism of microRNA-145 to suppress invasion-metastasis cascade in gastric cancer. Oncogene 2012 Feb 27;10.

[54] Sachdeva M, Mo YY. MicroRNA-145 suppresses cell invasion and metastasis by directly targeting mucin 1. Cancer Res 2010 Jan 1;70:378-87.

[55] Fan L, Wu Q, Xing X, Wei Y, Shao Z. MicroRNA-145 targets vascular endothelial growth factor and inhibits invasion and metastasis of osteosarcoma cells. Acta Biochim Biophys Sin (Shanghai) 2012 May;44(5):407-14.

[56] Liu C, Kelnar K, Liu B, Chen X, Calhoun-Davis T, Li H, et al. The microRNA miR-34a inhibits prostate cancer stem cells and metastasis by directly repressing CD44. Nat Med 2011 Feb;17(2):211-5.

[57] Huang Q, Gumireddy K, Schrier M, le SC, Nagel R, Nair S, et al. The microRNAs miR-373 and miR-520c promote tumour invasion and metastasis. Nat Cell Biol 2008 Feb;10:202-10.

[58] Wang CH, Lee DY, Deng Z, Jeyapalan Z, Lee SC, Kahai S, et al. MicroRNA miR-328 regulates zonation morphogenesis by targeting CD44 expression. PLoS One 2008 Jun 18;3(6):e2420.

[59] Li F, Tiede B, Massague J, Kang Y. Beyond tumorigenesis: cancer stem cells in metastasis. Cell Res 2007 Jan;17(1):3-14.

[60] Keklikoglou I, Koerner C, Schmidt C, Zhang JD, Heckmann D, Shavinskaya A, et al. MicroRNA-520/373 family functions as a tumor suppressor in estrogen receptor negative breast cancer by targeting NF-kappaB and TGF-beta signaling pathways. Oncogene 2011 Dec 12;10.

[61] Han M, Wang Y, Liu M, Bi X, Bao J, Zeng N, et al. MiR-21 regulates EMT phenotype and HIF-1alpha expression in third-sphereforming breast cancer stem cell-like cells. Cancer Sci 2012 Mar 21;10-7006.

[62] Noh H, Hong S, Dong Z, Pan ZK, Jing Q, Huang S. Impaired MicroRNA Processing Facilitates Breast Cancer Cell Invasion by Upregulating Urokinase-Type Plasminogen Activator Expression. Genes Cancer 2011 Feb;2(2):140-50.

[63] Li XF, Yan PJ, Shao ZM. Downregulation of miR-193b contributes to enhance urokinase-type plasminogen activator (uPA) expression and tumor progression and invasion in human breast cancer. Oncogene 2009 Nov 5;28(44):3937-48.

[64] Salvi A, Sabelli C, Moncini S, Venturin M, Arici B, Riva P, et al. MicroRNA-23b mediates urokinase and c-met downmodulation and a decreased migration of human hepatocellular carcinoma cells. FEBS J 2009 Jun;276(11):2966-82.

[65] Yu Z, Willmarth NE, Zhou J, Katiyar S, Wang M, Liu Y, et al. microRNA 17/20 inhibits cellular invasion and tumor metastasis in breast cancer by heterotypic signaling. Proc Natl Acad Sci U S A 2010 May 4;107(18):8231-6.

[66] Asangani IA, Rasheed SA, Nikolova DA, Leupold JH, Colburn NH, Post S, et al. MicroRNA-21 (miR-21) post-transcriptionally downregulates tumor suppressor Pdcd4 and stimulates invasion, intravasation and metastasis in colorectal cancer. Oncogene 2008 Apr 3;27:2128-36.

[67] Zhu S, Wu H, Wu F, Nie D, Sheng S, Mo YY. MicroRNA-21 targets tumor suppressor genes in invasion and metastasis. Cell Res 2008 Mar;18:350-9.

[68] Tsai WC, Hsu PW, Lai TC, Chau GY, Lin CW, Chen CM, et al. MicroRNA-122, a tumor suppressor microRNA that regulates intrahepatic metastasis of hepatocellular carcinoma. Hepatology 2009 May;49(5):1571-82.

[69] Coulouarn C, Factor VM, Andersen JB, Durkin ME, Thorgeirsson SS. Loss of miR-122 expression in liver cancer correlates with suppression of the hepatic phenotype and gain of metastatic properties. Oncogene 2009 Oct 8;28(40):3526-36.

[70] Hamada S, Satoh K, Fujibuchi W, Hirota M, Kanno A, Unno J, et al. MiR-126 acts as a tumor suppressor in pancreatic cancer cells via the regulation of ADAM9. Mol Cancer Res 2012 Jan;10(1):3-10.

[71] Feng R, Chen X, Yu Y, Su L, Yu B, Li J, et al. miR-126 functions as a tumour suppressor in human gastric cancer. Cancer Lett 2010 Dec 1;298(1):50-63.

[72] Fang JH, Zhou HC, Zeng C, Yang J, Liu Y, Huang X, et al. MicroRNA-29b suppresses tumor angiogenesis, invasion, and metastasis by regulating matrix metalloproteinase 2 expression. Hepatology 2011 Nov;54(5):1729-40.

[73] Steele R, Mott JL, Ray RB. MBP-1 upregulates miR-29b that represses Mcl-1, collagens, and matrix-metalloproteinase-2 in prostate cancer cells. Genes Cancer 2010 Apr 1;1(4):381-7.

[74] Sengupta S, den Boon JA, Chen IH, Newton MA, Stanhope SA, Cheng YJ, et al. MicroRNA 29c is down-regulated in nasopharyngeal carcinomas, up-regulating mRNAs encoding extracellular matrix proteins. Proc Natl Acad Sci U S A 2008 Apr 15;105(15):5874-8.

[75] Pujuguet P, Del ML, Gautreau A, Louvard D, Arpin M. Ezrin regulates E-cadherin-dependent adherens junction assembly through Rac1 activation. Mol Biol Cell 2003 May;14(5):2181-91.

[76] Lowery AJ, Miller N, Dwyer RM, Kerin MJ. Dysregulated miR-183 inhibits migration in breast cancer cells. BMC Cancer 2010 Sep 21;10:502.:502.

[77] Zhu J, Feng Y, Ke Z, Yang Z, Zhou J, Huang X, et al. Down-Regulation of miR-183 Promotes Migration and Invasion of Osteosarcoma by Targeting Ezrin. Am J Pathol 2012 Apr;%20.

[78] Wang G, Mao W, Zheng S. MicroRNA-183 regulates Ezrin expression in lung cancer cells. FEBS Lett 2008 Oct 29;582(25-26):3663-8.

[79] Li X, Zhang Y, Zhang H, Liu X, Gong T, Li M, et al. miRNA-223 promotes gastric cancer invasion and metastasis by targeting tumor suppressor EPB41L3. Mol Cancer Res 2011 Jul;9(7):824-33.

[80] Kurashige J, Watanabe M, Iwatsuki M, Kinoshita K, Saito S, Hiyoshi Y, et al. Overexpression of microRNA-223 regulates the ubiquitin ligase FBXW7 in oesophageal squamous cell carcinoma. Br J Cancer 2012 Jan 3;106(1):182-8.

[81] Ma L, Teruya-Feldstein J, Weinberg RA. Tumour invasion and metastasis initiated by microRNA-10b in breast cancer. Nature 2007 Oct 11;449:682-8.

[82] Nakata K, Ohuchida K, Mizumoto K, Kayashima T, Ikenaga N, Sakai H, et al. MicroRNA-10b is overexpressed in pancreatic cancer, promotes its invasiveness, and correlates with a poor prognosis. Surgery 2011 Nov;150(5):916-22.

[83] Liu Z, Zhu J, Cao H, Ren H, Fang X. miR-10b promotes cell invasion through RhoC-AKT signaling pathway by targeting HOXD10 in gastric cancer. Int J Oncol 2012 May;40(5):1553-60.

[84] Nishida N, Yamashita S, Mimori K, Sudo T, Tanaka F, Shibata K, et al. MicroRNA-10b is a Prognostic Indicator in Colorectal Cancer and Confers Resistance to the Chemotherapeutic Agent 5-Fluorouracil in Colorectal Cancer Cells. Ann Surg Oncol 2012 Feb 10.

[85] Kong W, Yang H, He L, Zhao JJ, Coppola D, Dalton WS, et al. MicroRNA-155 is regulated by the transforming growth factor beta/Smad pathway and contributes to epithelial cell plasticity by targeting RhoA. Mol Cell Biol 2008 Nov;28(22):6773-84.

[86] Valastyan S, Reinhardt F, Benaich N, Calogrias D, Szasz AM, Wang ZC, et al. A pleiotropically acting microRNA, miR-31, inhibits breast cancer metastasis. Cell 2009 Jun 12;137(6):1032-46.

[87] Valastyan S, Chang A, Benaich N, Reinhardt F, Weinberg RA. Activation of miR-31 function in already-established metastases elicits metastatic regression. Genes Dev 2011 Mar 15;25(6):646-59.

[88] Calin GA, Sevignani C, Dumitru CD, Hyslop T, Noch E, Yendamuri S, et al. Human microRNA genes are frequently located at fragile sites and genomic regions involved in cancers. Proc Natl Acad Sci U S A 2004 Mar 2;101:2999-3004.

[89] Zhang L, Huang J, Yang N, Greshock J, Megraw MS, Giannakakis A, et al. microRNAs exhibit high frequency genomic alterations in human cancer. Proc Natl Acad Sci USA 2006 Jun 13;103:9136-41.

[90] Yan LX, Huang XF, Shao Q, Huang MY, Deng L, Wu QL, et al. MicroRNA miR-21 overexpression in human breast cancer is associated with advanced clinical stage, lymph node metastasis and patient poor prognosis. RNA 2008 Nov;14:2348-60.

[91] Schaefer A, Jung M, Mollenkopf HJ, Wagner I, Stephan C, Jentzmik F, et al. Diagnostic and prognostic implications of microRNA profiling in prostate carcinoma. Int J Cancer 2010 Mar 1;126(5):1166-76.

[92] Creighton CJ, Fountain MD, Yu Z, Nagaraja AK, Zhu H, Khan M, et al. Molecular profiling uncovers a p53-associated role for microRNA-31 in inhibiting the proliferation of serous ovarian carcinomas and other cancers. Cancer Res 2010 Mar 1;70(5):1906-15.

[93] Guo J, Miao Y, Xiao B, Huan R, Jiang Z, Meng D, et al. Differential expression of microRNA species in human gastric cancer versus non-tumorous tissues. J Gastroenterol Hepatol 2009 Apr;24(4):652-7.

[94] Zhang Y, Guo J, Li D, Xiao B, Miao Y, Jiang Z, et al. Down-regulation of miR-31 expression in gastric cancer tissues and its clinical significance. Med Oncol 2010 Sep;27(3):685-9.

[95] Veerla S, Lindgren D, Kvist A, Frigyesi A, Staaf J, Persson H, et al. MiRNA expression in urothelial carcinomas: important roles of miR-10a, miR-222, miR-125b, miR-7 and miR-452 for tumor stage and metastasis, and frequent homozygous losses of miR-31. Int J Cancer 2009 May 1;124(9):2236-42.

[96] Bandres E, Cubedo E, Agirre X, Malumbres R, Zarate R, Ramirez N, et al. Identification by Real-time PCR of 13 mature microRNAs differentially expressed in colorectal cancer and non-tumoral tissues. Mol Cancer 2006 Jul;%19;5:29.:29.

[97] Motoyama K, Inoue H, Takatsuno Y, Tanaka F, Mimori K, Uetake H, et al. Over- and under-expressed microRNAs in human colorectal cancer. Int J Oncol 2009 Apr;34(4):1069-75.

[98] Wong QW, Lung RW, Law PT, Lai PB, Chan KY, To KF, et al. MicroRNA-223 is commonly repressed in hepatocellular carcinoma and potentiates expression of Stathmin1. Gastroenterology 2008 Jul;135(1):257-69.

[99] Liu X, Chen Z, Yu J, Xia J, Zhou X. MicroRNA profiling and head and neck cancer. Comp Funct Genomics 2009.

[100] Liu CJ, Tsai MM, Hung PS, Kao SY, Liu TY, Wu KJ, et al. miR-31 ablates expression of the HIF regulatory factor FIH to activate the HIF pathway in head and neck carcinoma. Cancer Res 2010 Feb 15;70(4):1635-44.

[101] Wong TS, Liu XB, Wong BY, Ng RW, Yuen AP, Wei WI. Mature miR-184 as Potential Oncogenic microRNA of Squamous Cell Carcinoma of Tongue. Clin Cancer Res 2008 May 1;14(9):2588-92.

[102] Valastyan S, Weinberg RA. Tumor metastasis: molecular insights and evolving paradigms. Cell 2011 Oct 14;147(2):275-92.

[103] Zheng B, Liang L, Wang C, Huang S, Cao X, Zha R, et al. MicroRNA-148a suppresses tumor cell invasion and metastasis by downregulating ROCK1 in gastric cancer. Clin Cancer Res 2011 Dec 15;17(24):7574-83.

[104] Wong CC, Wong CM, Tung EK, Au SL, Lee JM, Poon RT, et al. The microRNA miR-139 suppresses metastasis and progression of hepatocellular carcinoma by down-regulating Rho-kinase 2. Gastroenterology 2011 Jan;140(1):322-31.

[105] Lujambio A, Calin GA, Villanueva A, Ropero S, Sanchez-Cespedes M, Blanco D, et al. A microRNA DNA methylation signature for human cancer metastasis. Proc Natl Acad Sci U S A 2008 Sep 9;105(36):13556-61.

[106] Dews M, Fox JL, Hultine S, Sundaram P, Wang W, Liu YY, et al. The myc-miR-17~92 axis blunts TGF{beta} signaling and production of multiple TGF{beta}-dependent antiangiogenic factors. Cancer Res 2010 Oct 15;70(20):8233-46.

[107] Liu S, Goldstein RH, Scepansky EM, Rosenblatt M. Inhibition of rho-associated kinase signaling prevents breast cancer metastasis to human bone. Cancer Res 2009 Nov 15;69(22):8742-51.

[108] Valladares-Ayerbes M, Blanco M, Haz M, Medina V, Iglesias-Diaz P, Lorenzo-Patino MJ, et al. Prognostic impact of disseminated tumor cells and microRNA-17-92 cluster deregulation in gastrointestinal cancer. Int J Oncol 2011 Nov;39(5):1253-64.

[109] Oskarsson T, Acharyya S, Zhang XH, Vanharanta S, Tavazoie SF, Morris PG, et al. Breast cancer cells produce tenascin C as a metastatic niche component to colonize the lungs. Nat Med 2011 Jun 26;17(7):867-74.

[110] Tavazoie SF, Alarcon C, Oskarsson T, Padua D, Wang Q, Bos PD, et al. Endogenous human microRNAs that suppress breast cancer metastasis. Nature 2008 Jan 10;451:147-52.

[111] Png KJ, Halberg N, Yoshida M, Tavazoie SF. A microRNA regulon that mediates endothelial recruitment and metastasis by cancer cells. Nature 2011 Dec 14;481(7380):190-4.

[112] Okamoto K, Ishiguro T, Midorikawa Y, Ohata H, Izumiya M, Tsuchiya N, et al. miR-493 induction during carcinogenesis blocks metastatic settlement of colon cancer cells in liver. EMBO J 2012 Feb 28;31(7):1752-63.

[113] Dangi-Garimella S, Yun J, Eves EM, Newman M, Erkeland SJ, Hammond SM, et al. Raf kinase inhibitory protein suppresses a metastasis signalling cascade involving LIN28 and let-7. EMBO J 2009 Feb 18;28(4):347-58.

[114] Elsarraj HS, Stecklein SR, Valdez K, Behbod F. Emerging Functions of microRNA-146a/b in Development and Breast Cancer : MicroRNA-146a/b in Development and Breast Cancer. J Mammary Gland Biol Neoplasia 2012 Mar;17(1):79-87.

[115] Hurst DR, Welch DR. Unraveling the enigmatic complexities of BRMS1-mediated metastasis suppression. FEBS Lett 2011 Oct;%20;585(20):3185-90.

[116] Bhaumik D, Scott GK, Schokrpur S, Patil CK, Campisi J, Benz CC. Expression of microRNA-146 suppresses NF-kappaB activity with reduction of metastatic potential in breast cancer cells. Oncogene 2008 Sep 18;27(42):5643-7.

[117] O'Day E, Lal A. MicroRNAs and their target gene networks in breast cancer. Breast Cancer Res 2010;12(2):201.

[118] Piepoli A, Tavano F, Copetti M, Mazza T, Palumbo O, Panza A, et al. Mirna expression profiles identify drivers in colorectal and pancreatic cancers. PLoS One 2012;7(3):e33663.

[119] Ueda T, Volinia S, Okumura H, Shimizu M, Taccioli C, Rossi S, et al. Relation between microRNA expression and progression and prognosis of gastric cancer: a microRNA expression analysis. Lancet Oncol 2010 Feb;11(2):136-46.

[120] Martens-Uzunova ES, Jalava SE, Dits NF, van Leenders GJ, Moller S, Trapman J, et al. Diagnostic and prognostic signatures from the small non-coding RNA transcriptome in prostate cancer. Oncogene 2012 Feb 23;31(8):978-91.

[121] Schaefer A, Jung M, Miller K, Lein M, Kristiansen G, Erbersdobler A, et al. Suitable reference genes for relative quantification of miRNA expression in prostate cancer. Exp Mol Med 2010 Nov 30;42(11):749-58.

[122] Landi MT, Zhao Y, Rotunno M, Koshiol J, Liu H, Bergen AW, et al. MicroRNA expression differentiates histology and predicts survival of lung cancer. Clin Cancer Res 2010 Jan 15;16(2):430-41.

[123] Busacca S, Germano S, De CL, Rinaldi M, Comoglio F, Favero F, et al. MicroRNA signature of malignant mesothelioma with potential diagnostic and prognostic implications. Am J Respir Cell Mol Biol 2010 Mar;42(3):312-9.

[124] Volinia S, Galasso M, Sana ME, Wise TF, Palatini J, Huebner K, et al. Breast cancer signatures for invasiveness and prognosis defined by deep sequencing of microRNA. Proc Natl Acad Sci U S A 2012 Feb 21;109(8):3024-9.

[125] Farazi TA, Horlings HM, Ten Hoeve JJ, Mihailovic A, Halfwerk H, Morozov P, et al. MicroRNA sequence and expression analysis in breast tumors by deep sequencing. Cancer Res 2011 Jul 1;71(13):4443-53.

[126] du Rieu MC, Torrisani J, Selves J, Al ST, Souque A, Dufresne M, et al. MicroRNA-21 is induced early in pancreatic ductal adenocarcinoma precursor lesions. Clin Chem 2010 Apr;56(4):603-12.

[127] Heneghan HM, Miller N, Kerin MJ. Circulating miRNA signatures: promising prognostic tools for cancer. J Clin Oncol 2010 Oct 10;28:e573-e574.

[128] Huang Z, Huang D, Ni S, Peng Z, Sheng W, Du X. Plasma microRNAs are promising novel biomarkers for early detection of colorectal cancer. Int J Cancer 2010 Jul 1;127(1):118-26.

[129] Xing L, Todd NW, Yu L, Fang H, Jiang F. Early detection of squamous cell lung cancer in sputum by a panel of microRNA markers. Mod Pathol 2010 Aug;23(8):1157-64.

[130] Boeri M, Verri C, Conte D, Roz L, Modena P, Facchinetti F, et al. MicroRNA signatures in tissues and plasma predict development and prognosis of computed tomography detected lung cancer. Proc Natl Acad Sci USA 2011 Mar 1;108:3713-8.

[131] Lu Y, Govindan R, Wang L, Liu PY, Goodgame B, Wen W, et al. MicroRNA profiling and prediction of recurrence/relapse-free survival in stage I lung cancer. Carcinogenesis 2012 May;33(5):1046-54.

[132] Donnem T, Fenton CG, Lonvik K, Berg T, Eklo K, Andersen S, et al. MicroRNA signatures in tumor tissue related to angiogenesis in non-small cell lung cancer. PLoS One 2012;7(1):e29671.

[133] Heinzelmann J, Henning B, Sanjmyatav J, Posorski N, Steiner T, Wunderlich H, et al. Specific miRNA signatures are associated with metastasis and poor prognosis in clear cell renal cell carcinoma. World J Urol 2011 Jun;29(3):367-73.

[134] Iorio MV, Croce CM. MicroRNA dysregulation in cancer: diagnostics, monitoring and therapeutics. A comprehensive review. EMBO Mol Med 2012 Mar;4(3):143-59.

Chapter 5

Is *CCDC26* a Novel Cancer-Associated Long-Chain Non-Coding RNA?

Tetsuo Hirano

Additional information is available at the end of the chapter

1. Introduction

Large-scale analysis of total genome transcripts (transcriptome) in organisms including human and mouse has revealed that many RNAs are transcribed from genomic regions that encode no proteins (referred to as ncRNA) (1-5). Among such ncRNAs, microRNAs (miRNAs), small molecule RNAs 18-28 bases long, have been extensively studied over the past decade, and a gene regulatory system called "RNA silencing" has been revealed. In humans, more than 400 miRNAs are known to regulate at least one-third of protein-encoding genes (6-10). Most miRNAs are generated by processing of long miRNA precursors (pri-miRNAs) (6, 9). Pri-miRNAs are transcribed by RNA polymerase II and 5′ cap structures and poly A tails are added, similarly to protein-encoding mRNAs. Pri-miRNAs are further processed in the nucleus into pre-miRNAs with an approximately 70 base hairpin structure and are then exported to the cytoplasm. pre-miRNAs are finally processed into mature miRNAs by the enzyme, Dicer. It is noteworthy that miRNAs are sometimes encoded in the introns of other genes. A mature miRNA is incorporated into the RNA-induced silencing complex to act on its target mRNA. Broadly speaking, miRNAs can act on mRNAs in two ways. If there is limited homology between an miRNA and a target mRNA, the miRNA suppresses translation of the mRNA. However, if the miRNA has complete or nearly complete homology with a target mRNA, the mRNA is rapidly degraded. In animal cells, the former scenario usually occurs (7, 10-12). Many miRNAs have been reported to be associated with tumors, including AML and glioma; however, it is still unclear how predominant miRNAs are in tumorigenesis.

Relatively large ncRNAs of over several hundred bases, which are longer than pri-miRNAs whose length is usually 200-300 bases, are called long-chain non-coding RNAs (lncRNAs). Despite their somewhat unclear definition and their largely undetermined functions (13), the public databases for lncRNAs, for example, lncRNAdb (http://www.lncrnadb.org/) (14)

or NONCODE (http://www.noncode.org) (15), contain several hundred mammalian lncRNAs, including more than 100 from human (16). The RNAs included are heterologous; some localize in the nucleus to form certain structures, others interact with chromatin modifying enzymes such as p300, while others function in the cytoplasm (Fig. 1).

Both miRNAs and lncRNAs are physiologically important in many biological processes, including development and cell differentiation. Their association with disease, especially cancers, is of great interest (5). Association of miRNAs with various tumors, including different types of leukemia (Table 1) and glioma (Table 2), has been demonstrated. They sometimes act as tumor-promoting factors and sometimes as tumor suppressors. Expression of many lncRNAs, including *NDM29* (neuroblastoma) (17, 18) and *MALAT-1* (lung cancer) (19) are correlated with tumor progression, while *MEG3* (pituitary tumor) (20, 21), *HOTAIR* (breast carcinoma) (22), *H19* (Wilms' tumor) (23), *AK023948* (papillary thyroid tumor) (24) and *LOC285194* (osteosarcoma) (25) are putative tumor suppressors (Table 3). These lncRNAs seem to control cancer cell growth by regulating other genes (*NDM29*, *HOTAIR*, *H19*) or by adjusting the mRNA splicing mechanism (*MALAT-1*) (Fig. 1) (14).

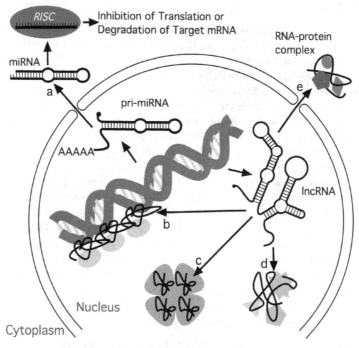

Figure 1. Classification of ncRNAs. (a) Pri-miRNAs are synthesized and processed in the nucleus, then exported to the cytoplasm. They are incorporated in the RISC complex to degrade or inhibit transcription of target mRNAs. However, some synthesized lncRNAs associate with chromatin (b) to silence certain genes. Some lncRNAs are incorporated in intranuclear bodies (c) or make complexes with specific proteins (d). Some are exported to the cytoplasm to work in the RNA-protein complex (e).

Name	Loci	Name	Loci
Oncogenic or Increased Expression in AML		*Tumor Suppressive or Decreased Expression in AML*	
let-7b	*22q13.31*	let-7	*9q22.32*
let-7e	*19q13.41*	let-7b	*22q13.31*
miR-10a	*17q21.32*	miR-9*	*1q22*
miR-10b	*2q31.1*	miR-15a	*13q14.2*
miR-27a	*19p13.13*	miR-15b	*3q25.33*
miR-30d	*8q24.22*	miR-16	*13q14.2*
miR-126	*9q34.3*	miR-19a	*13q31.3*
miR-129-5p	*7q32.1*	miR-20a	*13q31.3*
miR-130b	*22*	miR-26a	*3p22.2*
miR-142-5p	*17q22*	miR-29a	*7q32.3*
miR-155	*21q21.3*	miR-29b	*7q32.3*
miR-181a	*1q31.3/9q33.3*	miR-29c	*1q32.2*
miR-181b	*1q31.3/9q33.3*	miR-30a-3p	*6q13*
miR-181c	*19p13.13*	miR-34b	*11q23.1*
miR-181d	*19p13.13*	miR-34c	*11q23.1*
miR-195	*17p13.1*	miR-124	*8p23.1*
miR-221	*Xp11.3*	miR-128-1	*2q21.3*
miR-223	*Xq12*	miR-145	*5q32*
miR-221/222	*Xp11.3*	miR-147	*9q33.2*
miR-324-5p	*17p13.1*	miR-148a	*7p15.2*
miR-326	*11q13.4*	miR-151	*8q24.3*
miR-328	*16q22.1*	miR-181a	*1q31.3/9q33.3*
miR-331	*12q22*	miR-181b	*1q31.3/9q33.3*
miR-340	*5q35.3*	miR-182	*7q32.2*
miR-374	*Xq13.2*	miR-184	*15q25.1*
miR-424	*Xq26.3*	miR-194	*1q41*
		miR-196a	*17q21.32*
		miR-196a	*17q21.32*
		miR-199a	*19p13.2*
		miR-204	*9q21.12*
		miR-219-5p	*6q21.32*
		miR-220a	*Xq25*
		miR-302b*	*4q25*
		miR-302d	*4q25*
		miR-320	*8q21.3*
		miR-320	*8q21.3*
		miR-325	*Xq21.1*

Data are chosen from references 54, 55, 62, 63, 65, 66. Data confined to cytogenetically normal AML where possible. Note some miRNA appeared both oncogenic and tumor-suppressive.

Table 1. Examples of miRNAs associated with AML that change expression level

Name	Genetic Locus	Name	Genetic Locus
Oncogenic or Increased Expression in Glioma		*Tumor Suppressive or Decreased Expression in Glioma*	
miR-9*	*1q22*	let-7 family	*9q22.32*
miR-10a*	*17q21.32*	miR-7	*9q21.32*
miR-10b	*2q31.1*	miR-15b	*3q25.33*
miR-17/92 cluster	*13q31.3*	miR-17	*13q31.3*
miR-21	*17q23.1*	miR-26b	*2q35*
miR-25	*7q22.1*	miR-29b	*7q32.3*
miR-26a	*3p22.2*	miR-34a	*1p36.22*
miR-93	*7q22.1*	miR-101	*1p31.3*
miR-125b	*11q24.1*	miR-106a	*Xq26.2*
miR-182	*7q32.2*	miR-124	*8p23.1*
miR-195	*17p13.1*	miR-125a	*19q13.41*
miR-196a	*17q21.32*	miR-128	*2q21.3*
miR-196b	*7p15.2*	miR-137	*1p21.3*
miR-221/222	*Xp11.3*	miR-146b/146b-5p	*10q24.32*
miR-296	*20q13.32*	miR-153	*2q35*
miR-381	*14q32.31*	miR-181	*1q31.3/9q33.3*
miR-455-3p	*9q32*	miR-184	*15q25.1*
miR-486	*8p11.21*	miR-195	*17p13.1*
		miR-199b-5p	*9q34.11*
		miR-218	*4p15.31*
		miR-326	*11q13.4*
		miR-451	*17q11.2*

Data are chosen from references 67 and 68. Data confined to cases of low grade gliomas but exclusion of data from high grade glioblastoma is not necessarily complete. Note some miRNAs appeared both oncogenic and tumor-suppressive.

Table 2. miRNAs that show altered expression levels in glioma cells

Name	Alias	Mouse Homolog	Genetic Locus	Product Length (bp)	Tumor	Function	Refs
Tumor promoting or Increased Expression							
AIRN		Airn	6q26	NA	Wilms' tumor	NA	(59)
BC200	BCYRN1	Bc1	2p21	200	Breast cancer	Regulation of protein biosynthesis	(70)
HIF1A-AS2	aHIF	NA	14q23.2	2051	Multiple cancers	Decoy of mRNA	(71)
HOTAIR	Gm16258	Hotair	12q13.3	2364	Multiple cancers	Epigenetic silencing of HOXD gene through histoneH3K27 methylation	(72)
HULC		NA	6p24.3	500	Hepatocellular carcinoma	Post-transcriptional regulation	(73)
IGF2AS	PEG8	Igh2as	11p15.5	2091	Wilms' tumor	NA	(74)
KRASP1		NA	6p12-p11	5178	Prostate cancer	Decoy of miRNA	(75)
L1PA16		VL30-1ᵃ⁾	3q26.3	833	Many tumor cell lines	Activation of proto-oncogene	(76)
MALAT1	Neat2	Malat1	11q13.1	8708	Multiple cancer	Control of RNA procession	(19, 77)
MER11C	HERVK11	VL30-1ᵃ⁾	11p11.1	1060	Many tumor cell lines	Activation of proto-oncogene	(76)
PCA3	DD3	NA	9q21-q22	3735	Prostate cancer	NA	(78)
PCGEM1		NA	2q32	1603	Prostate cancer	NA	(79)
PRNCR1		NA	8q24	>12756	Prostate cancer	NA	(80)
SRA1		Sra1	5q31.3	1955	Breast cancer	Activation of nuclear receptors	(81)
TERC		Terc	3q26	451	Multiple cancer	Telomere template	(82)
UCA1	CUDR	NA	19p13.12	1591	Bladder cancer	Regulation of cell cycle	(83)
WT1-AS	WIT1	NA	11p13	1333	Wilms' tumor AML	Downregulation of WT1, tumor suppressor	(84)
XIST		Xist	Xq13.2	19271	Multiple cancers	Xinactivation	(56, 85)
Tumor Suppressing or Decreased Expression in Tumor							
AK023948		NA	8q24	2807	Papillary thyroid carcinoma	NA	(24)
ANRIL	CDK2BAS, p15AS	NA	9q21	944	Prostate cancer, breast cancer, melanoma, and other tumors	Regulation of epigenetic transcriptional repression	(58)
BC040587		NA	3q13.31	NA	Osteosarcoma	NA	(25)
DLEU2		Dleu2	13q14.3	2768	Chronic lymphocytic leukemia	pri-miRNA for miR15a and miR16	(86)

Name	Alias	Mouse Homolog	Genetic Locus	Product Length (bp)	Tumor	Function	Refs
GAS5		Gas5	1q25.1	651	Breast cancer	Decoy of glucocorticoid receptor	(87)
H19		H19	11p15.5	2322	Wilms' tumor	Epigenetic regulation through DNA methylation	(88)
KCNQ1OT1	LIT1, KvLQT1-AS, KvLQT1OT1	Kcnq1ot1	11p15	91671	Embryonal cancer associated with Beckwith-Wiedemann syndrome	Epigenetic imprinting through H3K27 methylation	(57)
LOC285194		NA	3q13.31	NA	Osteosarcoma	NA	(25)
MEG3	Gtl2	Meg3	14q32	1595	Glioma, pituitary adenoma and other tumor	Regulation of p53 target proteins	(89)
NDM29	29A	NA	11p15.3	131	Neuroblastoma	Induction the appearance of neuronal-like properties	(18)
p53 mRNA		Tp53	17p13.1	19144	Multiple cancer	RNA protein binding, MDM3	(90)
PTENP1		NA	9p21	3932	Prostate cancer	Decoy for PTEN-targeting miRNAs	(75)
RMRP		Rmrp	9p21-p12	267	Leukemia and lymphoma	Mitochondrial RNA processing endoribonuclease, hTERT-dependent	(91)
TERRA		TelRNAs	telomere repeats	NA	Many cancer cell lines	Interaction with the TRF1	(92)
vtRNA2-1		NA	5q31.1	100	AML, papillary thyroid cancer	Regulation of RNA dependent protein kinase (pPKR)	(93)
ZNFX1-AS1	Zfas1	1500012 F01Rik	20q13.13	1020	Breast cancer	NA	(94)

(a) no homologous RNA but binds to PSF, a transcriptional repressor. NA, not available.

Table 3. Human lncRNAs associated with tumors described in public data bases.

2. Genetic abnormality observed in acute myeloid leukemia (AML)

AML, which comprises approximately 25% of hematopoietic malignancies, has heterogeneous clinical features and variable responses to contemporary therapy (26). Genetic alterations are often observed in AML cells and the clinical heterogeneity of the disease is considered to reflect the genetic diversity of these cells (27, 28). It is very important to study the genetic mutations in AML cells to fully understand the cause of the disease. However, genetic lesion(s) responsible for AML, such as the loss or gain of a certain gene, have not yet been fully elucidated. Indeed, the complex features of AML suggest that the genetic cause of this disease is multifactorial (29). Several protein-encoding genes have been identified that are useful for indicating the prognosis of the disease (30-32). These include *RUNX1* (*AML1*)-*RUNX1T1* (*ETO*) and *CBFB-MYH11*, which are associated with specific chromosomal mutations, *t(8;21)(q22;q22)* and *inv(16)(p13;q12)/t(16;16)(p13;q22)*, respectively. AML with these cytogenetic features (singly or together) represents about 15% of *de novo* AML. The patients with these diagnostic criteria are classified in the favorable clinical outcome group (standard-risk group). Several other chromosomal abnormalities have been recurrently observed, as described in the WHO classification. AML with balanced or unbalanced translocations involving the *MLL* gene located on chromosome 11 are also well documented and are mostly classified in the intermediate-risk group. Meanwhile, AML patients with a normal karyotype and no cytological abnormality include cases classified in the unfavorable (adverse-risk) or intermediate-risk group. Moreover, a genetic abnormality of the *FL3* gene (internal tandem repeat) is found in many AML subtypes and, in combination with a wild-type *NPM* gene, contributes to poor prognosis (31). Recently, Paschka and colleagues have revealed that the genes encoding the metabolic enzymes, isocitrate dehydrogenase 1 and 2 (*IDH1/2*) are important for diagnosis and prognosis prediction of AML patients (33). These mutations of *IDH1/2* change the activity of the enzymes to reduce α-ketoglutarate levels and to elevate 2-hydroxyglutarate levels. This results in changes to chromatin structure and destabilization of certain gene-regulatory proteins, including *HIF-1* (34). While cytogenetically normal AML patients with an *NPM* mutation and a normal *FL3* gene tend to show favorable outcomes, AML patients with the same genetic profile but also with *IDH1/2* mutation showed adverse prognosis with poorer remission. *IDH1/2* mutation was also found in several other tumors, including glioma (35). Therefore, a combination of genetic alterations resulting in mutation of specific genes as well as cytogenetically apparent chromosomal changes are important for AML malignancy.

3. AML and *CCDC26*

In HL-60 cells derived from AML, a small part of chromosome 8 is excised and amplified as an extrachromosomal element, or double minute chromosome (dmin). Dmin is a cytogenetic abnormality infrequently observed in AML. The dmin of HL-60 cells consists of several repeats of an amplification unit (referred as amplicon) of about 2 million base pairs. The amplicon, which is derived from several areas of an approximately 4.6 million base pair region of chromosome *8q24*, contains an intact *MYC* oncogene. Besides *MYC*, several other genes, including *CCDC26* and tribbles homolog 1 (*TRIB1*), are also encoded on the amplicon (Fig. 2). All are actively transcribed in HL-60 cells. The drug-induced differentiation of HL-60 cells suppressed the expression of all these genes, indicating that they might be related to the cancerous nature of the cells. Some types of cancer cell respond to the anticancer drug hydroxyurea by excluding unstable extrachromosomal elements, which then lose their proliferative nature. In HL-60 cells, the original *MYC* genetic locus remained intact after dmin was excluded, but was no longer transcribed (36). These observations suggest that the expression of genes from dmin, with its altered DNA structure, and from the intact chromosome are different, and can be interpreted as being due to aberrant gene expression from dmin (including the *MYC* oncogene). Interestingly, in HL-60 cells, the *CCDC26* gene on dmin is rearranged as a result of chromosomal rejoining and is amplified in an incomplete form to produce abnormal transcripts (37).

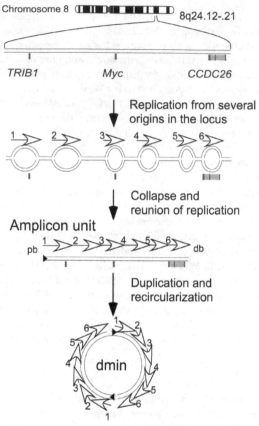

Figure 2. Depiction of the generation of the discontinuous amplicon unit of dmin in HL-60 cells. Several replication initiation bubbles collapse and "corrupted" bubbles reunite to form an amplicon unit. Excision of an initial large amplicon (possibly as an episome) might precede replication. The arrows numbered 1 through 6 indicate regions reunited in the amplicon. Note that the lengths of the various regions are not to scale. Once the amplicon unit has formed, its multimerization results in a dmin.

A common change occurs at the *CCDC26* locus in cytologically dmin-positive AML patients. This chromosomal change occurs at a position consistent with the amplified region observed in HL-60 cells (38, 39). Furthermore, destruction of the internal structure of the *CCDC26* gene seems to underlie the common mechanism behind the generation of dmin-positive AML cells.

A comprehensive genome-wide study of a group of childhood AML patients revealed that *CCDC26* was one of the genes with the highest increase in copy number in AML cells. Radtke and colleagues investigated chromosome number alteration (CNA) in pediatric AML using a comprehensive single nucleotide polymorphism (SNP) array analysis. They found the most common CNA, in 14% (15 in 111) of pediatric AML patients, to be in chromosome band 8q24 with a low-burden copy number increase (2.83-3.77 copies) (40). These included cases of trisomy 8, which frequently occurs in AML (41). The minimum altered region common in all 15 of these patients was located in a 20-megabase region of *8q24*, which contains *CCDC26*.

Originally, *CCDC26* was reported as a gene associated with differentiation and apoptosis of PLB985 cells (an HL-60 subclone) following induction by treatment with retinoic acid (*CCDC26* is also known as *RAM*, retinoic acid modifying). In cells that have become resistant to differentiation and apoptosis after infection of retrovirus, the viral genome was seen to be inserted in the intron of *CCDC26*. Retinoic acid promotes differentiation and apoptosis of not only many leukemia cells but also of neuroblastoma and glioblastoma cells through transcriptional regulation of many other genes. *CCDC26* may have a role with retinoic acid in differentiation and growth arrest of these cells (42).

4. Glioma and *CCDC26*

Primary brain tumor (PBT) is a disease with an incidence of 12 in 100,000 per year. Glioma accounts for a major part of PBT, and contains cases with different grades of malignancy, namely (I) benign glioma, (II) diffuse astrocytoma, (III) anaplastic astrocytoma and (IV) glioblastoma (43). Although many genetic abnormalities have been reported in gliomas, a single critical lesion responsible for tumorigenesis has not been found. Among these abnormalities, mutations occur in genes for DNA repair enzymes, including *PRKDC*, *XRCC*, *PARP1*, *MGMT*, *ERCC1*, *ERCC2*, epidermal growth factor and the inflammatory cytokine, *IL-13*. Furthermore, over-expression or amplification of the epidermal growth factor receptor gene and deletion of *p16INK* are correlated with poor survival (43). A genome wide association study using SNPs revealed the association of several genes with glioma, including telomerase regulating gene *TERT*, *RTEL1*, tumor suppressor gene *CDKN2A/2B*, pleckstrin homology-like domain family B member 1 (a protein with unknown function) and *CCDC26* (44). The *CCDC26* gene locus was strongly linked with this glioma by several SNPs, including rs4295627, rs16904140, rs6470745, rs891835, and rs10464870 (see Fig. 3a). A different SNP in the intergenic region bordering *CCDC26*, rs987525, was linked to cleft palate (45). Notably, cleft palate is also a risk factor of PBT. *CCDC26* is, therefore, a potential common factor of both conditions. *CCDC26* is just one of the risk factors for glioma and other genetic risk factors increase glioma incidence cumulatively. Therefore, there might be a synergistic effect with other genetic risk factors (46). *CCDC26* is not necessarily a risk factor of high grade (III-IV) glioma (47). Interestingly, in concordance with the situation for AML, the *CCDC26* genotype is associated with *IDH1/2* mutation in low grade glioma. Considering the synergy of *CCDC26* with *IDH1/2*, *CCDC26* may have linkage to a subpopulation of gliomas with relatively lower grade (46, 48).

The Gene Expression Omnibus database (GEO; http://www.ncbi.nlm.nih.gov/geo/) (49) contains data showing altered *CCDC26* expression between normal and tumorigenic cells. Expression of *CCDC26* is higher in myeloid leukemia cell lines, namely KG-1, THP-1 and U937, compared with normal monocytes (GEO dataset accession ID; GDS2251), and is higher in sporadic basal-like cancer compared with normal cells (GD2250). On the other

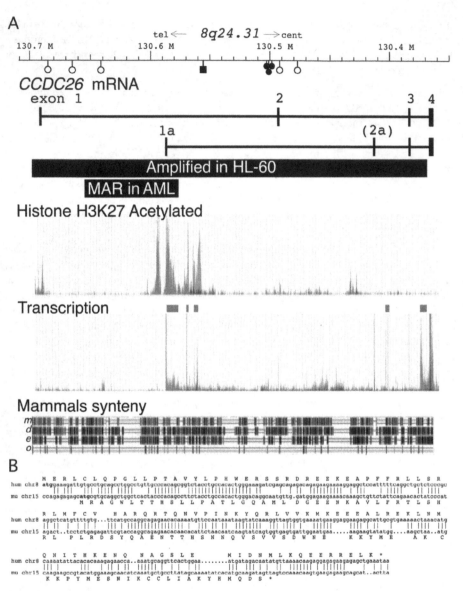

Figure 3. (A) Summary of genetic locus 8q24.31. The scale indicates the region 8q24.31 (130.35 Mb to 130.71 Mb; numbering is based on human genome assembly 37.1). Marks on the scale indicate the locations of five SNPs that are linked to glioma (open circles; rs4295627, rs16904140, rs6470745, rs891835 and rs10464870, left to right), three miRNAs registered in the public database (filled circles; mir-3669, mir-3673 and mir-3686, left to right) and a retrovirus insertion site (filled square) within the introns of CCDC26. Below the scale, which covers a 350-kb region, major variants of CCDC26 mRNA (long and

short) are shown. The long transcript consists of four (1-2-3-4) exons, and the short transcripts consist of three (1a-3-4) or four (1a-2a-3-4) exons. All variants share exon 3 and 4, in which the hypothetical open reading frame is encoded. Locations of the amplified region in HL-60 cells and the commonly amplified region (MAR) in childhood AML are shown with filled rectangles. The hypothetical open reading frame encoded in exons 3 and 4 is not included in the region amplified in HL-60 cells. The pattern of histone H3K27 acetylation, activity of transcription in leukemia cell lines, and bar plots for conserved synteny between human and each organism (m: mouse, d: dog, e: elephant and o: opossum) obtained from the UCSC Genome Browser (95) are shown. Actively transcribed regions that are not the major exons of CCDC26 mRNA are indicated by grey rectangles. (B) Optimal alignment of the CCDC26 exon 3-4 encoded ORF and the region of conserved synteny on mouse chromosome 15. A possible ORF (94 amino acids) in the mouse sequence is totally mismatched with that of human by frameshift changes.

hand, CCDC26 expression is decreased in hyperplastic enlarged lobular units considered as the earliest precursors of breast cancer compared with normal units (GDS2739). Increased CCDC26 expression is associated with malignancy progression in some cancerous cells. CCDC26 expression was increased in CD133 positive neurosphere-like glioma cell lines compared with CD133 negative adherent glioma cell lines (GDS2728), and was increased in alveolar macrophages of cigarette smokers comparison with macrophages of non-smokers (GDS3496). Increased expression of CCDC26 might mean this gene is tumorigenic or oncogenic. However, the relationship of altered CCDC26 expression to malignancy is still ambiguous.

5. Overview of the CCDC26 genetic locus

As described in the previous section, all SNPs associated with glioma, and a retrovirus insertion site where virus insertion makes AML cells resistant to retinoic acid (42) are located in the intron of CCDC26 (Fig. 3a). Exon 4, which encodes the majority of a hypothetical open reading frame (ORF), is not amplified in pediatric AML or in AML-derived HL-60 cells. The exonic sequence of CCDC26 is not well conserved in other species, including mouse, and an ORF has no homology with known proteins. These data strongly suggest that CCDC26 does not function as a protein-encoding RNA; rather it functions as a ncRNA. Highly conserved regions in the intron sequence of CCDC26 suggest the existence of another intronic ncRNA. As mentioned above, the CCDC26 locus is rearranged in the genome of HL-60 cells. It is plausible that the ncRNA encoded by this locus is important for the growth of these cells.

A short putative ORF encoding a protein or with a length of 109 amino acids is present in the CCDC26 exons; there is no other ORF of more than 50 amino acids. This actual protein, however, has not been observed. Moreover, orthologous proteins are not found in any other organism. For example, a loosely homologous sequence of human exon 4, found in the mouse chromosome 15 region of conserved synteny, with an ORF of 94 amino acids is actively transcribed in mouse leukemia cells (T. Hirano unpublished observation). However, this ORF is completely different from the human sequence and even contains frame shift alterations (Fig. 3b). This indicates that the putative protein encoded by CCDC26 has no conserved function among species. Although this ORF may be coincidental due to the absence of stop codons, an interesting possibility is that this unique protein has newly emerged during human evolution. mRNA stability is influenced by whether an ORF is encoded because nonsense mediated RNA decay, a mechanism associated with quality control of mRNA, rapidly degrades mRNAs that are not useful as templates for protein synthesis. Absence of an ORF in an mRNA promotes degradation by this mechanism, however, the existence of a *CCDC26* protein will prolong the lifetime of *CCDC26* mRNA and may maintain the function (if any) of the RNA itself.

Because of the considerable length of the *CCDC26* intron (330 kbp versus 1200 bp exons), it is very difficult to ignore the possibility that there is another transcript(s) within this intron with important function. Possible encoded ncRNAs within the *CCDC26* exon-intron region are summarized in Fig. 4 and include, mRNA (a), intronic encoded ncRNA (b), intronic lariat RNA (c-d) and miRNA independently transcribed or processed from the precursor of the *CCDC26* mRNA (e). Actually there are several regions in the *CCDC26* intron where nucleosomal histones undergo high levels of methylation and acetylation, meaning that these locations may be actively transcribed (Fig.3a). Furthermore, most of these regions are

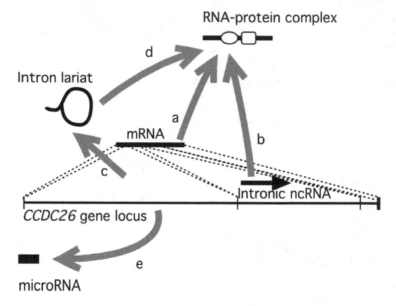

Figure 4. A possible function of *CCDC26*. The 330-kb precursor RNA transcribed from the gene is processed into mature mRNA. It then forms a complex with proteins to perform its biological function, for example, silencing a certain genetic locus (a). Alternatively, the ncRNA independently encoded in the intronic region (b) or the processed intron lariat (c-d) could have biological functions. The intronic microRNA could be transcribed directly from the genome using its own promoter or processed from the precursor of the *CCDC26* mRNA(e). Note that lengths of nucleic acid chains are not to scale. Length of the precursor RNA is approximately 330 kb; *CCDC26* mRNA is 1.3 kb; the spliced lariat is more than 100 kb; intronic microRNA is 18-23 bases.

highly conserved among mammals, suggesting that function is encoded. Also, expressed sequence tags other than known spliced *CCDC26* mRNAs have been reported in the intron. There are three miRNAs (miR-3669, 3673 and 3686) in the intron of *CCDC26* that are registered in the miRNA database (miRBase; http://www.mirbase.org/)(50). Although their functions are unknown, they may act as oncogenic or tumor suppressive ncRNAs.

6. Hypothetical function of *CCDC26* as a non-coding RNA

Although many ncRNAs are registered in databases, only a few have clearly demonstrated functions and detailed mechanisms of action. *CCDC26* might be a new ncRNA that is associated with cancer, including AML. Interestingly, expression of an miRNA, miR-21, is observed in many malignant cells, including AML cells (51). Also phorbol ester-induced differentiation of HL-60 cells into macrophage-like cells is accompanied by up-regulation of miR-21 (52). There are several reports suggesting that miRNAs act as oncogenic or tumor suppressive miRNAs in AML, as reviewed in (53, 54). Recently, Marcucci and colleagues used 305 different probes to search for miRNA expression in favorable and adverse-risk groups of normal karyotype AML (monocytic leukemia). They then used these data to link expression profiles with the cohort analysis of the patients. They identified a certain pattern of miRNA expression in the adverse-risk group and linked the expression level of eight types of miRNA to AML prognosis (55). It is possible that an unknown miRNA in the *CCDC26* locus affects cancer malignancy through the regulation of other genes. But all miRNAs described so far in the *CCDC26* locus (mir-3669, mir-3673 and mir-3686) show no expression in leukemia cells and no conservation among mammals in contrast to other oncogenic miRNAs; for example miR21 and let7, are actively transcribed and strongly conserved.

Within the CCDC26 intronic region, there are some long regions (>10 kb) that are actively transcribed in leukemia cells (Fig. 3a). They seem to be too long for pri-miRNAs but could encode lncRNAs. Indeed, active transcription occurs in the *CCDC26* region in cells derived from AML (T. Hirano unpublished observation), meaning that these transcripts might function as a tumor promoting or oncogenic lncRNAs. In contrast, if the original function of *CCDC26*, or of lncRNAs associated with *CCDC26*, was lost by chromosomal abnormality (for example in dmin of HL-60 cells), then they might function naturally as tumor suppressors. Some lncRNAs including *XIST* (56), *KCNQ1OT1* (57), *ANRIL* (58) and *AIRN* (59) are known to suppress (in cis) the expression of neighboring gene. It is well known that genes located in extrachromosomal elements such as dmin are actively transcribed, but the mechanism behind this phenomenon is not well understood (60, 61). Differences between dmin and an intact chromosome are caused by differences in chromatin structure, which is indicated by differences in DNase I hypersensitivity (36). Similarly to other gene silencing lncRNAs, an ncRNA encoded by the *CCDC26* locus might suppress the expression of other nearby genes. The hypothesis that neighboring genes, including the *MYC* oncogene, are activated when the normal *CCDC26* locus structure is destroyed by a chromosomal abnormality could explain the high transcriptional activity of genes in extrachromosomal elements (Fig.5). Further evidence is needed to determine whether *CCDC26* mRNA and/or its transcripts encoded in its intron are oncogenic or tumor suppressive.

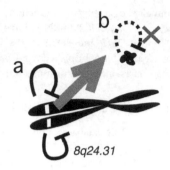

Figure 5. Hypothetical mechanism by which an oncogene (for example *MYC*) is inactivated in an intact chromosome (a) by *CCDC26* regulation. This suppression does not function on extrachromosomal chromatin (b).

7. Future perspectives

The size of the *CCDC26* locus, spanning over 330,000 base pairs, makes it difficult to study. If the ORF of the gene is not functional then it is unclear which part(s) of the locus are functional. Therefore, to study this gene, it is first necessary to determine all transcripts produced by the *CCDC26* locus and then to analyze their function. Comprehensive analysis of transcriptome of the relevant region using tiling microarray analysis is needed. Although lncRNA orthologs are frequently not found between species, homology analysis of this region between human and mouse could be helpful to identify functional sequences. Once transcripts are identified, we will be able to perform *in situ* hybridization to determine subcellular localization. Knock-down of transcripts will be useful to investigate their functions. Proteins interacting with the RNA transcripts will be identifiable by pull-down assays and mass spectrometry analysis. Finally, gene targeting should be used to investigate the effects of disruption of the region encoding the transcript. It will be of special interest if transcription of neighboring genes is activated or inactivated (in particular *MYC*), suggesting a regulatory function of the ncRNA encoded in the *CCDC26* locus. If an ortholog of the gene is found in mice, making a knock-out mouse of the ncRNA or a transgenic mouse with forced expression of the ncRNA will help to demonstrate its relationship to disease.

8. Conclusion

As a conclusion, the *CCDC26* locus is considered to encode an lncRNA involved in tumorigenesis. *CCDC26* itself might be an lncRNA or its intron might contain a functional miRNA or lncRNA. The study of this gene will bring new knowledge to gene regulation and to cancer treatment strategies targeting lncRNAs. Further *in vitro* and *in vivo* study is needed to prove the relationship between transcripts from the locus and disease, such as leukemia and glioma.

Author details

Tetsuo Hirano
Life Science Group, Graduate School of Integrated Arts and Sciences, Hiroshima University,
Kagamiyama, Higashihiroshima, Hiroshima, Japan

9. References

[1] Wilusz JE, Sunwoo H, Spector DL. Long noncoding RNAs: functional surprises from the RNA world. Genes Dev. 2009;23:1494-504.

[2] Mattick JS. The genetic signatures of noncoding RNAs. PLoS Genet. 2009;5:e1000459.

[3] Alexander RP, Fang G, Rozowsky J, Snyder M, Gerstein MB. Annotating non-coding regions of the genome. Nat Rev Genet. 2010;11:559-71.

[4] Chen L-L, Carmichael GG. Decoding the function of nuclear long non-coding RNAs. Curr Opin Cell Biol. 2010;22:357-64.

[5] Wapinski O, Chang HY. Long noncoding RNAs and human disease. Trends in Cell Biol. 2011;21:354-61

[6] Liu N, Okamura K, Tyler DM, Phillips MD, Chung W-j, Lai EC. The evolution and functional diversification of animal microRNA genes. Cell Res. 2008;18:985-96.

[7] Kutter C, Svoboda P. miRNA, siRNA, piRNA. RNA Biology. 2008;5:181-8.

[8] Vaz C, Ahmad HM, Sharma P, Gupta R, Kumar L, Kulshreshtha R, et al. Analysis of microRNA transcriptome by deep sequencing of small RNA libraries of peripheral blood. BMC Genomics. 2010;11:288.

[9] Czech B, Hannon GJ. Small RNA sorting: matchmaking for Argonautes. Nat Rev Genet. 2011;12:19-31.

[10] Varol N, Konac E, Gurocak OS, Sozen S. The realm of microRNAs in cancers. Mol Biol Rep. 2011;38:1079-89.

[11] Valeri N, Vannini I, Fanini F, Calore F, Adair B, Fabbri M. Epigenetics, miRNAs, and human cancer: a new chapter in human gene regulation. Mammalian Genome. 2009;20:573-80.

[12] Lujambio A, Lowe SW. The microcosmos of cancer. Nature. 2012;482:347-55.

[13] Brosnan CA, Voinnet O. The long and the short of noncoding RNAs. Curr Opin Cell Biol. 2009;21:416-25.

[14] Amaral PP, Clark MB, Gascoigne DK, Dinger ME, Mattick JS. lncRNAdb: a reference database for long noncoding RNAs. Nucleic Acids Res. 2011;39:D146-51.

[15] Bu D, Yu K, Sun S, Xie C, Skogerbø G, Miao R, et al. NONCODE v3.0: integrative annotation of long noncoding RNAs. Nucleic Acids Res. 2012;40:D210-5.

[16] Spizzo R, Almeida MI, Colombatti A, Calin Ga. Long non-coding RNAs and cancer: a new frontier of translational research? Oncogene. 2012:1-11.

[17] Castelnuovo M, Massone S, Tasso R, Fiorino G, Gatti M, Robello M, et al. An Alu-like RNA promotes cell differentiation and reduces malignancy of human neuroblastoma cells. FASEB J. 2010;24:4033-46.

[18] Gavazzo P, Vella S, Marchetti C, Nizzari M, Cancedda R, Pagano A. Acquisition of neuron-like electrophysiological properties in neuroblastoma cells by controlled expression of NDM29 ncRNA. J Neurochem. 2011;119:989-1001.

[19] Bernard D, Prasanth KV, Tripathi V, Colasse S, Nakamura T, Xuan Z, et al. A long nuclear-retained non-coding RNA regulates synaptogenesis by modulating gene expression. The EMBO J. 2010;29:3082-93.

[20] Zhang X, Gejman R, Mahta A, Zhong Y, Rice Ka, Zhou Y, et al. Maternally expressed gene 3, an imprinted noncoding RNA gene, is associated with meningioma pathogenesis and progression. Cancer Res. 2010;70:2350-8.

[21] Zhou Y, Zhang X, Klibanski A. MEG3 non-coding RNA: a tumor suppressor. J Mol Endocrinol. 2012:45-53.

[22] Gupta Ra, Shah N, Wang KC, Kim J, Horlings HM, Wong DJ, et al. Long non-coding RNA HOTAIR reprograms chromatin state to promote cancer metastasis. Nature. 2010;464:1071-6.

[23] Yoshimizu T, Miroglio A, Ripoche M-A, Gabory A, Vernucci M, Riccio A, et al. The H19 locus acts in vivo as a tumor suppressor. Proc Natl Acad Sci USA. 2008;105:12417-22.

[24] He H, Nagy R, Liyanarachchi S, Jiao H, Li W, Suster S, et al. A susceptibility locus for papillary thyroid carcinoma on chromosome 8q24. Cancer Res. 2009;69:625-31.

[25] Pasic I, Shlien A, Durbin AD, Stavropoulos DJ, Baskin B, Ray PN, et al. Recurrent focal copy-number changes and loss of heterozygosity implicate two noncoding RNAs and one tumor suppressor gene at chromosome 3q13.31 in osteosarcoma. Cancer Res. 2010;70:160-71.

[26] Estey E, Döhner H. Acute myeloid leukaemia. Lancet. 2006;368:1894-907.

[27] Walter MJ, Payton JE, Ries RE, Shannon WD, Deshmukh H, Zhao Y, et al. Acquired copy number alterations in adult acute myeloid leukemia genomes. Proc Natl Acad Sci USA. 2009;106:12950-5.

[28] Akagi T, Ogawa S, Dugas M, Kawamata N, Yamamoto G, Nannya Y, et al. Frequent genomic abnormalities in acute myeloid leukemia/myelodysplastic syndrome with normal karyotype. Haematologica. 2009;94:213-23.

[29] Renneville A, Roumier C, Biggio V, Nibourel O, Boissel N, Fenaux P, et al. Cooperating gene mutations in acute myeloid leukemia: a review of the literature. Leukemia. 2008;22:915-31.

[30] Vardiman JW, Thiele J, Arber Da, Brunning RD, Borowitz MJ, Porwit A, et al. The 2008 revision of the World Health Organization (WHO) classification of myeloid neoplasms and acute leukemia: rationale and important changes. Blood. 2009;114:937-51.

[31] Mrózek K, Radmacher MD, Bloomfield CD, Marcucci G. Molecular signatures in acute myeloid leukemia. Curr Opin Hematol. 2009;16:64-9.

[32] Döhner H, Estey EH, Amadori S, Appelbaum FR, Büchner T, Burnett AK, et al. Diagnosis and management of acute myeloid leukemia in adults: recommendations from an international expert panel, on behalf of the European LeukemiaNet. Blood. 2010;115:453-74.

[33] Paschka P, Schlenk RF, Gaidzik VI, Habdank M, Krönke J, Bullinger L, et al. IDH1 and IDH2 mutations are frequent genetic alterations in acute myeloid leukemia and confer

adverse prognosis in cytogenetically normal acute myeloid leukemia with NPM1 mutation without FLT3 internal tandem duplication. J Clin Oncol. 2010;28:3636-43.

[34] Xu W, Yang H, Liu Y, Yang Y, Wang P, Kim S-H, et al. Oncometabolite 2-hydroxyglutarate is a competitive inhibitor of α-ketoglutarate-dependent dioxygenases. Cancer Cell. 2011;19:17-30.

[35] Dang L, Jin S, Su SM. IDH mutations in glioma and acute myeloid leukemia. Trends Mol Med. 2010;16:387-97.

[36] Kitajima K, Haque M, Nakamura H, Hirano T, Utiyama H. Loss of irreversibility of granulocytic differentiation induced by dimethyl sulfoxide in HL-60 sublines with a homogeneously staining region. Biochem Biophys Res Commun. 2001;288:1182-7.

[37] Hirano T, Ike F, Murata T, Obata Y, Utiyama H, Yokoyama KK. Genes encoded within 8q24 on the amplicon of a large extrachromosomal element are selectively repressed during the terminal differentiation of HL-60 cells. Mutat Res. 2008;640:97-106.

[38] Storlazzi CT, Fioretos T, Paulsson K, Strömbeck B, Lassen C, Ahlgren T, et al. Identification of a commonly amplified 4.3 Mb region with overexpression of C8FW, but not MYC in MYC-containing double minutes in myeloid malignancies. Hum Mol Genet. 2004;13:1479-85.

[39] Storlazzi CT, Fioretos T, Surace C, Lonoce A, Mastrorilli A, Strömbeck B, et al. MYC-containing double minutes in hematologic malignancies: evidence in favor of the episome model and exclusion of MYC as the target gene. Hum Mol Genet. 2006;15:933-42.

[40] Radtke I, Mullighan CG, Ishii M, Su X, Cheng J, Ma J, et al. Genomic analysis reveals few genetic alterations in pediatric acute myeloid leukemia. Proc Natl Acad Sci USA. 2009;106:12944-9.

[41] Paulsson K, Johansson B. Trisomy 8 as the sole chromosomal aberration in acute myeloid leukemia and myelodysplastic syndromes. Pathologie-biologie. 2007;55:37-48.

[42] Yin W, Rossin A, Clifford JL, Gronemeyer H. Co-resistance to retinoic acid and TRAIL by insertion mutagenesis into RAM. Oncogene. 2006;25:3735-44.

[43] Liu Y, Shete S, Hosking F, Robertson L, Houlston R, Bondy M. Genetic advances in glioma: susceptibility genes and networks. Curr Opin Genet Dev. 2010;20:239-44.

[44] Shete S, Hosking FJ, Robertson LB, Dobbins SE, Sanson M, Malmer B, et al. Genome-wide association study identifies five susceptibility loci for glioma. Nat Genet. 2009;41:899-904.

[45] Boehringer S, van der Lijn F, Liu F, Günther M, Sinigerova S, Nowak S, et al. Genetic determination of human facial morphology: links between cleft-lips and normal variation. Eu J Hum Genet. 2011;19:1192-7.

[46] Lasho TL, Tefferi A, Pardanani A, Finke CM, Fink SR, Caron aa, et al. Differential distribution of CCDC26 glioma-risk alleles in myeloid malignancies with mutant IDH1 compared with their IDH2R140-mutated or IDH-unmutated counterparts. Leukemia. 2012;26:1406-7.

[47] Wrensch M, Jenkins RB, Chang JS, Yeh R-f, Xiao Y, Decker PA, et al. Variants in the CDKN2B and RTEL1 regions are associated with high-grade glioma susceptibility. Nat Genet. 2009;41:905-8.

[48] Melin B. Genetic causes of glioma: new leads in the labyrinth. Curr Opin Oncol. 2011;23:643-7.

[49] Barrett T, Troup DB, Wilhite SE, Ledoux P, Evangelista C, Kim IF, et al. NCBI GEO: archive for functional genomics data sets--10 years on. Nucleic Acids Res. 2011;39:D1005-10.

[50] Kozomara A, Griffiths-Jones S. miRBase: integrating microRNA annotation and deep-sequencing data. Nucleic Acids Res. 2011;39:D152-7.

[51] Volinia S, Calin Ga, Liu C-G, Ambs S, Cimmino A, Petrocca F, et al. A microRNA expression signature of human solid tumors defines cancer gene targets. Proc Natl Acad Sci USA. 2006;103:2257-61.

[52] Fujita S, Ito T, Mizutani T, Minoguchi S, Yamamichi N, Sakurai K, et al. miR-21 Gene expression triggered by AP-1 is sustained through a double-negative feedback mechanism. J Mol Biol. 2008;378:492-504.

[53] Havelange V, Garzon R, Croce CM. MicroRNAs: new players in acute myeloid leukaemia. Br J Cancer. 2009;101:743-8.

[54] Larson RA. Micro-RNAs and copy number changes: new levels of gene regulation in acute myeloid leukemia. Chem Biol Interact. 2010;184:21-5.

[55] Marcucci G, Radmacher MD, Maharry K, Mrózek K, Ruppert AS, Paschka P, et al. MicroRNA expression in cytogenetically normal acute myeloid leukemia. New Eng J Med. 2008;358:1919-28.

[56] Agrelo R, Wutz A. X inactivation and disease. Semin Cell Dev Biol. 2010;21:194-200.

[57] DeBaun MR, Niemitz EL, McNeil DE, Brandenburg Sa, Lee MP, Feinberg AP. Epigenetic alterations of H19 and LIT1 distinguish patients with Beckwith-Wiedemann syndrome with cancer and birth defects. Am J Hum Genet. 2002;70:604-11.

[58] Aguilo F, Zhou M-M, Walsh MJ. Long noncoding RNA, polycomb, and the ghosts haunting INK4b-ARF-INK4a expression. Cancer Res. 2011;71:5365-9.

[59] Yotova IY, Vlatkovic IM, Pauler FM, Warczok KE, Ambros PF, Oshimura M, et al. Identification of the human homolog of the imprinted mouse Air non-coding RNA. Genomics. 2008;92:464-73.

[60] Haque MM, Hirano T, Itoh N, Utiyama H. Evolution of large extrachromosomal elements in HL-60 cells during culture and the associated phenotype alterations. Biochem Biophys Res Commun. 2001;288:592-6.

[61] Haque MM, Hirano T, Nakamura H, Utiyama H. Granulocytic differentiation of HL-60 cells, both spontaneous and drug-induced, might require loss of extrachromosomal DNA encoding a gene(s) not c-MYC. Biochem Biophys Res Commun. 2001;288:586-91.

[62] Garzon R, Garofalo M, Martelli MP, Briesewitz R, Wang L, Fernandez-Cymering C, et al. Distinctive microRNA signature of acute myeloid leukemia bearing cytoplasmic mutated nucleophosmin. Proc Natl Acad Sci USA. 2008;105:3945-50.

[63] Dixon-McIver A, East P, Mein CA, Cazier J-b, Molloy G, Chaplin T, et al. Distinctive patterns of microRNA expression associated with karyotype in acute myeloid leukaemia. PloS One. 2008;3:e2141.

[64] Langer C, Marcucci G, Holland KB, Radmacher MD, Maharry K, Paschka P, et al. Prognostic importance of MN1 transcript levels, and biologic insights from MN1-

associated gene and microRNA expression signatures in cytogenetically normal acute myeloid leukemia: a cancer and leukemia group B study. J Clin Oncol. 2009;27:3198-204.

[65] Zhao H, Wang D, Du W, Gu D, Yang R. MicroRNA and leukemia: tiny molecule, great function. Crit Rev Oncol Hematol. 2010;74:149-55.

[66] Marcucci G, Radmacher MD, Mrózek K, Bloomfield CD. MicroRNA expression in acute myeloid leukemia. Cur Hematol Malignancy Reports. 2009;4:83-8.

[67] Chistiakov Da, Chekhonin VP. Contribution of microRNAs to radio- and chemoresistance of brain tumors and their therapeutic potential. Eur J Pharmacol. 2012.

[68] Zhang X, Yang H, Lee JJ, Kim E, Lippman SM, Khuri FR, et al. MicroRNA-related genetic variations as predictors for risk of second primary tumor and/or recurrence in patients with early-stage head and neck cancer. Carcinogenesis. 2010;31:2118-23.

[69] Hummel R, Maurer J, Haier J. MicroRNAs in brain tumors : a new diagnostic and therapeutic perspective? Mol Neurobiol. 2011;44:223-34.

[70] Iacoangeli A, Lin Y, Morley EJ, Muslimov Ia, Bianchi R, Reilly J, et al. BC200 RNA in invasive and preinvasive breast cancer. Carcinogenesis. 2004;25:2125-33.

[71] Bertozzi D, Iurlaro R, Sordet O, Marinello J, Zaffaroni N, Capranico G. Characterization of novel antisense HIF-1α transcripts in human cancers. Cell Cycle. 2011;10:3189-97.

[72] Niinuma T, Suzuki H, Nojima M, Nosho K, Yamamoto H, Takamaru H, et al. Upregulation of miR-196a and HOTAIR Drive Malignant Character in Gastrointestinal Stromal Tumors. Cancer Res. 2012;72:1126-36.

[73] Panzitt K, Tschernatsch MMO, Guelly C, Moustafa T, Stradner M, Strohmaier HM, et al. Characterization of HULC, a novel gene with striking up-regulation in hepatocellular carcinoma, as noncoding RNA. Gastroenterol. 2007;132:330-42.

[74] Vu TH, Chuyen NV, Li T. Loss of Imprinting of IGF2 Sense and Antisense Transcripts in Wilms ' Tumor. Cancer Res. 2003;63:1900-5.

[75] Poliseno L, Salmena L, Zhang J, Carver B, Haveman WJ, Pandolfi PP. A coding-independent function of gene and pseudogene mRNAs regulates tumour biology. Nature. 2010;465:1033-8.

[76] Li L, Feng T, Lian Y, Zhang G, Garen A, Song X. Role of human noncoding RNAs in the control of tumorigenesis. Proc Natl Acad Sci USA. 2009;106:12956-61.

[77] Zong X, Tripathi V, Prasanth KV. RNA splicing control: yet another gene regulatory role for long nuclear noncoding RNAs. RNA Biology. 2011;8:968-77.

[78] Schalken Ja. Towards Early and More Specific Diagnosis of Prostate Cancer? Beyond PSA: New Biomarkers Ready for Prime Time. Eur Urol Supple. 2009;8:97-102.

[79] Srikantan V, Zou Z, Petrovics G, Xu L, Augustus M, Davis L, et al. PCGEM1, a prostate-specific gene, is overexpressed in prostate cancer. Proc Natl Acad Sci USA. 2000;97:12216-21.

[80] Chung S, Nakagawa H, Uemura M, Piao L, Ashikawa K, Hosono N, et al. Association of a novel long non-coding RNA in 8q24 with prostate cancer susceptibility. Cancer Science. 2011;102:245-52.

[81] Cooper C, Guo J, Yan Y, Chooniedass-Kothari S, Hube F, Hamedani MK, et al. Increasing the relative expression of endogenous non-coding Steroid Receptor RNA

Activator (SRA) in human breast cancer cells using modified oligonucleotides. Nucleic Acids Res. 2009;37:4518-31.

[82] Cao Y, Bryan TM, Reddel RR. Increased copy number of the TERT and TERC telomerase subunit genes in cancer cells. Cancer Science. 2008;99:1092-9.

[83] Yang C, Li X, Wang Y, Zhao L, Chen W. Long non-coding RNA UCA1 regulated cell cycle distribution via CREB through PI3-K dependent pathway in bladder carcinoma cells. Gene. 2012;496:8-16.

[84] Dallosso AR, Hancock AL, Malik S, Salpekar A, King-Underwood L, Pritchard-Jones K, et al. Alternately spliced WT1 antisense transcripts interact with WT1 sense RNA and show epigenetic and splicing defects in cancer. RNA. 2007;13:2287-99.

[85] Agrelo R, Wutz A. Cancer progenitors and epigenetic contexts: an Xisting connection. Epigenetics. 2009;4:568-70.

[86] Klein U, Lia M, Crespo M, Siegel R, Shen Q, Mo T, et al. The DLEU2/miR-15a/16-1 cluster controls B cell proliferation and its deletion leads to chronic lymphocytic leukemia. Cancer Cell. 2010;17:28-40.

[87] Mourtada-Maarabouni M, Pickard MR, Hedge VL, Farzaneh F, Williams GT. GAS5, a non-protein-coding RNA, controls apoptosis and is downregulated in breast cancer. Oncogene. 2009;28:195-208.

[88] Schofield PN, Joyce Ja, Lam WK, Grandjean V, Ferguson-Smith a, Reik W, et al. Genomic imprinting and cancer; new paradigms in the genetics of neoplasia. Toxicol Lett. 2001;120:151-60.

[89] Wang X-S, Gong J-N, Yu J, Wang F, Zhang X-H, Yin X-L, et al. MicroRNA-29a and microRNA-142-3p are regulators of myeloid differentiation and acute myeloid leukemia. Blood. 2012.

[90] Candeias MM, Malbert-Colas L, Powell DJ, Daskalogianni C, Maslon MM, Naski N, et al. P53 mRNA controls p53 activity by managing Mdm2 functions. Nat Cell Biol. 2008;10:1098-105.

[91] Maida Y, Yasukawa M, Furuuchi M, Lassmann T, Possemato R, Okamoto N, et al. An RNA-dependent RNA polymerase formed by TERT and the RMRP RNA. Nature. 2009;461:230-5.

[92] Azzalin CM, Reichenbach P, Khoriauli L, Giulotto E, Lingner J. Telomeric repeat containing RNA and RNA surveillance factors at mammalian chromosome ends. Science. 2007;318:798-801.

[93] Treppendahl MB, Qiu X, Søgaard A, Yang X, Nandrup-Bus C, Hother C, et al. Allelic methylation levels of the noncoding VTRNA2-1 located on chromosome 5q31.1 predict outcome in AML. Blood. 2012;119:206-16.

[94] Askarian-Amiri ME, Crawford J, French JD, Smart CE, Smith Ma, Clark MB, et al. SNORD-host RNA Zfas1 is a regulator of mammary development and a potential marker for breast cancer. RNA. 2011;17:878-91.

[95] Kent WJ, Sugnet CW, Furey TS, Roskin KM, Pringle TH, Zahler AM, et al. The human genome browser at UCSC. Genome Res. 2002;12:996-1006.

Oncogenes for Transcription Factors

Chapter 6

The MYCN Oncogene

Leanna Cheung, Jayne E. Murray, Michelle Haber and Murray D. Norris

Additional information is available at the end of the chapter

1. Introduction

MYCN is a member of the *MYC* family of oncogenes, which also includes *c-MYC* and *MYCL*. Despite knowing about the existence of MYCN for nearly thirty years, the majority of functional studies involving MYC family members have focused on c-MYC due to the limited expression profile of MYCN in human cancers, and also in part due to the existence of highly conserved functional domains between c-MYC and MYCN [1]. MYCN is normally expressed during embryonal development and orchestrates cell proliferation and differentiation in the developing peripheral neural crest [2]. However, the deregulated expression of MYCN has been shown to contribute to tumorigenesis and neuronal transformation [3]. Thus, MYCN represents a highly desirable therapeutic target. Previous studies have shown that downregulating *MYCN* expression, via antisense oligonucleotides, resulted in lower tumour incidence and decreased tumour mass in a murine neuroblastoma tumour model [4]. However, to date, no molecularly targeted therapies have been developed that are able to mimic this response in the clinic, and further studies are required to help elucidate the mechanisms that drive *MYCN* tumour formation and progression.

2. The MYC family and the discovery of MYCN

The eventual discovery of *MYC* oncogenes arose from early pioneering work on the Rous sarcoma virus (RSV), a transforming retrovirus able to cause sarcomas in infected chicken cells. Using the information provided by RSV, hybridisation studies were performed on a specific group of avian tumours involving a retrovirus responsible for inducing myeloid leukaemia. This led to the identification of a sequence that was named *v-gag-myc*, or *v-myc* for myelocytomatosis (the leukaemia that is induced following the transduction of avian cells with this virus) and supported the idea that viral integration into a host genome could activate a nearby host oncogene [5, 6]. As it transpired, the human homologue of *v-myc*, termed *c-MYC* (cellular-*MYC*) was the first cellular oncogene whose overexpression was shown to be activated through retroviral insertional mutagenesis [7]. Deregulated expression of *c-MYC* has since been implicated in a range of cancers, and allowed the discovery of other important *MYC* family members including *MYCN* and *MYCL*.

Neuroblastoma is the most common extracranial solid tumour of early childhood and accounts for approximately 15% of all cancer related deaths in children. Aggressive drug refractory neuroblastoma cells have been frequently observed to contain genomic aberrations referred to as double-minute chromatin bodies and homogeneously staining regions. Both of these types of aberrations were found to contain multiple copies or amplification of specific genes, and in particular, the critical gene within these regions was later identified to be the *c-MYC*-related oncogene, *MYCN*, so-called because of its identification in neuroblastoma cells [8]. Amplification of the *MYCN* oncogene has also been demonstrated in retinoblastoma, glioblastoma, medulloblastoma, astrocytoma and small cell lung cancer cells [9]. In addition, another member of the *MYC*-oncogene family, *MYCL*, was identified in small cell lung cancer (SCLC), and demonstrated homology to a small region of both *c-MYC* and *MYCN*. Gene mapping studies assigned *MYCL* to human chromosome region 1p32, a location that is distinct from that of either *c-MYC* or *MYCN* (regions 8q24 and 2p24 respectively) but is also associated with cytogenetic abnormalities in certain human tumours such as thyroid cancer and lung cancer [10, 11]. *MYCL* was found to be amplified in some SCLC cells [12]. In mammals, a fourth member of the *MYC* family, *s-Myc* has been identified, however only *c-MYC*, *MYCN* and *MYCL* have been implicated in the tumorigenesis of specific human cancers [13].

All three tumour-associated *MYC* genes have the same characteristic three-exon structure with the major polypeptide open reading frame residing in the second and third exons. The first exon is not conserved between the genes, but rather possesses regulatory functions, whereas the two coding exons produce highly homologous sections of amino acids interspersed with areas of diminished conservation, leading to the suggestion that individual MYC polypeptides have discrete, independent, functional domains [14]. In tumour biology, many cancers have been shown to exhibit increased levels of MYC protein in tumour tissue relative to the surrounding normal tissues, and this has been shown to contribute to the aggressiveness of the tumour [15]. Importantly, the MYC family of proteins share functionally similar roles, acting as transcription factors to drive cellular proliferation and vasculogenesis, promote metastasis and genomic instability, as well as inhibit cell differentiation and reduce cell adhesion [13, 16]. However, recent findings have also raised the possibility of transcriptionally-independent functions of the MYC proteins [17].

3. The functional activity of MYCN

MYC proteins are well established as nuclear phosphoproteins that act as regulators of transcription, and can both activate and repress the expression of its target genes [16]. *MYCN* encodes a 60kDa protein that has affinity for and binds to DNA, and is phosphorylated by casein kinase II [18, 19]. Phosphorylation is important for the transforming abilities of MYC family members and also for the regulation of MYC protein stability and activity [20]. The affinity of MYCN protein for DNA relies on the presence of certain motifs, comprising a basic DNA binding region, an α-helical protein-protein interaction domain or helix-loop-helix (HLH), and a leucine zipper motif (Zip) encompassing the bHLH-Zip domain at the carboxy or C-terminus of the protein [9]. The mechanism that mediates the DNA-binding capacity of MYC proteins was confirmed via the identification of MAX, also a bHLH-Zip protein [21]. MYCN and MAX (Figure 1) interact to form a complex that binds to DNA in a sequence specific manner [22]. MYCN binds to MAX protein via its bHLH-LZ region. Several other proteins have also been shown to interact with the C-terminus of MYCN, including YY-1, AP-2, TFII-I and BRCA1 [23], or with the central region of MYCN such as NMi [24], all of which are associated with MYCN's function as a transcriptional regulator.

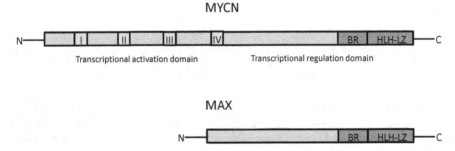

Figure 1. Domains of the MYCN and MAX proteins. The N-terminus of MYCN has three elements, known as MYC homology boxes I-III, which are highly conserved in MYC proteins. The C-terminus contains the basic-region/helix-loop-helix/leucine-zipper that is responsible for interaction with the MAX protein.

The amino or N-terminus of MYCN acts as a transactivation domain that contains two highly conserved regions called Myc Homology Boxes I and II (MBI and MBII) [1]. This region has been shown to bind to nuclear cofactors, including TRRAP, p107, BIN1, MM-1, AMY-1, PAM, α-Tubulin, TIP48 and TIP49, to assist the targeting of protein to specific gene promoters [23, 25]. Another protein YAF2, has been demonstrated to bind to the central region of MYCN to further stimulate transcription upon MYCN-MAX transactivation [26]. All of these interacting proteins are a part of a transcription factor complex by which target genes are activated. Myc Homology Box III (MBIII) is conserved only within c-MYC and MYCN, but not MYCL, and is necessary for cellular transformation [27]. A fourth Myc Homology Box (MBIV) is also necessary for MYC transforming activity [28].

Recent studies have provided evidence of a function of MYCN that is independent from its role as a classical transcription factor. MYCN was shown to remodel large domains of euchromatin, regions of lightly packaged chromatin that contain active, functioning genes, by regulating histone acetylation [29, 30]. Two possibilities have been suggested for this role. The first is that MYCN maintains the activity of euchromatin, whilst the second is that MYCN maintains euchromatin at remote sites to act as an enhancer and regulator of genes at a distance. Novel functions of other MYC proteins have been identified through mutational analyses that have uncoupled the transforming ability of c-MYC from its role as a transcription factor [28, 31]. c-MYC was found to increase the translation of specific mRNAs by promoting the methylation of the 5′ mRNA guanine "cap", including mRNAs encoding cyclin T1 and CDK9 [31]. A role for c-MYC has also been described in the initiation of DNA replication by binding to various components of the pre-replicative complex and localising to early sites of DNA replication [32]. These observations suggest that c-MYC may play a role in controlling initiation of the S phase of the cell cycle and contribute to replicative stress and genomic instability, to further accelerate tumorigenesis [17]. Even though the evidence has yet to be provided, given the high level of homology between c-MYC and MYCN, the described transcription-independent roles of c-MYC suggest similar roles will be identified for MYCN in contributing to tumour cell biology.

4. MYCN as a transcriptional activator

As indicated above, MYCN heterodimerises with MAX and binds with high affinity to a CACA/GTG E-box sequence found upstream of promoter target sequences [13]. The MYCN-MAX heterodimer activates transcription via several mechanisms. TRRAP (or TRansactivation/tRansformation Associated Protein) binds to the N-terminal region of MYCN and is essential for MYCN transformation. Through TRRAP, MYCN recruits histone acetylation (HAT) complexes to chromatin, including the 1.8 megaDalton SAGA complex (SPT/ADA/GCN5/Acetyltransferase) [33]. Histone acetylation is associated with gene activation by chromatin modification influencing histone-DNA and histone-histone contact [34]. TRRAP is involved with another HAT complex, TIP60, an H2A/H4 acetylase [35]. Interestingly, *in vivo* acetylation of histone H4 is highly associated with MYC target gene activation [36]. Two other proteins, TIP48 and TIP49 that are found in the TIP60 complex also bind to the N-terminus of MYCN [25]. Both proteins are highly conserved hexameric ATPases that are involved in chromatin remodelling involving the movement or displacement of nucleosomes, as opposed to chromatin modification [37].

The MYC family represents a particularly unusual set of transcription factors in that they can bind to and regulate approximately 10-15% of the entire genome [14]. Some MYCN target genes have been shown to be activated independently of TRRAP and HAT complexes. Investigation into HAT independent activation has revealed the involvement of RNA polymerase II at the promoter regions of target genes. c-MYC protein binding has been shown to stimulate the clearance of RNA polymerase II from the promoter region to allow for efficient transcription elongation by the RNA pol II kinases, TFIIH and positive transcription elongation factor b (PTEFb) [38]. c-MYC also regulates RNA pol II promoter clearance by controlling the expression of RNA pol II kinases via mRNA cap methylation, polysome loading, and the rate of translation [31].

5. MYCN as a transcriptional repressor

Most studies have focused on the role of MYC proteins as transcriptional activators. However, cells transformed by constitutive expression of c-MYC are characterised by the loss of expression of numerous genes such as those involved in cell adhesion and cell cycle regulation, and even loss of *c-MYC* itself [39-41]. An early indicator of the transcriptional repressor role of MYC proteins was the involvement of c-MYC in a negative feedback loop, where the introduction of ectopic c-MYC or MYCN was able to downregulate endogenous expression of c-MYC in mouse fibroblast cells [42]. Structure and function analyses found that the regions of c-MYC that are required for transformation are also required for negative autoregulation [43] and led to the idea that the repression of target genes by MYC proteins could also contribute to transformation.

The understanding of transcriptional repression by MYC proteins was greatly advanced via the identification of repressed target genes such as *transglutaminase-2* (*TG2*) and *interleukin-6* (*IL-6*) [44]. Genomic studies have now revealed that MYC proteins repress as many targets as they activate, emphasising the role of gene repression by these oncoproteins during cellular transformation [14]. One recent example is the identification of *TG2* repression by MYCN in neuroblastoma, which occurs via the interaction between MYCN with Specificity Protein I (SP1) [45]. *TG2* is a multifunctional enzyme that catalyses the transamidation and multimerisation of proteins, but also promotes programmed cell death and induces neuritic differentiation in neuroblastoma cells [46]. Hence downregulation of *TG2* by MYCN would allow neuroblastoma cells to overcome apoptosis and continue to proliferate. Similarly, MYCN has been shown to interact with SP1 to downregulate the expression of *MRP3* (also known as *ABCC3*), the gene encoding an intermembrane transporter which is involved in the transport of organic anions, prostaglandins, leukotrienes and selected chemotherapeutics [47-49]. Another important gene that is downregulated by MYCN is *IL-6*, which has been shown to play an important anti-angiogenic role by inhibiting vascular endothelial cell proliferation [50]. The transcriptional repression by MYCN is also supported by the interaction between MYC proteins and another transcription factor MIZ-1 (Myc-interacting zinc finger protein-1) [51]. MIZ-1 is a POZ/BTB (poxvirus and zinc finger/bric-a-brac, tramtrack and broad complex) domain protein that transactivates genes involved in cell cycle regulation as well as tumour suppressor genes via the recruitment of the p300 histone acetyltransferase [52]. Interestingly, high-level MIZ-1 expression is associated with a favourable disease outcome of neuroblastoma [53]. MIZ-1 interacts with the carboxy-terminal HLH region of c-MYC and MYCN, where the binding of the MYC-MAX heterodimer to MIZ-1 disrupts the interaction between MIZ-1 and p300, causing the transcriptional repression of tumour suppressor genes [54]. MYC has also been shown to recruit a DNA methyltransferase, DNMT3a to the MYC-MIZ-1 complex, suggesting that repression can be mediated by the methylation of target gene promoters [55].

6. Mechanisms of regulating MYCN expression

Due to the gross transforming ability of deregulated expression of MYC proteins, the expression of these protooncogenes is tightly regulated in normal cells at both the transcriptional and protein level. For example, MYC mRNA transcripts and proteins have very short half-lives and are expressed at constant levels as cells enter the cell cycle [56, 57]. Furthermore, anti-proliferative signals trigger rapid down-regulation in expression, and the phosphorylation patterns of MYC proteins are known to influence their stability. In addition to these mechanisms, expression of MYCN is particularly tightly regulated with regards to timing and tissue specificity. Thus, MYCN is normally expressed during embryonal development of the peripheral nervous system in neural crest cells [2]. Neural crest cells migrate during mid-gestation to populate the entire peripheral nervous system, including autonomic and peripheral ganglia and the adrenal gland. These migrating progenitor cells represent a highly proliferative population, and during normal development exit the cell-cycle and undergo differentiation following the colonisation to the ganglia and spinal cord area. This event is orchestrated by extracellular signalling molecules such as mitogens and cytokines and coincides with decreased expression of MYCN [56, 58]. Without this strict control, dysregulated MYCN expression impairs the ability of progenitor cells to undergo differentiation. Studies which sustained MYCN expression in murine neural crest cells under the control of a tyrosine hydroxylase promoter, demonstrated the capacity to cause neuroblastoma in transgenic mice [3]. Despite this transforming ability, MYCN is vital for normal embryonic development, and murine embryos lacking MYCN exhibit profound hypoplasia, particularly in the central and peripheral nervous system, disorganized architecture of the brain, defective heart development and defects in the lung, genitourinary system, stomach, intestines and limb buds [59].

In order to understand how extracellular stimuli controlled MYC expression in cells, gene mapping studies in association with *MYC* transcription studies were undertaken, and these identified response elements within the *MYC* transcript as well as their regulators. In neuronal cells, *MYCN* has been shown to be regulated in its promoter region as well as in an enhancer region upstream of the coding region. The elongation transcription factor, E2F binds to the promoter region of *MYCN* in response to different mitogenic signals [60]. The promoter region also contains positive transcription factor binding sites for SP1, SP3 and TGFβ [61]. However, the presence of a retinoic acid response element (RARE) within this region allows for negative regulation of *MYCN* by retinoic acid [62].

A key finding was made in 1986 which identified *c-MYC* as the first eukaryotic gene to be negatively regulated by transcriptional elongation control, where a block in the elongation of mRNA during transcription occurred during cellular differentiation [63]. This finding was later confirmed in *MYCN* studies where transcription elongation pausing sites were identified in exon 1 and intron 1 of human *MYCN* [64, 65]. Furthermore, there is *in vivo* evidence that the downregulation of *MYCN* during mouse embryogenesis is partly regulated by the control of transcriptional elongation [66].

Transcription alone cannot account for the large difference in mRNA levels following the introduction of proliferative or anti-proliferative stimuli. The rapid turnover of mRNA was also associated with the discovery of two distinct mechanisms of *MYC* mRNA decay. The first involves a translation-independent mechanism involving poly(A) tail shortening of the untranslated region of the transcript, while the second represents a translation-dependent mechanism that is regulated by a region of mRNA which corresponds to the C-terminus of the protein, called the coding region determinant [67-69]. This region is bound to a 75kDa protein that protects the region of mRNA from endonuclease attack, in response to growth signals that induce c-MYC stabilisation. In the case of *MYCN*, RNA stability factors have also been identified which bind to the untranslated region of *MYCN* mRNA. In addition, an internal ribosomal entry segment (IRES) in the transcript acts to enhance neuronal specific translation [70, 71].

7. Regulation of MYCN protein expression

The regulation of MYCN protein levels has also been investigated and phosphopeptide analysis has revealed that specific serine and threonine residues of MYCN are phosphorylated *in vivo*. Two residues in particular, Threonine 58 (Thr58) and Serine 62 (Ser62) have been demonstrated as important determinants of transformation and MYCN protein stability and activity [20]. Proliferative stimuli activate phosphorylation of Ser62 by cyclin B and Cdk1 during prophase to increase MYCN protein stability [7?]. Phospho Ser62 via a feedback mechanism, then serves as a platform for the phosphorylation of Thr58 by glycogen synthase kinase 3 (GSK3), allowing the tumour suppressor FBW7 to bind and recruit a ubiquitylation complex, directing MYCN protein for degradation. Mitotic degradation of MYCN in the absence of growth factor-dependent signals allows cell cycle exit and the commencement of differentiation [73]. Another kinase, Aurora A, has recently been identified and shown to inhibit degradation of ubiquitinated MYCN by supporting the synthesis of non-degradable ubiquitin chains [74].

8. MYCN downstream target genes

The first transcriptional target for a MYC protein was discovered ten years after the identification of human *c-MYC*. The development of a conditionally expressed *c-MYC* construct, via the fusion of human *c-MYC* to the hormone-binding domain of the oestrogen receptor, led to the identification of a downstream target involved in cell cycle progression, α-prothymosin [75]. This approach was then used to identify additional targets including ornithine decarboxylase 1 (ODC1), the rate-limiting enzyme involved in polyamine synthesis [76]. A different method of identifying MYC targets utilised *MYC*-null models to determine whether the regulation of expression of genes was dependent on the presence of a *MYC* oncogene. Such examples of labour-intensive techniques were invaluable in determining single *bona fide* MYC targets, however recent advances in technology have allowed for large-scale analyses of MYC-regulated genes [77, 78].

Expression microarrays and chromatin immunoprecipitation assays (ChIP) have helped researchers identify MYC-regulated targets as well as link MYC-target expression to functional cellular pathways which are associated with transformation [79, 80]. MYC and MYCN-regulated targets have since been linked to a number of transforming activities involving the cell cycle (eg. cyclin D2, CDK4, p21), cell proliferation (e.g. MDM2), growth, metabolism (e.g. ribosomal proteins, proteins involved in nucleotide biosynthesis such as thymidylate synthase and ODC1), cell adhesion and migration (e.g. integrins) and angiogenesis (e.g. thrombospondin) [81-86]. Indeed, the activation and repression of MYC target genes is a well-coordinated event. Time course studies using microarray have identified differences between early and delayed gene expression responses, following MYC activation in a MYC-inducible cell system [87]. Early-response MYC target genes are primarily involved in MAPK signalling, RNA metabolism and transcription factors, which suggests a program that prepares cells for entry into the S phase. On the other hand, delayed-response MYC target genes are involved in ribosomal biogenesis, nucleotide metabolism and energy metabolism, suggesting subsequent maintenance of cells during the S phase. Finally, late steady-state MYC-mediated transcription involved genes that regulate the cell cycle, nucleotide metabolism and DNA replication. Most genes that were activated in the early response were then repressed during this late steady-state phase. Furthermore, sustained MYC activation led to the silencing of differentiation-related genes and upregulation of genes that are involved cell proliferation.

During tumorigenesis, MYCN promotes cell cycle progression by the activation of cyclins (such as cyclin D1 and D2) as well as cyclin-dependent kinase 4 (CDK4), and represses the expression of mediators of cell cycle arrest such as p21 [73]. One important MYCN-regulated metabolic pathway involves the synthesis of polyamines, which are organic cations that enhance transcription, translation and replication [88]. *MYCN* expression is strongly correlated with *ODC1* expression in neuroblastoma, and the high levels of *ODC1* expression that are driven by *MYCN*-amplification and over-expression are strongly associated with poor clinical outcome of this disease [89].

Another gene whose expression is strongly correlated with *MYCN* expression in neuroblastoma is that encoding the multidrug resistance-associated protein, MRP1, a glycoprotein that belongs to the superfamily of ATP-binding cassette (ABC) transmembrane transporters [90-92]. MRP1, also known as ABCC1, is able to confer resistance to a broad range of structurally unrelated chemotherapeutic drugs [93]. MRP1 has since been shown to be a downstream transcriptional target of MYCN in neuroblastoma, whose expression is highly predictive of outcome in this disease [91, 94, 95]. The expression of another gene that is also a member of the ABC family of transporters, *MRP4* (or *ABCC4*), has also been demonstrated to be positively correlated to *MYCN* expression in neuroblastoma and like *MRP1*, its over-expression is a prognostic indicator of neuroblastoma outcome [95, 96]. In fact, it has recently been shown that MYCN can coordinate the transcription of a large set of *ABC* genes, and the expression profiles of these genes correlate with MYCN function [48].

9. MYCN tumorigenesis

The evidence for a clinical role of MYCN in the tumorigenesis of neuroblastoma was first recognised when the amplification of the *MYCN* oncogene was identified in 24 out of 63 primary untreated neuroblastoma tumour samples and appeared to correlate with more advanced stage of disease [97]. *MYCN*-amplification was subsequently associated with rapid disease progression as well as poor patient outcome in this disease [98]. Importantly, the progression-free survival of neuroblastoma patients was then shown to be dose-dependent on *MYCN* where higher copy number resulted in lower survival. This association was independent of patient age and disease stage. *MYCN*-amplification was later confirmed in numerous studies to be a powerful prognostic marker for predicting neuroblastoma patient outcome, independent of other clinical variables [99-102]. Determination of *MYCN* amplification status is now routinely determined in primary neuroblastomas and is one of the most powerful prognostic markers yet identified for this disease.

The MYCN oncogene is normally located on the distal short arm of chromosome 2 (2p24). This region was found to be amplified across a panel of neuroblastoma cell lines [8], and although the exact mechanism by which this occurs is unknown, the process of amplification usually results in 50 to 400 copies of the gene per cell, leading to the production of abnormally high levels of MYCN RNA and protein, presumably conferring a selective advantage to the tumour cell [103].

The potent transforming ability of MYCN has been demonstrated by several studies, while MYCN transfection studies have demonstrated that the oncoprotein plays a crucial role in neuroblastoma progression [104, 105]. Conditional overexpression of MYCN in neuroblastoma cell lines was shown to dramatically increase the growth rates and metastatic ability of these tumour cells, increase DNA synthesis, and inhibit exit from the cell cycle and neuronal differentiation [106, 107]. Furthermore, targeted expression of the MYCN oncogene in neuroectodermal cells of transgenic mice resulted in the development of neuroblastoma [3]. In these animals, human MYCN (hMYCN) oncogene expression was targeted to neural crest cells via an upstream rat tyrosine hydroxylase promoter. Tyrosine hydroxylase is the first and rate-limiting step in catecholamine synthesis. In contrast, reduction in the MYCN RNA levels via introduction of MYCN antisense oligonucleotides in vitro as well as in vivo led to reduced rates of growth and of tumorigenicity [4, 108, 109].

Whilst MYCN-amplification has been shown to be associated with a highly malignant neuroblastoma phenotype, the precise role of this oncogene in non-amplified tumours remains controversial. Approximately 40% of those neuroblastomas that lack MYCN-amplification are nevertheless still clinically aggressive, and the clinical significance of MYCN expression in the absence of MYCN-amplification, remains elusive with evidence both for and against an association with adverse outcome [110, 111]. One study that analysed both MYCN mRNA and protein levels in a cohort of non-amplified tumours, found no prognostic significance attributable to expression of this oncogene [110]. Rather, since the survival rates for older children with or without high MYCN expression were poor, the results suggested that additional factors contribute to tumour aggressiveness in this subgroup. Furthermore, in a more recent study involving 91 neuroblastoma patients, high MYCN expression was found to be associated with a favourable outcome in neuroblastomas lacking MYCN-amplification [111]. Interestingly, in this study, the forced expression of MYCN significantly suppressed growth of non-amplified neuroblastoma cells by inducing apoptosis. It is possible that the prognostic value of MYCN gene expression in neuroblastoma may be an artefact of the different biology of neuroblastoma in infants compared to older children, and further well-controlled, large cohort studies will be needed in order to clarify the precise role of MYCN in non-amplified neuroblastoma.

Although the majority of the literature investigating MYCN in cancer comes from studies on neuroblastoma, this oncogene has also been shown to play a role in the tumorigenesis of other cancers, both adult and paediatric. For example, MYCN amplification and/or overexpression has been observed in high grade C5 serous ovarian tumours, small cell lung cancer, rhabdomyosarcoma and neuroendocrine prostate cancer [112-115], while gain of 2p (and *MYCN*) plays a role in chronic lymphocytic leukaemia [116]. In childhood medulloblastoma, MYCN, c-MYC, and to a lesser extent MYCL, appear to be involved in the biology of this disease [117]. *MYCN* amplification occurs in up to 10% of medulloblastoma patients and is associated with poor clinical outcome, and like neuroblastoma, the risk of death increases with increasing copy number [117]. Furthermore, *MYCN* expression was found to be high in foetal cerebella, with the levels decreasing to almost absent in adult cerebella, suggesting that MYCN is essential to normal foetal development [118]. Interestingly, in this study, *MYCN* expression was absent from the medulloblastoma cell lines tested, which differed from the expression pattern observed in the primary tumours [118]. Finally, as with neuroblastoma, the association of *MYCN* mRNA levels with clinical outcome remains unclear [119] and it has been postulated that mRNA levels of both *c-MYC* and *MYCN* may only be clinically relevant in subgroups of medulloblastoma [117].

The most compelling evidence for a role of MYCN in the biology of medulloblastoma comes from two mouse models of this disease. Firstly, targeted expression of MYCN to the cerebellum in transgenic mice has demonstrated the importance of MYCN in contributing to the initiation and progression of medulloblastoma and also in the metastatic spread of disease to the spinal and paraspinal tissues via cerebral spinal fluid. Furthermore, the MYCN downstream targets Odc1, MDM2 and Fb1 were upregulated and correlated with *MYCN* mRNA levels [118]. The second model used targeted Smoothened (SmoA1) to the cerebella of transgenic mice, which were then crossed with mice harbouring conditional knock-out of MYCN, to demonstrate that MYCN was essential for medulloblastoma tumorigenesis [120]. These two models thus serve to demonstrate the importance of MYCN in the initiation and progression of this disease.

10. Molecular targeting of MYCN for therapeutic benefit

Molecular targeted therapy involves targeting malignant cell growth by directly inhibiting the function of specific molecules within a cell, namely those that are responsible for driving cancer progression. Such agents aim to block or exploit various aspects of cancer biology, such as genetic instability, proliferative signal transduction, aberrant cell cycle control, deregulated survival, angiogenesis and metastasis [121]. Numerous methods of molecular targeted therapy have been investigated, including antisense oligonucleotides (ASOs) that hybridise to and inhibit the mRNA of a specific gene; peptide nucleic acids (PNAs), which are DNA analogues that specifically hybridise to DNA and/or RNA in a complementary manner to inhibit transcription/translation of a target gene; and small interfering RNA (siRNA), which silences gene expression by inducing the sequence specific degradation of complementary mRNA or by inhibiting translation [122]. However, such technologies although useful in the laboratory, have had limited success in the clinic due to problems associated with their delivery.

Immunotherapy has also generated interest, and utilises the body's immune system to target and remove cancer cells by the recognition of certain molecular markers, or block specific cell receptor pathways. Another approach to molecular targeting, involves the development of synthetic small molecule inhibitors which potentially have the ability to interfere with a molecular target at multiple levels [122]. These small molecules may diffuse into cells to act directly on intracellular targets, such as inhibiting the expression of a target gene at the transcriptional or translational level, or inhibiting the function of a protein by directly binding to the protein and inducing conformational changes that prevent its interaction with other factors [123]. Synthetic small molecules are generally defined by a molecular weight cut-off of <500Da. They are favoured by the pharmaceutical industry because of their attractive pharmacokinetic properties, especially tumour cell penetration, and their relative ease of development and pharmaceutical production [123]. At present, strategies to develop novel small molecule inhibitors as viable therapies are aimed at using these technologies in combination with other cytotoxic drugs, with the hope of reducing drug dosages, and thus overcoming drug resistance associated with intensive chemotherapy, and reducing drug-related toxicity and side effects.

A number of molecular mechanisms have been identified as possible targets for the treatment of neuroblastoma. However, the prominent deregulated expression and amplification of *MYCN* suggests that this oncogene represents an ideal target for therapeutic inhibition [124]. In addition, normal MYCN expression is restricted to the early stages of embryonic development and is virtually undetectable in normal post-natal tissues, therefore weighing in its favour as a target for inhibition. Inhibition of *MYCN* expression by antisense treatment against *MYCN* mRNA or by retinoic acid has been demonstrated to decrease proliferation and induce neuronal differentiation in neuroblastoma cells [125-127]. Furthermore, the introduction of *MYCN* antisense oligonucleotides in the human *MYCN* (*hMYCN*) trangenic mouse model led to reduced rates of tumour growth in these animals [4, 108, 109].

Inhibition of MYCN protein through its protein-protein interactions and protein-DNA interactions was previously seen as too difficult to target by small molecules [128]. However, it has been reported that small-molecule antagonists of MYC/MAX dimerisation interfered with c-MYC-induced oncogenic transformation of chicken embryo fibroblasts *in vitro* [129]. In addition, a number of endogenous MYCN/MAX antagonists such as MAX/MAX have been found to compete for binding to E-box sequences and repress transcription [130], causing cell cycle arrest, terminal differentiation or apoptosis. More recently, inhibition of c-MYC transcription via a Bromodomain and Extra Terminal Domain (BET) inhibitor, JQ1, has been described [131]. This inhibitor has been shown to disrupt c-MYC mRNA synthesis by preventing the recruitment of coactivator proteins required for c-MYC transcriptional initiation and mRNA elongation [131]. Furthermore, this molecule was able to decrease the tumour burden in an orthotopic mouse model of multiple myeloma. Treatment of several MYCN-amplified neuroblastoma cell lines with JQ1, resulted in a decrease in MYCN expression, although this effect was far less dramatic that that observed in a c-MYC driven cell line [132]. Despite promising evidence for targeting MYCN as a therapeutic strategy, no MYC or MYCN inhibitors have yet entered clinical trial, and further studies are required to develop effective MYCN inhibitors.

11. Future perspectives

The validity for targeting MYCN for therapeutic benefit relies on the gross transforming ability of this transcription factor. MYCN represents a particularly attractive target due to its lack of expression in adult and normal paediatric tissues. Although MYCN, and MYC proteins in general are commonly viewed as "undruggable" due to the nature of these proteins, MYCN offers potential advantages at a number of levels for therapeutic inhibition, either upstream, or downstream along the MYCN transcriptional pathway. If clinically useful MYCN inhibitors can be successfully developed, they are likely to find application in combination therapies involving conventional chemotherapeutic drugs and be used as an improved approach to target aggressive cancers that are driven by this oncoprotein.

Author details

Leanna Cheung, Jayne E. Murray, Michelle Haber and Murray D. Norris
Children's Cancer Institute Australia for Medical Research, Lowy Cancer Research Centre, UNSW, Sydney, Australia

12. References

[1] Cowling, V.H. and M.D. Cole, *Mechanism of transcriptional activation by the Myc oncoproteins.* Semin Cancer Biol, 2006. 16(4): p. 242-52.

[2] Grimmer, M.R. and W.A. Weiss, *Childhood tumors of the nervous system as disorders of normal development.* Curr Opin Pediatr, 2006. 18(6): p. 634-8.

[3] Weiss, W.A., et al., *Targeted expression of MYCN causes neuroblastoma in transgenic mice.* EMBO J, 1997. 16(11): p. 2985-95.

[4] Burkhart, C.A., et al., *Effects of MYCN antisense oligonucleotide administration on tumorigenesis in a murine model of neuroblastoma.* J Natl Cancer Inst, 2003. 95(18): p. 1394-403.

[5] Varmus, H.E., *The molecular genetics of cellular oncogenes.* Annu Rev Genet, 1984. 18: p. 553-612.

[6] Hayward, W.S., B.G. Neel, and S.M. Astrin, *Activation of a cellular onc gene by promoter insertion in ALV-induced lymphoid leukosis.* Nature, 1981. 290(5806): p. 475-80.

[7] Payne, G.S., J.M. Bishop, and H.E. Varmus, *Multiple arrangements of viral DNA and an activated host oncogene in bursal lymphomas.* Nature, 1982. 295(5846): p. 209-14.

[8] Schwab, M., et al., *Amplified DNA with limited homology to myc cellular oncogene is shared by human neuroblastoma cell lines and a neuroblastoma tumour.* Nature, 1983. 305(5931): p. 245-8.

[9] Schwab, M., *MYCN in neuronal tumours.* Cancer Lett, 2004. 204(2): p. 179-87.

[10] Yaylim-Eraltan, I., et al., *L-myc gene polymorphism and risk of thyroid cancer.* Exp Oncol, 2008. 30(2): p. 117-20.

[11] Kumimoto, H., et al., *L-myc genotype is associated with different susceptibility to lung cancer in smokers.* Jpn J Cancer Res, 2002. 93(1): p. 1-5.

[12] Nau, M.M., et al., *L-myc, a new myc-related gene amplified and expressed in human small cell lung cancer.* Nature, 1985. 318(6041): p. 69-73.

[13] Adhikary, S. and M. Eilers, *Transcriptional regulation and transformation by Myc proteins.* Nat Rev Mol Cell Biol, 2005. 6(8): p. 635-45.

[14] Meyer, N. and L.Z. Penn, *Reflecting on 25 years with MYC.* Nat Rev Cancer, 2008. 8(12): p. 976-90.

[15] Pelengaris, S., M. Khan, and G.I. Evan, *Suppression of Myc-induced apoptosis in beta cells exposes multiple oncogenic properties of Myc and triggers carcinogenic progression.* Cell, 2002. 109(3): p. 321-34.

[16] Marcu, K.B., S.A. Bossone, and A.J. Patel, *myc function and regulation.* Annu Rev Biochem, 1992. 61: p. 809-60.

[17] Cole, M.D. and V.H. Cowling, *Transcription-independent functions of MYC: regulation of translation and DNA replication.* Nat Rev Mol Cell Biol, 2008. 9(10): p. 810-5.

[18] Ramsay, G., et al., *Human proto-oncogene N-myc encodes nuclear proteins that bind DNA.* Mol Cell Biol, 1986. 6(12): p. 4450-7.

[19] Hamann, U., et al., *The MYCN protein of human neuroblastoma cells is phosphorylated by casein kinase II in the central region and at serine 367.* Oncogene, 1991. 6(10): p. 1745-51.

[20] Vervoorts, J., J. Luscher-Firzlaff, and B. Luscher, *The ins and outs of MYC regulation by posttranslational mechanisms.* J Biol Chem, 2006. 281(46): p. 34725-9.

[21] Blackwood, E.M. and R.N. Eisenman, *Max: a helix-loop-helix zipper protein that forms a sequence-specific DNA-binding complex with Myc.* Science, 1991. 251(4998): p. 1211-7.

[22] Wenzel, A., et al., *The N-Myc oncoprotein is associated in vivo with the phosphoprotein Max(p20/22) in human neuroblastoma cells.* EMBO J, 1991. 10(12): p. 3703-12.

[23] Sakamuro, D. and G.C. Prendergast, *New Myc-interacting proteins: a second Myc network emerges.* Oncogene, 1999. 18(19): p. 2942-54.

[24] Bannasch, D., I. Weis, and M. Schwab, *Nmi protein interacts with regions that differ between MycN and Myc and is localized in the cytoplasm of neuroblastoma cells in contrast to nuclear MycN.* Oncogene, 1999. 18(48): p. 6810-7.

[25] Wood, M.A., S.B. McMahon, and M.D. Cole, *An ATPase/helicase complex is an essential cofactor for oncogenic transformation by c-Myc.* Mol Cell, 2000. 5(2): p. 321-30.

[26] Bannasch, D., B. Madge, and M. Schwab, *Functional interaction of Yaf2 with the central region of MycN.* Oncogene, 2001. 20(41): p. 5913-9.

[27] Herbst, A., et al., *A conserved element in Myc that negatively regulates its proapoptotic activity.* EMBO Rep, 2005. 6(2): p. 177-83.

[28] Cowling, V.H., et al., *A conserved Myc protein domain, MBIV, regulates DNA binding, apoptosis, transformation, and G2 arrest.* Mol Cell Biol, 2006. 26(11): p. 4226-39.

[29] Cotterman, R., et al., *N-Myc regulates a widespread euchromatic program in the human genome partially independent of its role as a classical transcription factor.* Cancer Res, 2008. 68(23): p. 9654-62.

[30] Knoepfler, P.S., *Myc goes global: new tricks for an old oncogene.* Cancer Res, 2007. 67(11): p. 5061-3.

[31] Cowling, V.H. and M.D. Cole, *The Myc transactivation domain promotes global phosphorylation of the RNA polymerase II carboxy-terminal domain independently of direct DNA binding.* Mol Cell Biol, 2007. 27(6): p. 2059-73.

[32] Dominguez-Sola, D., et al., *Non-transcriptional control of DNA replication by c-Myc.* Nature, 2007. 448(7152): p. 445-51.

[33] McMahon, S.B., M.A. Wood, and M.D. Cole, *The essential cofactor TRRAP recruits the histone acetyltransferase hGCN5 to c-Myc.* Mol Cell Biol, 2000. 20(2): p. 556-62.

[34] Strahl, B.D. and C.D. Allis, *The language of covalent histone modifications.* Nature, 2000. 403(6765): p. 41-5.

[35] Ikura, T., et al., *Involvement of the TIP60 histone acetylase complex in DNA repair and apoptosis.* Cell, 2000. 102(4): p. 463-73.

[36] Frank, S.R., et al., *Binding of c-Myc to chromatin mediates mitogen-induced acetylation of histone H4 and gene activation.* Genes Dev, 2001. 15(16): p. 2069-82.

[37] Shen, X., et al., *A chromatin remodelling complex involved in transcription and DNA processing.* Nature, 2000. 406(6795): p. 541-4.

[38] Eberhardy, S.R. and P.J. Farnham, *Myc recruits P-TEFb to mediate the final step in the transcriptional activation of the cad promoter.* J Biol Chem, 2002. 277(42): p. 40156-62.

[39] Marhin, W.W., et al., *Myc represses the growth arrest gene gadd45.* Oncogene, 1997. 14(23): p. 2825-34.

[40] Wu, S., et al., *Myc represses differentiation-induced p21CIP1 expression via Miz-1-dependent interaction with the p21 core promoter.* Oncogene, 2003. 22(3): p. 351-60.

[41] Judware, R. and L.A. Culp, *Over-expression of transfected N-myc oncogene in human SKNSH neuroblastoma cells down-regulates expression of beta 1 integrin subunit.* Oncogene, 1995. 11(12): p. 2599-607.

[42] Cleveland, J.L., et al., *Negative regulation of c-myc transcription involves myc family proteins.* Oncogene Res, 1988. 3(4): p. 357-75.

[43] Grignani, F., et al., *Negative autoregulation of c-myc gene expression is inactivated in transformed cells.* EMBO J, 1990. 9(12): p. 3913-22.

[44] Bell, E., et al., *MYCN oncoprotein targets and their therapeutic potential.* Cancer Lett, 2010. 293(2): p. 144-57.

[45] Liu, T., et al., *Activation of tissue transglutaminase transcription by histone deacetylase inhibition as a therapeutic approach for Myc oncogenesis.* Proc Natl Acad Sci U S A, 2007. 104(47): p. 18682-7.

[46] Tucholski, J., M. Lesort, and G.V. Johnson, *Tissue transglutaminase is essential for neurite outgrowth in human neuroblastoma SH-SY5Y cells.* Neuroscience, 2001. 102(2): p. 481-91.

[47] Zeng, H., et al., *Transport of amphipathic anions by human multidrug resistance protein 3.* Cancer Res, 2000. 60(17): p. 4779-84.

[48] Porro, A., et al., *Direct and coordinate regulation of ATP-binding cassette transporter genes by Myc factors generates specific transcription signatures that significantly affect the chemoresistance phenotype of cancer cells.* J Biol Chem, 2010. 285(25): p. 19532-43.

[49] Paumi, C.M., et al., *Multidrug resistance protein (MRP) 1 and MRP3 attenuate cytotoxic and transactivating effects of the cyclopentenone prostaglandin, 15-deoxy-Delta(12,14)prostaglandin J2 in MCF7 breast cancer cells.* Biochemistry, 2003. 42(18): p. 5429-37.

[50] Hatzi, E., et al., *N-myc oncogene overexpression down-regulates IL-6; evidence that IL-6 inhibits angiogenesis and suppresses neuroblastoma tumor growth.* Oncogene, 2002. 21(22): p. 3552-61.

[51] Schneider, A., et al., *Association of Myc with the zinc-finger protein Miz-1 defines a novel pathway for gene regulation by Myc.* Curr Top Microbiol Immunol, 1997. 224: p. 137-46.

[52] Peukert, K., et al., *An alternative pathway for gene regulation by Myc.* EMBO J, 1997. 16(18): p. 5672-86.

[53] Ikegaki, N., et al., *De novo identification of MIZ-1 (ZBTB17) encoding a MYC-interacting zinc-finger protein as a new favorable neuroblastoma gene.* Clin Cancer Res, 2007. 13(20): p. 6001-9.

[54] Wanzel, M., S. Herold, and M. Eilers, *Transcriptional repression by Myc.* Trends Cell Biol, 2003. 13(3): p. 146-50.

[55] Brenner, C., et al., *Myc represses transcription through recruitment of DNA methyltransferase corepressor.* EMBO J, 2005. 24(2): p. 336-46.

[56] Schwab, M., *Human neuroblastoma: from basic science to clinical debut of cellular oncogenes.* Naturwissenschaften, 1999. 86(2): p. 71-8.

[57] Laird-Offringa, I.A., *What determines the instability of c-myc proto-oncogene mRNA?* Bioessays, 1992. 14(2): p. 119-24.

[58] Mirsky, R., et al., *Novel signals controlling embryonic Schwann cell development, myelination and dedifferentiation.* J Peripher Nerv Syst, 2008. 13(2): p. 122-35.

[59] Stanton, B.R., et al., *Loss of N-myc function results in embryonic lethality and failure of the epithelial component of the embryo to develop.* Genes Dev, 1992. 6(12A): p. 2235-47.

[60] Strieder, V. and W. Lutz, *E2F proteins regulate MYCN expression in neuroblastomas.* J Biol Chem, 2003. 278(5): p. 2983-9.

[61] Morrow, M.A., et al., *Interleukin-7 induces N-myc and c-myc expression in normal precursor B lymphocytes.* Genes Dev, 1992. 6(1): p. 61-70.

[62] Wada, R.K., et al., *Cell type-specific expression and negative regulation by retinoic acid of the human N-myc promoter in neuroblastoma cells.* Oncogene, 1992. 7(4): p. 711-7.

[63] Bentley, D.L. and M. Groudine, *A block to elongation is largely responsible for decreased transcription of c-myc in differentiated HL60 cells.* Nature, 1986. 321(6071): p. 702-6.

[64] Sivak, L.E., et al., *A novel intron element operates posttranscriptionally To regulate human N-myc expression.* Mol Cell Biol, 1999. 19(1): p. 155-63.

[65] Keene, R.G., et al., *Transcriptional pause, arrest and termination sites for RNA polymerase II in mammalian N- and c-myc genes.* Nucleic Acids Res, 1999. 27(15): p. 3173-82.

[66] Xu, L., S.D. Morgenbesser, and R.A. DePinho, *Complex transcriptional regulation of myc family gene expression in the developing mouse brain and liver.* Mol Cell Biol, 1991. 11(12): p. 6007-15.

[67] Brewer, G. and J. Ross, *Poly(A) shortening and degradation of the 3' A+U-rich sequences of human c-myc mRNA in a cell-free system.* Mol Cell Biol, 1988. 8(4): p. 1697-708.

[68] Ross, J., *mRNA stability in mammalian cells.* Microbiol Rev, 1995. 59(3): p. 423-50.

[69] Bernstein, P.L., et al., *Control of c-myc mRNA half-life in vitro by a protein capable of binding to a coding region stability determinant.* Genes Dev, 1992. 6(4): p. 642-54.

[70] Chagnovich, D. and S.L. Cohn, *Activity of a 40 kDa RNA-binding protein correlates with MYCN and c-fos mRNA stability in human neuroblastoma.* Eur J Cancer, 1997. 33(12): p. 2064-7.

[71] Jopling, C.L. and A.E. Willis, *N-myc translation is initiated via an internal ribosome entry segment that displays enhanced activity in neuronal cells.* Oncogene, 2001. 20(21): p. 2664-70.

[72] Sjostrom, S.K., et al., *The Cdk1 complex plays a prime role in regulating N-myc phosphorylation and turnover in neural precursors.* Dev Cell, 2005. 9(3): p. 327-38.

[73] Knoepfler, P.S., P.F. Cheng, and R.N. Eisenman, *N-myc is essential during neurogenesis for the rapid expansion of progenitor cell populations and the inhibition of neuronal differentiation.* Genes Dev, 2002. 16(20): p. 2699-712.

[74] Kim, H.T., et al., *Certain pairs of ubiquitin-conjugating enzymes (E2s) and ubiquitin-protein ligases (E3s) synthesize nondegradable forked ubiquitin chains containing all possible isopeptide linkages.* J Biol Chem, 2007. 282(24): p. 17375-86.

[75] Eilers, M., S. Schirm, and J.M. Bishop, *The MYC protein activates transcription of the alpha-prothymosin gene.* EMBO J, 1991. 10(1): p. 133-41.

[76] Bello-Fernandez, C., G. Packham, and J.L. Cleveland, *The ornithine decarboxylase gene is a transcriptional target of c-Myc.* Proc Natl Acad Sci U S A, 1993. 90(16): p. 7804-8.

[77] Grandori, C. and R.N. Eisenman, *Myc target genes.* Trends Biochem Sci, 1997. 22(5): p. 177-81.

[78] Cole, M.D. and S.B. McMahon, *The Myc oncoprotein: a critical evaluation of transactivation and target gene regulation.* Oncogene, 1999. 18(19): p. 2916-24.

[79] Zeller, K.I., et al., *An integrated database of genes responsive to the Myc oncogenic transcription factor: identification of direct genomic targets.* Genome Biol, 2003. 4(10): p. R69.

[80] Guccione, E., et al., *Myc-binding-site recognition in the human genome is determined by chromatin context.* Nat Cell Biol, 2006. 8(7): p. 764-70.

[81] McMahon, S.B., *Control of nucleotide biosynthesis by the MYC oncoprotein.* Cell Cycle, 2008. 7(15): p. 2275-6.

[82] Bell, E., J. Lunec, and D.A. Tweddle, *Cell cycle regulation targets of MYCN identified by gene expression microarrays.* Cell Cycle, 2007. 6(10): p. 1249-56.

[83] Lastowska, M., et al., *Identification of candidate genes involved in neuroblastoma progression by combining genomic and expression microarrays with survival data.* Oncogene, 2007. 26(53): p. 7432-44.

[84] Dang, C.V., et al., *The c-Myc target gene network.* Semin Cancer Biol, 2006. 16(4): p. 253-64.

[85] Nesbit, C.E., J.M. Tersak, and E.V. Prochownik, *MYC oncogenes and human neoplastic disease.* Oncogene, 1999. 18(19): p. 3004-16.

[86] Slack, A., G. Lozano, and J.M. Shohet, *MDM2 as MYCN transcriptional target: implications for neuroblastoma pathogenesis.* Cancer Lett, 2005. 228(1-2): p. 21-7.

[87] Fan, J., et al., *Time-dependent c-Myc transactomes mapped by Array-based nuclear run-on reveal transcriptional modules in human B cells.* PLoS One, 2010. 5(3): p. e9691.

[88] Pegg, A.E., *Polyamine metabolism and its importance in neoplastic growth and a target for chemotherapy.* Cancer Res, 1988. 48(4): p. 759-74.

[89] Hogarty, M.D., et al., *ODC1 is a critical determinant of MYCN oncogenesis and a therapeutic target in neuroblastoma.* Cancer Res, 2008. 68(23): p. 9735-45.

[90] Bordow, S.B., et al., *Expression of the multidrug resistance-associated protein (MRP) gene correlates with amplification and overexpression of the N-myc oncogene in childhood neuroblastoma.* Cancer Res, 1994. 54(19): p. 5036-40.

[91] Norris, M.D., et al., *Expression of the gene for multidrug-resistance-associated protein and outcome in patients with neuroblastoma.* N Engl J Med, 1996. 334(4): p. 231-8.

[92] Haber, M., et al., *Altered expression of the MYCN oncogene modulates MRP gene expression and response to cytotoxic drugs in neuroblastoma cells.* Oncogene, 1999. 18(17): p. 2777-82.

[93] Munoz, M., et al., *Role of the MRP1/ABCC1 multidrug transporter protein in cancer.* IUBMB Life, 2007. 59(12): p. 752-7.

[94] Manohar, C.F., et al., *MYCN-mediated regulation of the MRP1 promoter in human neuroblastoma.* Oncogene, 2004. 23(3): p. 753-62.

[95] Henderson, M.J., et al., *ABCC multidrug transporters in childhood neuroblastoma: clinical and biological effects independent of cytotoxic drug efflux.* J Natl Cancer Inst, 2011. 103(16): p. 1236-51.

[96] Norris, M.D., et al., *Expression of multidrug transporter MRP4/ABCC4 is a marker of poor prognosis in neuroblastoma and confers resistance to irinotecan in vitro.* Mol Cancer Ther, 2005. 4(4): p. 547-53.

[97] Brodeur, G.M., et al., *Amplification of N-myc in untreated human neuroblastomas correlates with advanced disease stage.* Science, 1984. 224(4653): p. 1121-4.

[98] Seeger, R.C., et al., *Association of multiple copies of the N-myc oncogene with rapid progression of neuroblastomas.* N Engl J Med, 1985. 313(18): p. 1111-6.

[99] Bartram, C.R. and F. Berthold, *Amplification and expression of the N-myc gene in neuroblastoma.* Eur J Pediatr, 1987. 146(2): p. 162-5.

[100] Nakagawara, A., et al., *Amplification of N-myc oncogene in stage II and IVS neuroblastomas may be a prognostic indicator.* J Pediatr Surg, 1987. 22(5): p. 415-8.

[101] Brodeur, G.M., et al., *International criteria for diagnosis, staging, and response to treatment in patients with neuroblastoma.* J Clin Oncol, 1988. 6(12): p. 1874-81.

[102] Brodeur, G.M. and C.T. Fong, *Molecular biology and genetics of human neuroblastoma.* Cancer Genet Cytogenet, 1989. 41(2): p. 153-74.

[103] Amler, L.C. and M. Schwab, *Multiple amplicons of discrete sizes encompassing N-myc in neuroblastoma cells evolve through differential recombination from a large precursor DNA.* Oncogene, 1992. 7(4): p. 807-9.

[104] Brodeur, G.M., *Neuroblastoma: clinical significance of genetic abnormalities.* Cancer Surv, 1990. 9(4): p. 673-88.

[105] Xu, L., et al., *Loss of transcriptional attenuation in N-myc is associated with progression towards a more malignant phenotype.* Oncogene, 1995. 11(9): p. 1865-72.

[106] Bogenmann, E., M. Torres, and H. Matsushima, *Constitutive N-myc gene expression inhibits trkA mediated neuronal differentiation.* Oncogene, 1995. 10(10): p. 1915-25.

[107] Lutz, W., et al., *Conditional expression of N-myc in human neuroblastoma cells increases expression of alpha-prothymosin and ornithine decarboxylase and accelerates progression into S-phase early after mitogenic stimulation of quiescent cells.* Oncogene, 1996. 13(4): p. 803-12.

[108] Whitesell, L., A. Rosolen, and L.M. Neckers, *Antisense suppression of N-myc expression inhibits the transdifferentiation of neuroectoderm tumor cell lines.* Prog Clin Biol Res, 1991. 366: p. 45-54.

[109] Whitesell, L., A. Rosolen, and L.M. Neckers, *In vivo modulation of N-myc expression by continuous perfusion with an antisense oligonucleotide.* Antisense Res Dev, 1991. 1(4): p. 343-50.

[110] Cohn, S.L., et al., *MYCN expression is not prognostic of adverse outcome in advanced-stage neuroblastoma with nonamplified MYCN.* J Clin Oncol, 2000. 18(21): p. 3604-13.

[111] Tang, X.X., et al., *The MYCN enigma: significance of MYCN expression in neuroblastoma.* Cancer Res, 2006. 66(5): p. 2826-33.

[112] Tonelli, R., et al., *Antitumor activity of sustained N-myc reduction in rhabdomyosarcomas and transcriptional block by antigene therapy.* Clin Cancer Res, 2012. 18(3): p. 796-807.

[113] Helland, A., et al., *Deregulation of MYCN, LIN28B and LET7 in a molecular subtype of aggressive high-grade serous ovarian cancers.* PLoS One, 2011. 6(4): p. e18064.

[114] Kim, Y.H., et al., *Combined microarray analysis of small cell lung cancer reveals altered apoptotic balance and distinct expression signatures of MYC family gene amplification.* Oncogene, 2006. 25(1): p. 130-8.

[115] Beltran, H., et al., *Molecular Characterization of Neuroendocrine Prostate Cancer and Identification of New Drug Targets.* Cancer Discov, 2011. 1(6): p. 487-495.

[116] Ma, D., et al., *Array Comparative Genomic Hybridization Analysis Identifies Recurrent Gain of Chromosome 2p25.3 Involving the ACP1 and MYCN Genes in Chronic Lymphocytic Leukemia.* Clinical Lymphoma Myeloma and Leukemia, 2011. 11, Supplement 1(0): p. S17-S24.

[117] Ryan, S.L., et al., *MYC family amplification and clinical risk-factors interact to predict an extremely poor prognosis in childhood medulloblastoma.* Acta Neuropathol, 2012. 123(4): p. 501-13.

[118] Swartling, F.J., et al., *Pleiotropic role for MYCN in medulloblastoma.* Genes Dev, 2010. 24(10): p. 1059-72.

[119] Eberhart, C.G., et al., *Histopathological and molecular prognostic markers in medulloblastoma: c-myc, N-myc, TrkC, and anaplasia.* J Neuropathol Exp Neurol, 2004. 63(5): p. 441-9.

[120] Hatton, B.A., et al., *N-myc is an essential downstream effector of Shh signaling during both normal and neoplastic cerebellar growth.* Cancer Res, 2006. 66(17): p. 8655-61.

[121] Garrett, M.D. and P. Workman, *Discovering novel chemotherapeutic drugs for the third millennium.* Eur J Cancer, 1999. 35(14): p. 2010-30.

[122] Vita, M. and M. Henriksson, *The Myc oncoprotein as a therapeutic target for human cancer.* Semin Cancer Biol, 2006. 16(4): p. 318-30.

[123] Jain, R.K., *Delivery of novel therapeutic agents in tumors: physiological barriers and strategies.* J Natl Cancer Inst, 1989. 81(8): p. 570-6.

[124] Lu, X., A. Pearson, and J. Lunec, *The MYCN oncoprotein as a drug development target.* Cancer Lett, 2003. 197(1-2): p. 125-30.

[125] Negroni, A., et al., *Decrease of proliferation rate and induction of differentiation by a MYCN antisense DNA oligomer in a human neuroblastoma cell line.* Cell Growth Differ, 1991. 2(10): p. 511-8.

[126] Marshall, G.M., et al., *Increased retinoic acid receptor gamma expression suppresses the malignant phenotype and alters the differentiation potential of human neuroblastoma cells.* Oncogene, 1995. 11(3): p. 485-91.

[127] Thiele, C.J., C.P. Reynolds, and M.A. Israel, *Decreased expression of N-myc precedes retinoic acid-induced morphological differentiation of human neuroblastoma.* Nature, 1985. 313(6001): p. 404-6.

[128] Soucek, L., et al., *Modelling Myc inhibition as a cancer therapy.* Nature, 2008. 455(7213): p. 679-83.

[129] Berg, T., et al., *Small-molecule antagonists of Myc/Max dimerization inhibit Myc-induced transformation of chicken embryo fibroblasts.* Proc Natl Acad Sci U S A, 2002. 99(6): p. 3830-5.

[130] Facchini, L.M. and L.Z. Penn, *The molecular role of Myc in growth and transformation: recent discoveries lead to new insights.* FASEB J, 1998. 12(9): p. 633-51.

[131] Delmore, J.E., et al., *BET bromodomain inhibition as a therapeutic strategy to target c-Myc.* Cell, 2011. 146(6): p. 904-17.

[132] Mertz, J.A., et al., *Targeting MYC dependence in cancer by inhibiting BET bromodomains.* Proc Natl Acad Sci U S A, 2011. 108(40): p. 16669-74.

Chapter 7

STAT Transcription Factors in Tumor Development and Targeted Therapy of Malignancies

Gordana Konjević, Sandra Radenković, Ana Vuletić,
Katarina Mirjačić Martinović, Vladimir Jurišić and Tatjana Srdić

Additional information is available at the end of the chapter

1. Introduction

The signal transducers and activators of transcription, STAT proteins, were originally discovered in interferon (IFN)-regulated gene transcription in the early 1990's. Since then, a number of cytokines have been recognized to activate various STAT proteins. STATs constitute a family of seven transcription factors, STAT1α/β, STAT2, STAT3α/β, STAT4, STAT5A, STAT5B and STAT6, that transduce signals from a variety of extracellular stimuli initiated by different cytokine families that aside from interferons (interferon α, β and γ) include gp130 cytokines, i.e., IL-6, IL-12, IL-23 and γC cytokines that include IL-2, IL-15 and IL-21 [1].

Although structurally similar, the seven STAT family members possess diverse biological roles and are engaged in numerous processes from embryonic development, organogenesis, cell differentiation to regulation of immune processes. Awareness of their important role in regulation of cell proliferation, differentiation and survival has spurred interest in investigation of their activity in malignant transformation [2]. Evidence has now accumulated that confirms their role in pathogenesis of leukemias and numerous solid tumors [3] (Table1).

Aside from cytokine receptors, STATs are also activated by receptors for growth factors (family of tyrosine kinase receptors) that include receptors for epidermal growth factor - EGFR, platelet-derived growth factor - PDGF, hepatocyte growth factor - HGF and colony-stimulating factor 1- CSF-1 receptors that possess an intrinsic tyrosine kinase activity [4]. These receptors may activate STAT proteins either directly or indirectly by means of JAK kinase proteins. Also, free intracellular enzymes, i.e., non-receptor tyrosine kinases that include oncogenes *src* and *bcr-abl* activate various STATs [5].

Different biological processes regulated by STAT proteins
Embryonic development
Organogenesis and function
Cells proliferation
Cell differentiation, growth and apoptosis
Innate and adoptive immunity
Inflammation
Angiogenesis
Wound healing
Malignant transformation

Table 1. Role of STATs in the organism

Interaction of cytokines and their specific receptors directly activates free intracellular non-receptor enzymes, Janus kinases, and subsequently, latent STAT transcription factors that through the JAK/STAT signaling pathway lead to the expression of numerous genes that regulate important cellular processes. It is of importance that numerous cytokines, growth factors in different cell types activate STAT1, STAT3 and STAT5 and mediate broadly diverse biologic processes that control cell homeostasis. On the other hand, STATs such as STAT4 and STAT6 have a more specific role and they are engaged in T helper cell differentiation and maintenance of equilibrium between Th1 and Th2 immune response [6]. Defects in STAT molecules can lead to serious defects in development and to fetal death indicating the importance of JAK/STAT pathway in normal cell development. Defects in the JAK/STAT signaling pathway are often encountered in primary malignant tumors, as well as in peripheral blood lymphocytes [7,8,9] and STAT3 has been the first to be identified as a potential oncogene [2] (Fig.1).

Given the critical roles of STAT proteins such as activation of pro-inflammatory and anti-proliferative processes by STAT1 and control of cell-cycle progression and apoptosis by STAT3 and STAT5 it has been established in many studies that their dysregulation can contribute to oncogenesis [10] by increasing proliferation and slowing-down apoptosis. In this sense, studies show that STAT3 is activated in a majority of breast and prostate cancers, and that STAT3 inhibition using RNA interference or a dominant negative genotype leads to reduced cell proliferation, survival, and induces wound healing. Further, blocking STAT3 interaction with EGFR using peptide aptamers has been shown to reduce tumor growth. On the other hand, STAT1 has been primarily defined as a tumor suppressor gene and its inactivation was associated with malignant transformation. Initially STAT proteins were extensively studied in leukemias, but later their role in the development of different solid tumors has been shown.

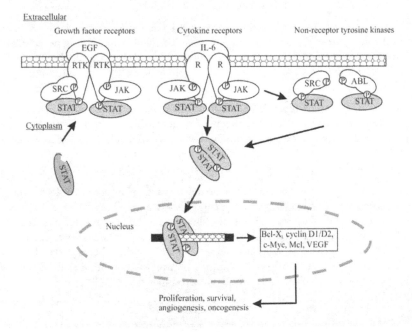

Figure 1. Mechanisms of STAT signaling upon activation of different tyrosine kinase (TK) signaling pathways that can induce activation of STAT proteins. In the case of growth factors like EGF that bind to receptor tyrosine kinases (RTKs), the receptor can directly phosphorylate STATs and/or indirectly induce STAT phosphorylation. Also, cytokines, like IL-6, that bind to cytokine receptors lacking intrinsic TK activity undergo ligand-induced dimerization of the receptor that results in phosphorylation of receptor-associated JAK kinases. JAKs in turn phosphorylate the receptor cytoplasmic tails on tyrosine, providing "docking sites" for recruitment of monomeric STATs. JAKs then phosphorylate the recruited STAT proteins on tyrosine, inducing dimerization, nuclear translocation, and DNA-binding activity. Other non-receptor bound free intracellular enzymes named non-receptor TKs such as SRC family kinases are also involved and can directly induce STAT activation. Once in the nucleus, activated STAT proteins bind to specific DNA sequences in the promoters of genes and induce their expression. In the context of oncogenesis, constitutive activation of TK-STAT signaling pathways induces elevated expression of genes involved in controlling cellular processes such as cell proliferation and survival.

Aside from their role in the development of tumors STAT1,3 and 5 can be considered as molecular markers for early detection of certain types of tumors, as well as prognostic factors for determining tumor aggressiveness and predictors of response to various types of therapy. Novel data also indicate functional interplay between several activated STATs and association of STAT5 with certain well differentiated tumors with favorable prognosis [11].Based on numerous new data it appears that dysregulation of STAT signaling pathway may serve as a basis for designing novel targeted molecular therapeutic strategies that hold great potential for the treatment of solid tumors and leukemias.

1.1. Structural and functional characteristics of STATs

STATs share structurally and functionally conserved domains that include the amino-terminal domain (NH2), the coiled-coiled domain (CCD), the DNA binding domain (DBD), the linker domain and the SH2/tyrosine activation domain [12]. In contrast, the carboxyl-terminal transcriptional activation domain (TAD) is quite divergent and contributes to STAT specificity (Table 2).

Functionally, the amino-terminal domain of STAT molecules is the oligomerization domain that interacts with other proteins and mediates oligomerization of STAT dimers to form tetramers [13]. The DNA binding domain defines the DNA-binding specificity to tandem GAS elements and each STAT component of the dimer recognizes bases in the most proximal half of GAS and mediates distinct signals for specific ligands.

SH2 domain, located near the C-terminal domain, plays an important role in signaling through its capacity to bind to specific phosphotyrosine motifs and to mediate specific interactions. Consistent with this, it is the most highly conserved STAT domain. The ability of this SH2 domain to recognize specific phosphotyrosine motifs plays an essential role in three STAT signaling events that include recruitment to the phosphorylated cytokine receptor through recognition of specific receptor phosphotyrosine motifs, association with the activating JAKs, as well as STAT homo- or heterodimerization [14].

Domain	Role
NH2-terminal domain Oligomerization domain	Interacts with other proteins and mediates oligomerization of STAT dimers to form tetramers
DNA binding domain	Defines the DNA-binding specificity and mediates distinct signals for specific ligands
SH2 domain	Mediates specific interactions between STAT and receptors, STAT and JAK and STAT homo or hetero dimerization
COOH-terminal domain Transcription activation domain (TAD)	TAD regulates the transcriptional activity of STATs and provides specificity
Tyrosine residue	Phosphorylation site in the COOH-terminal domain that regulates the DNA-binding activity of all STATs. On phosphorylation mediates STAT dimerization
Serine residue	A second phosphorylation site in the C-terminal domain

Table 2. STAT structure

Close to the SH2 domain the critical tyrosine residue is located that is required for SH-phosphotyrosine interaction and thus STAT activation. This tyrosine residue is then rapidly phosphorylated by the active JAK determining STAT dimerization by binding to the SH2 domain of the reciprocal STAT molecule.

A conserved serine residue in the C-terminal domain of STAT1,3, and 5 is a second phosphorylation site that enhances DNA binding affinity and transcriptional activity [15]. It has been determined that the transcriptional activity of several STATs can be modulated through serine phosphorylation. Serine phosphorylation appears to enhance the transcription of some, but not all target genes. It has been suggested that serine phosphorylation may alter the affinity for other transcriptional regulators like minichromosome maintenance complex component 5 (MCM5) and BRCA1 [12].

C-terminal domain also encodes transcriptional activation domain (TAD) that contributes to STAT specificity and is thought to be involved in communication with transcriptional complexes, to regulate the transcriptional activity of STATs and provide functional specificity. Altered serine phosphorylation site associated with the c-terminal transactivation domain truncation of STAT1 and STAT3 reduces their transcriptional capacity by 20% [16]. Moreover, a c-TAD truncation leads to the α and β isoforms of STAT proteins that are biologically significant and appear to affect the cell's fate [13].

1.2. Mechanism and regulation of STAT protein function

When ligands bind to their receptors they initiate a cascade of intracellular phosphorylation events. However, members of the hematopoietin receptor family possess no catalytic kinase activity. Rather, they rely on members of the JAK family of tyrosine kinases to provide this activity. JAKs are constitutively associated with a proline-rich domain of these receptors [17]. Upon ligand stimulation, receptors undergo the conformational changes that bring JAKs into proximity of each other, enabling activation by trans-phosphorylation [18]. Once activated, JAKs mediate the described signal transduction. Several studies have also suggested that JAKs associate with the receptor tyrosine kinases [12]. The phosphorylated JAKs, in turn, mediate phosphorylation at the specific receptor tyrosine residues, which then serve as docking sites for STATs and other signaling molecules. Once recruited to the receptor, STATs also become phosphorylated by JAKs, on a single tyrosine residue. The position of these tyrosines in STAT molecule is specific for each member of STAT family of proteins, such as Tyr 701 for STAT1, Tyr690 for STAT2, Tyr 705 for STAT3, Tyr 693 for STAT4, Tyr 694 for STAT5, and Tyr 641 for STAT6. Their phosphorylation mediates STAT dimerization which occurs by binding of the SH2 domain of one molecule with the domain containing the phosphotyrosine of another STAT molecule [19], so the resulting dimers are thus stabilized by bivalent bonds. STAT2 is the only STAT representative that does not act as a homodimer, forming instead a complex with STAT1 and p48. As a response to several cytokines, the heterodimers STAT1-2, STAT1-3 STAT5A-5B are formed, while no heterodimers with STAT 4 and STAT6 have been identified [20] (Table 3).

Activated STATs dissociate from the receptor, dimerize, translocate to the nucleus and bind to members of the GAS (gamma activated site) family of enhancers. There are several more recent developments regarding STAT signaling, structural studies, nuclear as well as mitochondrial translocation, gene targeting and newly identified regulatory molecules.

Classical activation of STATs occurs after cytokine binding to cell-surface receptors that initiates a cascade of intracellular phosphorylation events. The phosphorylation of STATs is essential not only for dimerization, but also for the concomitant translocation of the dimers into the nucleus. Binding of STAT1 and STAT5B to importin-α5, a part of the nucleocytoplasmic transport machinery, has been described [21].

Considering that a second phosphorylation site is serine residue in the c-terminal domain, STATs, in addition to tyrosine phosphorylation can be serine phosphorylated by various serine kinases [22] that regulate and increase STAT1,3 and 5 transcriptional activity. It is of interest that one of the kinases responsible for the phosphorylation of this serine in STAT1 and STAT3, belongs to the MAP kinases family (ERKs, JNK and p38) which emphasizes the important "cross-talk" occurring between the two transductional pathways [23]. Furthermore, there is also evidence of the activity of ERK-independent serine kinases [24], such as the role of protein kinase C (PKC) in serine phosphorylation of STATs [25] and mTOR of the PKI2 pathway. The relative contribution of each of these serine kinases to STAT signaling in vivo would depend on cell-type specific expression of kinases [22]. Therefore, STATs can be phosphorylated in great many serine/threonine residues, which may modulate DNA binding and/or their transcriptional activity [26].

One can envision a negative feedback mechanism in which serine phosphorylation of STATs promotes the induction of physiologic inhibitors of STAT signaling, such as those of the suppressor of cytokine signaling (SOCS) family that inhibit at the level of JAKs [27]. Assumingly dual functional role is thus implied for STAT serine phosphorylation events, whereby the same serine kinases can apparently both enhance and repress STAT signaling, the indirect negative effect being due to preferential association of STAT proteins with the serine kinases, precluding interaction with tyrosine kinases [2, 25].

In addition to classical, canonical activation by tyrosine phosphorylation, the noncanonical STAT activation includes, besides serine phosphorylation, other, phosphorylation-independent modifications that regulate their activity. In this sense, it has been shown that following stimulation of cells with IL-1 plus IL-6 unphosphorylated STAT3 affects gene expression in the nucleus through binding to NF-κB that mediates its nuclear import [28]. Furthermore, the classical IL-6 mediated activation of STAT3 induces tyrosine-phosphorylation of STAT3 and activates many genes, including the STAT3 gene itself that results in STAT3 synthesis that in its unphosphorylated form can induce not only the synthesis of IL-6 but also the expression of other genes such as *RANTES*, *IL-8*, *Met*, and *MRAS*.

Aside from this, the noncanonical STAT activation includes acetylation of lysine 685 in the SH2 STAT domain [29] that occurs in IL-6-induced acute phase reactions [30]. Novel findings indicate that acetylation of STAT3 is an important regulatory modification that influences protein–protein interaction and its transcriptional activity. Moreover, in oncogenesis new data regarding transmembrane glycoprotein CD44 [31], a marker of tumor metastatic phenotype, translocates into the nucleus in association with acetylated STAT3 and by regulating transcription of cyclin D enhances cell proliferation [32] (Fig. 2).

Also, many more posttranslational STAT modifications such as isgylation [33], sumoylation [34] and ubiquitination [35] are being explored in STAT-dependent tumor formation and metastasis. These noncanonical pathways include the many roles of nontyrosine phosphorylated STATs, which alter their stability, dimerization, nuclear localization, transcriptional activation function, and association with histone acetyltransferases (HAT), and histone deacetylases (HDAC) [36] (Fig. 2).

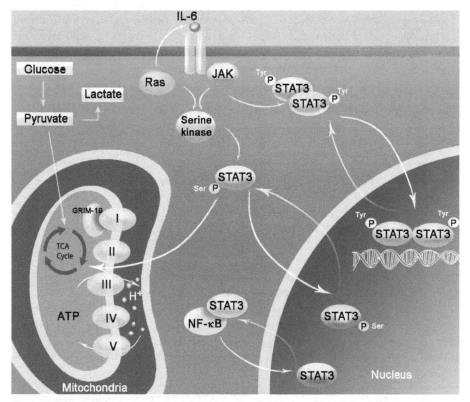

Figure 2. Different signaling pathways initiated by phosphorylation of STAT3 on tyrosine or serine residues. STAT3 is constitutively imported into and exported from the nucleus independent of its phosphorylation status. Oncogenic Ras can stimulate the autocrine production of IL-6, and the resulting phosphorylation of STAT3 Tyr705 promotes dimerization and the ability to bind specific DNA target sequences. STAT3 can also be phosphorylated on Ser727 and can mediate nuclear import of the NF-κB transcription factor. Serine phosphorylated STAT3 stimulates the electron transport chain in mitochondria and augments transformation by oncogenic Ras.

The duration of STATs activation is a temporary process, thus within hours the activating signals decay and the STATs are exported back to the cytoplasm. Negative nuclear regulators of STATs are nuclear tyrosine phosphatases that induce STAT dephosphorylation in the nucleus important for its export back to the cytoplasm. There is evidence that a specific nuclear tyrosine phosphatase (TC45), is a phosphatase relevant for STAT1 and STAT3 [37]. In addition, it has been reported that cells lacking this enzyme retain tyrosine phosphorylated STAT1 for much longer than normal cells, and overexpression of TC45 leads to dephosphorylation of STAT5 [38]. However, TC45 has also been implicated in regulating cytoplasmic dephosphorylation of JAK1 and JAK3 [39].

Recently, the negative activity on STAT protein of a group of nuclear proteins termed "proteins that inhibit activated STATs" (PIAS) has been discovered. Studies in cultured mammalian cells indicated that PIAS1 and PIAS3 interact only with tyrosine-phosphorylated STAT1 and STAT3, respectively [40]. PIAS prevents their binding to DNA, especially of STAT1, or it speeds-up their degradation in the proteasome.

Besides nuclear, other phosphatases in the cytoplasm also represent negative STAT regulators, they include phosphatases such as SH2-containing phosphatase-1 (SH1), SH2, and protein-tyrosine-phosphatase-1B (PTP1B) implicated as cytoplasmic regulators of JAKs or STATs' phosphorylation [38].

The activity of STAT proteins is also regulated by the inhibitors of the suppressors of the cytokine signal (SOCS) family, responsible for modulating the JAK-STAT pathway by acting on the JAK kinases. These cytokine-induced SOCS proteins are recruited to active receptor complexes to cause inhibition, and can also cause protein turnover of the receptor through a process of proteolytic degradation ubiquitine-proteasome mediated [41]. As SOCS belong to the family of target STAT genes they constitute with them a classical negative feedback mechanism [12] that can negatively regulate their own phosphorylation state [42]. Several members of this family have been identified, SOCS1,2,3,4,5,6 and 7. These regulatory proteins have an indirect negative effect on STATs by inhibiting their activating enzymes, especially Janus kinases (JAK1, JAK2, JAK3 and Tyk2), as well as, upstream receptors for growth factors [43]. Considering their negative regulatory role, SOCS proteins represent an important intracellular mechanism for limiting the potentially adverse effects of cytokines in immune reactions [44].

Aside from these mechanisms, mutations that augment the function of their activators or decreases the function of their inhibitors may lead to STAT hyperactivity and their engagement in malignant transformation.

Moreover, due to alternate splicing of STAT gene the short forms of STATs, i.e., inactive STATβ form, can potentially act as dominant-negative protein and by competitive inhibition occupy DNA as non-functional protein without transcriptional capability or by binding to wild-type STATs form [45] competitive inhibition, prevent binding of the STATα isoform and transcription of target genes. Aside from that, the truncated STATγ isoform of this molecule that is created by proteolysis, also competitively inhibits transcription mediated by the active α form (Table 3).

Positive regulation of STATs	Effects	
Canonical regulation of STATs		
Phosphorylation of tyrosine	STAT1 - Tyr 701	STAT4 - Tyr 693
	STAT2 - Tyr690	STAT5 - Tyr 694
	STAT3 - Tyr 705	STAT6 - Tyr 641
Noncannonical regulation of STATs		
Phosphorylation of serine	STAT3 - Ser727	
	STAT4 - Ser721	
	STAT5 - Ser725/730	
Unphosphorylated STAT	IL-6 gene dependant expression	
	IL-6 mediated acute phase reactions	
NFκB	Nuclear import of CD44	
Acetylation		
Isgylation		
Sumoylation		
Genetic regulation		
Mutations		
Hypermorphic allele of STAT3	Increased transcription	
Epigenetic regulation		
Histone acetyl transferase (HAT)		

Negative regulation of STATs		
Negative cytoplasmic regulators		
Tyrosine phosphatase (SHP1,2)	Dephosphorylation	
Protein-tyrosine-phosphatase-1B		
Suppressors of cytokine signals	Inhibit JAK	
(SOCS1-7)	degrade receptors	
Proteases	STAT inactive forms (β and γ)	
Negative nuclear regulators		
Nuclear tyrosine phosphatase	Dephosphorylation	
Proteins that inhibit activated STATs	Inhibits STAT1-3 DNA binding	
(PIAS1-3)	Proteasome degradation	
DNA methyltransferase (DNMT)	Decreased transcription	
Ubiquitination	Degradation	

Table 3. Regulation of STAT activity

2. STAT proteins in carcinogenesis

Aside from their essential role in mediating the effect of cytokines, it has been shown that STATs can have a significant role in tumor development and they are being considered as potential oncogenes. In normal cells, the activation of STAT proteins is transient, ranging from between a few minutes to a few hours. However, in a large group of different tumors constitutive activation of STAT family, especially STAT3 and STAT5 members, as well as the loss of

STAT1 signaling, has been detected [3, 46]. Novel results indicate that STAT proteins regulate numerous pathways that participate in oncogenesis, such as cell cycle progression, apoptosis, angiogenesis, tumor invasiveness, metastasis, and immune response evasion. Based on this STAT proteins have become significant target molecules in novel therapeutic approaches in oncology as blocking of these molecules, directly or indirectly, may arrest the malignant process [47].

Gough et al. [48] provide evidence that STAT3 has joined a set of transcription factors that in mitochondria exhibit noncanonical roles independent of classical STAT3-mediated transcription in the nucleus. In this sense, mitochondria have become important in cancer research because they regulate proapoptotic and antiapoptotic factors.

It is also of importance that according to their general principle of action STAT proteins may be divided into two groups that differ greatly. The group that comprises STAT2, STAT4 and STAT6 is activated by a limited number of cytokines and it is engaged in T cell development and the effect of interferons, while the other group that is comprised of STAT1, STAT3 and STAT5 is activated in numerous tissues and cell types by great many cytokines, different hormones and growth factors and aside from mediating immune reactions, regulates many important general processes such as cell proliferation, differentiation and survival in embryogenesis, as well as breast development [49]. In that sense, this second group of STAT proteins is of importance in malignant transformation. Aside from that, earlier results indicated that active STAT1 protein has tumor-suppressor characteristics as it down-regulates cell proliferation and induces apoptosis, so that its decreased activity is associated with numerous neoplasias. On the other hand, it has been shown for STAT3 and STAT5 that they are proto-oncogenes that activate oncogenes, *c-myc, cyklin D* and antiapoptotic Bcl-xL protein, facilitate passage through G1/S check-point and in that sense, aside from down-regulating apoptosis, enhance cell proliferation and transformation [12].

It has been shown that STAT3 is frequently activated in hematological and epithelial malignancies. Constitutive activation of STAT3 leads to proliferation of tumor cells and prevents apoptosis, down-regulates the production of numerous proinflamatory cytokines and chemokines and leads to secretion of factors that prevent dendritic cell (DC) maturation that suppresses adaptive antitumor immunity establishment. Aside from the disturbance of the JAK/STAT signaling pathway in primary tumors, a similar finding is frequently found in peripheral blood lymphocytes of patients with malignancies [3].

2.1. Constitutively activated STATs affect tumor microenvironment

It is known that invasive tumors need to modulate gene expression in a manner that impairs the activity of innate and adaptive immunity in immune surveillance [50, 51]. STAT3 positive tumors achieve this by preventing the production of proinflamatory cytokines, i.e., "danger signals". Activation of the transcription factor STAT3 in the tumor and adjacent immune cells, including tumor associated macrophages (TAMs),T regulatory cells (Treg cells), DCs, Th1 cells, Th2 cells, B regulatory cells (Bregs), myeloid derived suppressor cells (MDSCs), Th17 cells, as well as, normal epithelial cells, lead to production of cytokines IL-1β, IL-6, IL-10, IL-17, as well as VEGF creating a feedback loop that promotes tumor growth, angiogenesis, evasion of immune surveillance and metastasis [52].

It has been shown that especially tumor produced IL-6 through JAKs/STAT3 signaling has an important role in modulating the tumor-associated immune microenvironment. IL-6 has pleiotropic functions by activating numerous cell types expressing membrane-bound gp130 IL-6 receptor, i.e., classical IL-6 signaling, as well as, by soluble form of the IL-6 receptor (sIL-6 receptor) that after binding IL-6 and interaction with gp130 in the form of IL-6 *trans*-signaling modulates a broad spectrum of target cells including epithelial cells, neutrophils, macrophages, and T cells [53]. Upregulated STAT3 in TAM has been shown to enhance the expression of IL-23 that leads to the expansion of Tregs, while conversely, transcriptionally repressing IL-12 that supports proinflamatory cytokines and antitumor immune reactions within the tumor milieu [54]. Also, tumor-evoked Bregs express activated STAT3 and induce TGFβ conversion of Tregs from resting T cells [55] (Fig.3). Therefore, the production

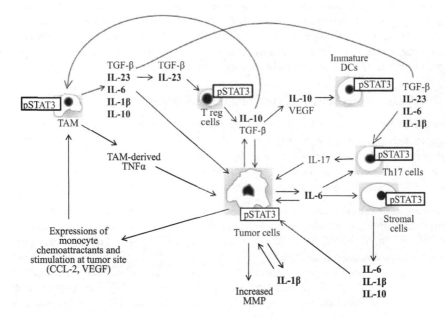

Figure 3. Interaction between tumor cells and tumor microenvironment mediated by cytokines. Tumor cells and different immune cells including TAMs, Treg cells, DC, Th17 cells, and non-tumor (normal epithelial) cells undergo STAT3 activation under the effect of various cytokines, and in turn produce more cytokines forming a feedback loop. STAT3 also regulates cell proliferation, cell cycle progression, apoptosis, angiogenesis together with immune evasion. Inhibition of STAT signaling could eliminate tumor cells while exerting minimal effect on the normal cells. Preclinical models have validated STAT3 as a target for cancer therapy, although only indirect JAK inhibitors have advanced to clinical trials (Cytokines that induce STAT3 activation are written in bold letters).

and release of various survival factors, including IL-6 as a major activator of STAT3, also serve to block apoptosis in cells during the inflammatory process, keeping them alive in very toxic environments. Unfortunately, at the same time these same pathways serve to maintain cells progressing towards neoplastic growth, protecting them from cellular apoptotic deletion and chemotherapeutic drugs.

It is of importance that activation of STAT3 within tumors is heterogeneous and it has been found that pSTAT3 are highest on the leading edge of tumors and that this is associated with stromal, immune, and endothelial cells. This follows from IL-6 from cancer-associated fibroblasts or myeloid cells that in a feedback loop induces autocrine production of IL-6 and pSTAT3 expression in tumor cells, thus also leading to heterogeneous levels of pSTAT3 [56].

Therefore tumor STAT3 activity can mediate tumor immune evasion and induce tolerance rather than immunity by blocking both the production and sensing of inflammatory signals by components of the innate and adaptive immune systems that have been recently defined as "extrinsic tumor suppressors" [57].

Regarding tumor microenvironment, in physiological conditions the activation of STAT3 is of paramount importance during tissue remodeling in the process of „wound healing" [58]. As tumor growth also includes tissue damage, the dysregulation of STAT3 in the context of tumor microenvironment has a detrimental effect that instead of wound healing leads to further tissue destruction, together with evasion of immune response.

2.2. STATs support oncogene-dependent cellular transformation

Oncogenes can only transform cells that have been immortalized by carcinogens or other oncogenes exemplifying the paradigm of multistep carcinogenesis. In this sense, mammal cells transformed by oncogenic *src* show constitutively active STAT3 and negative-dominant forms of STAT3 block the transforming ability of *src*, demonstrating a close correlation between STAT3 activation and the oncogenic transformation by this oncogene [59].

Moreover, recent studies have shown that constitutive activation of STAT3 in human breast cancer cells correlates with EGFR family kinase signaling and also with aberrant JAK and Src activity [60]. In addition to Src, many other transforming tyrosine kinases, such as Eyk, Ros and Lck, constitutively activate STAT3 in the context of oncogenesis. Another example of tumorigenic stimuli known to activate STAT proteins is Abl that may constitutively activate STAT3 and STAT5, whereas the fusion protein, Bcr-Abl, may activate them in the absence of constitutive JAK activation, showing that the presence of the JAK kinases is not always essential for STAT activation [2] (Table 4).

In addition to its previously characterized nuclear roles, transformation specific function for mitochondrial STAT3 has now been shown. Although previous data implicated a Ras-STAT3 axis in transformation, those cases were in the context of activated tyrosine kinases, such as NPM-ALK [61], RET [62], or autocrine cytokine signaling requiring STAT3 function in the nucleus. However, it has now been shown that for cellular transformation and anchorage-independent growth induced by activated H-, N- or K-Ras, STAT3 phosporylated on Serine727 and expressed exclusively in mitochondria was required. In contrast, recent findings also show that mitochondrially restricted STAT3 did not support *src*-driven anchorage-independent growth, consistent with former data that *src* requires nuclear functions of STAT3 [63].

Cell type	Oncogene	Activated STATs
Fibroblasts	v-Src	STAT3
	c-Src	STAT3
	v-Sis	STAT3
	v-Ras	
	v-Raf	
	IGF-1 receptor	STAT3
Myeloid	v-Src	STAT1, STAT3, STAT5
T cell	Lck	STAT3, STAT5
Mammary/Lung epithelial	v-Src	STAT3
Gallbladder adenocarcinoma	v-Src	STAT3
Pre-B lymphocytes	v-Abl	STAT1, STAT5
Erythroleukemia/blast cells/ basophils/mast cells	Bcr-Abl	STAT1, STAT5
Primary bone marrow	Bcr-Abl	STAT5

Table 4. STAT activation by oncogenes

Mitochondrial STAT3 contributes to Ras-dependent cellular transformation by augmenting electron transport chain activity, particularly that of complexes II and V, accompanied by energy production to favor cytoplasmatic glycolysis that represents a hallmark of cancer formulated in the 1950's by Warburg [64]. Additional analyses are required to understand the connections between glycolysis and oxidative phosphorylation affected by STAT3 in the presence or absence of oncogenic Ras.

STAT3 apparently enters mitochondria associated with GRIM-19 that was identified as a subunit of the mitochondrial complex I and Ser727 appears to be needed for their interaction [65].

Therefore, the "metabolic shift" important for tumor growth mediated by mitochondrial STAT3 may reflect exploitation of a normal function and in this sense mitochondrial STAT3 function could provide a new target for therapeutic approaches to cancer [65].

2.3. Anti-oncogenic and oncogenic characteristics of STAT1

STAT1 has been considered to be an anti-oncogene, i.e., tumor-suppressor protein that blocks proliferation and induces apoptosis [66]. Moreover, it has been shown that its dysfunction leads to the loss of immune surveillance [67]. Loss of STAT1 supports angiogenesis and metastasis of tumors.

It has been established that STAT1, the first STAT to be discovered, is required for signaling by the IFNs which in addition to their role in innate immunity, serve as potent inhibitors of proliferation and promoters of apoptosis. The involvement of STAT1 in growth arrest and apoptosis in many cell types may be explained by its capacity to induce caspase and p21 expression [68] and reduce c-myc expression. Although, normally, high p21 expression is associated with cell growth arrest, p21 increase has also been observed in some human neoplasias. This contradiction has been explained by Bowman et al. (2000) [2] with the fact that p21 is also responsible for the correct association of the cyclin D1/CDK cyclin complex, and thus its increase may be necessary for cell-cycle progression. Interestingly, in mammary cells p21 upregulation by STAT1 appears to involve BRCA1, which is often lost in familial and other forms of breast cancer. Effective STAT1-BRCA1 binding is mediated by serine phosphorylation of STAT1. More recently besides its role as tumor suppressor, new evidence has shown that STAT1 can be activated in some malignancies such as breast, lung, head and neck cancer and brain tumors [46]. In this sense, STAT1 tyrosine 701 phosphorylation increase was demonstrated in human breast tumor cells with elevated levels of HER-2/Neu as well as in cell lines transfected with HER-2/Neu gene [70]. However, it is of interest that breast cancer patients with higher levels of phosphorylated and DNA-bound STAT1 show better prognosis and live longer.

Besides increased STAT activation, high expression of the unphosphorylated form of STAT1 was also found in cancer cells. Moreover, it has been also shown that recurrent tumors express higher levels of unphosphorylated STAT1 compared to the original tumors [72], as well as cancer cells resistant to ionizing radiation and anticancer agents [73]. Recently, functions of some STAT1-induced genes in cancer cells have been investigated, and some have been shown to have pro-metastatic, pro-proliferative, or antiapoptotic properties [74]. In this sense it has been found in melanoma cells that high levels of STAT1 expression inhibits caspase 3/7 activation in response to doxorubicin which contributes to patients' resistance to this chemotherapeutic agent [75]. It has also been shown by Khodarev et al. (2007) [76] that ectopically increased expression of STAT1 can induce a radiation-resistant phenotype.

Both type I and type II IFNs increase STAT1 expression in many cell types, including normal fibroblasts and mammary epithelial cells, and the newly synthesized STAT1 protein persists for many days after IFN stimulation in unphosphorylated form [77]. Certain types of human tumors are unresponsive to IFNs due to defects in the STAT1 activation pathway.

Contrary to these findings, recent data states that the expression level of STAT1 does not influence the response to IFN adjuvant therapy in cancer [72] and that the overexpression of STAT1 in recurrent tumors might be caused by IFN treatment. In these tumor cells the found increase in STAT1 level does not result in enhanced anticancer effects of STAT1 as many IFN-induced pro-apoptotic and antiproliferative proteins as APO2L/TRAIL and IRF1 [78] are not upregulated in resistant cells. This strongly indicates that IFN signaling is not responsible for STAT1 upregulation in cancer cells. It has also been found that high level of unphosphorylated STAT1 in tumors protects cancer cells from DNA damage [79].

These observations suggest that increased levels of unphsphorylated STAT1 might participate in oncogenesis as well as resistance to cell death by inducing target genes that increase proliferation, decrease cell death, or increase repair of DNA damage. Increased DNA damage in cancer is due to oncogene-induced damage, chromosome instability, and other causes that are intrinsic to tumorigenesis. Therefore, evolving cancer cells must learn to resist the consequences of DNA damage, avoiding normal cellular responses such as cell cycle arrest or apoptosis, thus relying on support mechanisms that are characteristic for the tumor "stress phenotype". A working hypothesis that is now being formulated is that the increase in STAT1 expression in cancers is due to processes intrinsic to tumorogenesis [77].

2.4. Oncogenic characteristics of STAT3 and STAT5

Although STAT3 was originally identified as an acute phase response factor that is activated after stimulation by interleukin-6 (IL-6) [65], the biological functions of STAT3 are diverse, in part stemming from the activation of STAT3 by a wide range of cytokines, growth factors, as well as oncogenes. Among its many effects, it is now known to promote oncogenesis, while a hypermorphic allele of STAT3 can function as an oncogene [10].

It is established that the basic role of STAT3 in tumors is the prevention of apoptosis that is achieved by increased expression of antiapoptotic molecule, Bcl-2, or by affecting cell cycle progression by increased expression of c-myc and cyclin D1 engaged in the transition through G1/S check point. This is a characteristic of tumor cell lines with deleted STAT3 gene (STAT3 -,-) where the lack of STAT3 activity leads to the appearance of apoptosis due to an increase in the level of caspases, and a decrease in the level of Bcl-2, while down-regulated proliferation follows from decreased level of cycline D i c-myc oncogenes.

In contrast to normal cells, in which STAT tyrosine phosphorylation occurs transiently, it has been determined that STATs 1, 3, and 5 are persistently tyrosine phosphorylated in most malignancies (particularly STAT3) [2, 46]. The mechanisms by which STAT3 is persistently or constitutively tyrosine phosphorylated in cancers include increased production of cytokines and cytokine receptors, which is initiated by tumor cells in an autocrine, and by tumor microenvironment in a paracrine manner, by a decrease in the expression of the SOCS proteins through gene promoter methylation, as well as loss of tyrosine phosphatase activity [11].

Most of the described oncogenic functions of STAT3 depend on the phosphorylation status of Tyr705, however, another role of STAT3 is independent of tyrosine phosphorylation, as unphosphorylated STAT3 can also affect gene expression in the nucleus, one mechanism is through binding to NF-κB and mediating its nuclear import [80].

STAT3 has been directly linked to human cancer as it is required for cell transformation by the *src* oncogene [81], as well as in promoting cellular transformation by the *H-ras* oncogene. This function, which is dependent on the noncanonical serine phosphorylation of STAT3, takes place in mitochondria.

Unlike another member of STAT family, STAT1, that is imported in the nucleus only in phosphorylated form, STAT3 dynamically shuttles in and out of the nucleus independent of its tyrosine phosphorylation status [82, 83]. Nuclear import requires binding of STAT3 to an importin-α–importin-β dimer. On the other hand, mitochondrial import could be mediated in several ways, including by association with the cytosolic chaperones, heat shock proteins (Hsp70, Hsp90) [84] or associated with GRIM-19, a subunit of mitochondrial complex I of the electron transport chain [85] engaged in cell death processes in mitochondria that when overexpressed inhibits the activity of STAT3 by direct binding [86].

In light of this finding and the fact that STAT3 function has been linked to cancer, Gough et al. (2009) [48] evaluated the contribution of STAT3 to Ras oncogenic transformation. Ras protooncogenes become constitutively active oncogenes with the acquisition of specific point mutations [87], which stabilize Ras binding to guanosine 5′-triphosphate (GTP), thus allowing Ras in its GTP-bound state to stimulate numerous downstream effectors. However, Ras oncogenes can only transform cells that have been immortalized by carcinogens or other oncogenes, in the classical multistep carcinogenesis. Some of the signaling molecules activated in response to Ras can impact the STAT3 transcription factor. For example, mitogen-activated protein kinases (MAPKs) can phosphorylate STAT3 on Ser727 and downstream activation of the NF-κB transcription factor induces autocrine IL-6 production canonical tyrosine phosphorylation of STAT3 [88].

Cancer cells tend to have reduced oxidative phosphorylation in mitochondria, and have increased glycolysis in the cytoplasm leading to lactate production [89]. STAT3, inspite of its role in cellular transformation and cancer, promotes oxidative phosphorylation in mitochondria. New findings show that Ser727 phosphorylation of STAT3 contributed to oxidative phosphorylation in mitohondria. The effect of STAT3 on oxidative phosphorylation in mitochondria was investigated by comparing enzyme activity in STAT3+/+ to STAT3−/− cells [48]. Wegrzyn et al. (2009) [90] showed that STAT3+/+ cells had comparatively greater activity of electron transport complex I and complex II but no difference in the activities of complex III or complex VI. Comparing Ras-transformed STAT3+/+ and STAT3−/− cells revealed that, the presence of STAT3 increased activities of electron transport complex II and V. Analogous to cells that lack oncogenic Ras [90], STAT3 appears to stoke the powerhouse, i.e., mitochondria.

Unexpectedly, STAT3-expressing cells also had decreased mitochondrial membrane potential and increased lactate dehydrogenase production, indicating a shift to cytoplasmic glycolysis. Additional analyses are required to understand the complex connections between glycolysis and oxidative phosphorylation affected by STAT3 in the presence or absence of oncogenic Ras.

Originally, STAT5 was originally identified as a specific transcription factor that mediates the effects of prolactin [91]. STAT5A and STAT5B forms are 96% conserved at the protein level but they differ in their C terminal domain as STAT5A has 20 and STAT5B 8 unique amino acids in the C-terminus [92]. However, STAT5A transmits predominantly the signals initiated by the prolactin receptor, while STAT5B mediates the biological effects of growth hormone.

The most important role of STAT5A and STAT5B is in lymphoid, myeloid and erythroid cell development and function as they are activated by multiple cytokines, including IL-2, IL-3, IL-5, IL-7, IL-9, IL-15, GM-CSF and erythropoietin [93]. STAT5B serine 193 is a novel cytokine induced phospho-regulatory site that is constitutively activated in primary hematopoietic malignancies [94]. Following cytokine stimulation, human STAT5A and STAT5B are phosphorylated by JAK1, JAK2 or Tyk on the conserved tyrosine residues 694 and 699, respectively, which allows for their dissociation from the receptor complex, formation of hetero- or homo-dimers, and nuclear translocation to bind specific elements in the promoter of target genes and activate transcription [95]. While tyrosine phosphorylation is a part of activation signal, the serine 726 on STAT5A and 731 on STAT5B phosphorylation may abrogate the transcriptional activity of STAT5A/B [96].

In addition to the physiological role of STAT5 in hematopoietic cell development, dysregulation of the STAT5 signaling pathway plays a role in oncogenesis and leukemogenesis [97]. Specifically, STAT5 has been shown to be constitutively activated in several forms of lymphoid, myeloid and erythroid leukemia [98-100]. Persistent activation of STAT5 was found to be a result of deregulated cytokine signaling [101] or the presence of oncogenic tyrosine kinases. STAT5 proteins can activate many oncogenic tyrosine kinases, including Bcr-Abl, mutated forms of Flt-3 and Kit, and the JAK2 V617F mutant [102-104]. In acute promyelocytic leukemia (APL) beside the most common PML-RARα chromosomal translocation, RARα gene can be fused with STAT5B forming a fusion protein that blocks myeloid differentiation [105].

The most probable molecular mechanism by which STAT5 promotes tumorogenesis is upregulation of cyclin D and c-myc expression which promotes progression from the G1 to the S-phase of the cell cycle [2]. Aside from stimulating proliferation, STAT5 inhibits apoptosis by inducing the expression of anti-apoptotic Bcl-x₁ protein and promotes survival of tumor cells [106].

In addition to several types of leukemia and hematopoietic disorders [8], active STAT5A/B is also frequently detected in solid tumors, such as prostate cancer, breast cancer, uterine cancer, squamous cell carcinoma of the head and neck [107].

STAT5A/B controls viability and growth of prostate and breast cancer. The expression of nuclear, active STAT5A/B is often associated with high grade prostate cancer, predicts early disease recurrence and promotes metastatic dissemination. In prostate cancer, active STAT5A/B signaling pathway increases transcriptional activity of androgen receptors. Androgen receptor, in turn, increases transcriptional activity of STAT5A/B. STAT5A/B potentially contributes to castration resistant growth of prostate cancer [108]. The molecular mechanisms underlying constitutive activation of STAT5 in primary and recurrent human prostate cancers are currently unclear, and may involve the autocrine prolactine–JAK2 pathway [109], Src kinases, or Rho GTPases.

In breast cancer, the role of STAT5A/B is more complex. In rodent model systems STAT5A/B may promote malignant transformation and enhance growth of breast tumors [110], while in contrast, STAT5A/B activation in established human breast cancer positively correlates with tumor differentiation [111], prevents metastatic dissemination, and predicts favorable clinical outcome [112] of node-negative breast cancer. In addition, active STAT5A/B, induced by Akt-1, positively correlated with mammary epithelial cell differentiation and possibly a better response to endocrine therapy [113]. Collectively, these studies suggest a dual role for STAT5A/B in the mammary gland as an initiator of tumor formation, as well as a promoter of differentiations of established tumors.

2.5. STAT dysfunction associated with different malignancies

In addition to individual roles of each STAT, they may be coactivated in cancers. In this sense, STATs 1, 3, and 5 are simultaneously tyrosine phosphorylated in a number of human cancers including breast, lung, and head and neck tumors (Table5). The presence of pSTAT5 in addition to pSTAT3 in head and neck tumors can enhance tumor growth and invasion and may contribute to resistance to EGFR inhibitors and chemotherapy [114].

The functional interplay between activated STAT3 and STAT5 has also been described in breast cancers. Considering that STAT3 is included in breast development in association with EGFR, it has been shown on breast cancer cell lines and primary tumors that EGFR mutations, as well as the activity of *src* proto-oncogene, lead to hyperactivity and STAT3 oncogenic properties [115]. JAK/STAT3 signaling pathway is required for growth of CD44+CD23- breast cancer stem cells in tumors [116]. It has been shown that STAT1 blocking by EGFR in this tumor, unlike inhibition of STAT3, does not show any influence on cell proliferation [117].

Activated STAT3 and IL-6 are preferentially found in triple-negative breast cancers or in high-grade tumors and are associated with poor response to chemotherapy [118]. In human tumors, however, the presence of pSTAT5 is found predominantly in well-differentiated estrogen receptor (ER)–positive tumors and is associated with favorable prognosis. Furthermore, the presence of pSTAT5 is a predictive factor for endocrine therapy response and strong prognostic molecular marker in ER-positive breast cancer. Tumors expressing both activated STAT3 and STAT5 were more likely to be ER positive and human EGFR2 negative and of a lower stage.

Aside from the detected STAT dysregulation in tumors, more recent data report STAT status in peripheral blood lymphocytes (PBL). Results of an investigation of STATs in PBL of patients with breast cancer indicates constitutive, as well as stage-dependent, decrease in STAT1, STAT3, STAT5 expression and impaired induction of these proteins by Th1 cytokines [119]. The commonly found dysfunction of NK cells in breast cancer patients [120-122] is probably the consequence of cytokine dysbalance due to the prevalence of immunosuppressive cytokines such as IL-10 and TGFβ [123], as well as tumor-produced inhibitory factors [124]. This finding is in concordance with the only previous study published for breast cancer patients [125] and also with several other investigations showing STAT dysregulation in PBL of melanoma and renal cell carcinoma patients [126,127]. Moreover, we showed that breast cancer patients' T and NK cell subsets have lower pSTAT1 level that could be a biomarker of decreased NK cell cytotoxicity and IFNγ production associated with progression of this disease [120, 128,129].

Constitutively active STAT3 present in breast cancer and many human solid tumors, is associated with immunosuppression of the host immune response. STAT3 expression promotes the production of IL-1β, IL-6, IL-10, TGFβ and VEGF by tumor cells [130] leading to STAT3 activation in immune cells and in turn production of more cytokines forming a feedback loop. These cytokines also inhibit dendritic cell maturation, exerting a pro-tumor response. In this sense, evaluation of STATs in PBL is of importance in predicting the possibility of immunomodulatory and antitumor effect of immunotherapy with cytokines in patients with malignancies.

Constitutive activation of STATs has been detected in human head and neck squamous carcinoma cells [131]. In these cells, activation of STATs is dependent on TGFα induced activation of EGFR and studies utilizing antisense oligonucleotides have demonstrated that STAT3 mediates oncogenic growth of these cells. Activation of STATs in non-small cell lung carcinoma (NSCLC) increased production of TGFα by activating EGFR tyrosine kinase [132] induces downstream STAT3 activation and engages it in the pathogenesis of this malignancy. EGFR constitutive activation of STATs has also been detected in prostate, renal cell, lung, ovarian, and pancreatic cancers, as well as melanomas.

In addition, activation of *src* also occurs with elevated frequency during progression of human breast, ovarian and prostate cancer, and EGFR and Src have been shown to cooperate in human breast cancer [133]. Aside from that, it is of importance that in prostate cancer cell lines the role of BRCA1 gene has been shown in forming of hyperactive STAT3 [134]. When castration resistant disease develops in androgen receptor (AR) positive prostate cancer, these tumors often express higher levels of AR, possibly through activated STAT3, which can transcriptionally regulate AR. Thus, combining antiandrogens with anti-STAT3 drugs should be considered, rather than with chemotherapy in hormone-refractory metastatic prostate cancer [11]. Also, in B16 mouse melanoma cell line hyperactive STAT3 has also been detected [135] (Table 5).

STAT hyperactivity has been demonstrated in lymphomas and leukemias. In acute myeloid leukemia (AML), characterized by the presence of immature myeloid cells in the bone marrow, STAT3 and STAT5 hyperactivity has been found. This may follow from an overproduction of hematopoietic cytokines by tumor cells [136]. An increased level of STAT3β isoform in leuekimic blasts in the bone marrow has been found in patients with this leukemia that have an overall shorter time of survival [137]. It is presumed that STAT5 in AML is activated by mutations in the *flt-3* gene. It has also been shown that hyperactive STAT3 induces increased production of VEGF in bone marrow of acute and chronic leukemia. This is in accord with the common finding of increased blood vessel density in bone marrow in these malignancies [138]. Constitutive activation of STATs 1 and 5 has been additionally detected in acute myelogenous leukemia (AML) and chronic myelogenous leukemia (CML) cells possessing the activated Bcr-Abl tyrosine kinase [139]. Moreover, T cell leukemia that arise in HIV infections, as well as Hodgkin's disease, express active STAT3.

Tumor type	Activated STAT proteins
Solid tumors	
Breast cancer	STAT1,STAT3, STAT5
Head and neck cancer	STAT1,STAT3, STAT5
Melanoma	STAT3
Lung cancer	STAT3,STAT5
Ovarian cancer	STAT3
Pancreatic cancer	STAT3
Prostate cancer	STAT3,STAT5
Hematological malignancies	
Acute myelogenous leukemia	STAT1,STAT3
HTLV-1 dependent leukemia	STAT3,STAT5
Multiple myeloma	STAT1,STAT3, STAT5
Acute lymphoblastic leukemia	STAT5
LGL leukemia	STAT3
Chronic myelogenous leukemia	STAT5
Lymphomas	
Cutaneous T cell lymphoma	STAT3
EBV-related and Burkitt's lymphoma	STAT3
B-cell non-Hodgkin's lymphoma	STAT3
Anaplastic LGL lymphoma	STAT3

Table 5. Activated STAT proteins found in various solid and hematologic tumors

The constitutive activation of STAT3 is more striking than STAT5 in ALK+ anaplastic large T-cell lymphoma (ALCL). In Sezary Syndrome, a leukaemic form of cutaneous T cell lymphoma (CTCL), the JAK3-STAT3 pathway is constitutively activated, while STAT5 activation is inducible [140]. In APL, aside from characteristic RARα - PML chimeric fusion protein, the novel translocation resulting in STAT5B - RARα is considered to be responsible for the lack of response to ATRA-mediated prodifferentiation therapy [141]. Moreover, inadequate activity of STAT4 leads to T helper 2 (Th2) cytokine (IL-4, IL-5 and IL-10) production and prevents adequate antitumor immune response.

3. STATs as therapeutic targets

As malignant tumors are now treated, aside from standard chemo and radiation therapy, by novel therapeutic approaches based on tumor molecular profile, therapy of different tumors now includes agents for specific targeted therapy designed to neutralize pathogenic mutations, a goal that is complex and in development. For this reason, novel therapy has extended to transcription factors, such as STATs, and agents have been designed that directly or indirectly block oncogenic STAT3 and STAT5 activity.

Following extensive cell-based screening systems for these agents in different normal, gene modified and malignant cell lines, as well as studies in experimental animals, it has been established that oncogenic STATs may be inhibited in a direct manner. One of the means is by decreasing STAT gene expression by antisense oligonucleotides (DNA and RNA) or by blocking STAT3 and STAT5 activity by small inhibitory molecules and peptide analogues. These STAT inhibitory agents have been most commonly designed to target the domains responsible for STAT dimerization , i.e., the N-terminus domain and the Src homology (SH2) domain, as well as the DNA-binding domain that makes physical contact with the STAT-responsive elements in the promoters of target genes [142] (Figure 4).

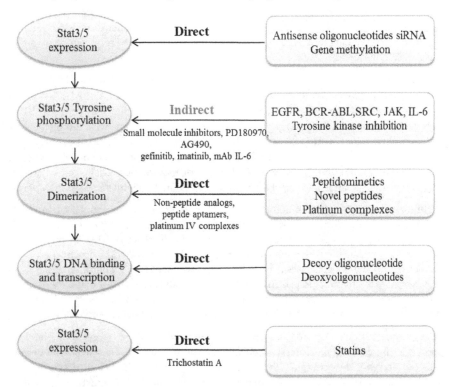

Figure 4. Available approaches and strategies to target STAT signaling pathways. These approaches target directly or indirectly STAT signaling in tumors and include interfering with STAT3 and/or STAT5 expression, phosphorylation, degradation, inhibition of receptor and non-receptor tyrosine kinases, direct interaction with STAT proteins intended to disrupt dimerization, and finally approaches to inhibit DNA-binding activity and gene transcription. These strategies should lead to a decrease in STAT signaling activity and even lower their level to normal values.

On the other hand, hyperactive STAT molecules can also be inhibited indirectly by inhibiting up-stream, either receptor or non-receptor tyrosine kinases that drive tyrosine phosphorylation and activate STATs leading to their hyperactive state [143]. In this sense, aside from JAK enzyme inhibitors, in use are also inhibitors of *src* oncogene and inhibitors of EGFR enzymatic activity, including tyrosine kinase inhibitor gefitinib, and imatinib, an inhibitor of *bcr-abl* oncogene characteristic for CML, as well as passive immunotherapy with antibody for IL-6 or its receptor [47].

JAK enzyme inhibitors, such as tyrphostine AG490, have been shown in clinical trials to be effective in the therapy of multiple myeloma and other hematological malignancies and solid tumors with aberrant activation of the JAK-STAT signaling pathway [144]. Other agents of this type, including ruxolitinib, by showing promising results in phase III clinical trials for myelofibrosis provide a basis for their study in solid tumors such as prostate cancer. In addition to improved outcome, many JAK inhibitors have been found to be tolerable with no adverse impact on the quality of life of patients possibly due to redundancies in signaling downstream of cytokine receptors, with STATs being only a part of the signaling network.

Considering both the crosstalk between STAT and other signaling pathways and activation of other pathways by STAT inhibiting agents, such as activation of Erk MAPK kinases during pimozide STAT5 inhibitor therapy, therapeutic modalities may include STAT inhibitors in combination with MEK inhibitors, an approach defined as complementary signaling pathway inhibition [145]. Although STAT inhibitors may decrease expression of pro-survival genes, this may not be sufficient to induce apoptosis, but may merely lower the threshold for apoptosis. In this sense, a STAT inhibitor may reduce resistance to cytotoxic agents or ionizing radiation and may best be used in combination with standard therapies.

Other indirect methods for inhibition include modulation of the activity of STAT molecule by using their natural negative regulators. Thus, the activity of these signaling molecules is suppressed by increased protease activity, especially for hyperactive STAT5, induction of nuclear and cytoplasmatic STAT inhibitory proteins, SOCS and PIAS, respectively, or up-regulation of tyrosine-phosphatases that dephosphorylate them [146]. Application of statins, as trichostatin A, leads to inhibition of enzyme histone deacetylase (HDAC) that by decreasing STAT transcriptional activity promotes apoptosis of malignant cells, whereas direct binding of statins to STATs leads to their covalent modification and enhanced degradation [147].

In this sense, different approaches in the context of modern targeted therapy of malignancies by decreasing expression, phosphorylation, dimerization or DNA binding of STATs can decrease the activity of these important signaling molecules or down-regulate them to almost normal level. Considering that inhibition of STAT3 and STAT5 leads to growth arrest and selective apoptosis of tumor cells, sparing benign cells, this approach may be of importance not only in the therapy, but also in chemoprevention of tumors. These aspects of molecular targeted therapy of cancer patients need to be validated in additional, properly designed clinical trials.

4. Conclusion

As STAT proteins are involved in regulating fundamental biological processes, including apoptosis and cell proliferation that are known to be dysregulated in tumors, it is not surprising to frequently find defects in STAT signaling pathways in malignancies. In the past few years advances have been made in understanding molecular mechanisms that are responsible for STAT protein dysregualtion in different malignant diseases. The critical role of constitutively active STAT3 and STAT5 in tumorogenesis has now been definitely established. Aside from that, STAT1, 3 and 5 can be considered as molecular markers for early detection of certain tumors, as well as prognostic parameters for evaluation of tumor aggressiveness and response to various types of therapies.

Obtained data that associate these molecules with tumor development support the use of STATs as molecular targets in the therapy and chemoprevention of malignancies. Inhibition of oncogenic STATs represents a comprehensive approach in tumor therapy that leads to decreased cell proliferation, survival, angiogenesis and evasion of immune response. Blocking of constitutively active STATs in tumors allows the destruction of tumor cells with minimal effect on normal cells. It is of importance that this type of molecular therapy that inhibits hyperactive STATs can potentiate response to chemo or radiation therapy and may have great potential in the therapy of solid tumors and leukemia. The efficacy of STAT inhibitors in oncological therapy remains still to be evaluated in numerous undergoing and future clinical trials.

Author details

Gordana Konjević
Institute of Oncology and Radiology of Serbia, Laboratory for Immunology
Medical Faculty, University of Belgrade, Serbia

Sandra Radenković, Ana Vuletić, Katarina Mirjačić Martinović and Tatjana Srdić
Institute of Oncology and Radiology of Serbia, Laboratory for Immunology

Vladimir Jurišić
Medical Faculty, University of Kragujevac, Serbia

Acknowledgement

This study was supported by the Ministry of Education, Science and Technological development of the Republic of Serbia through grants 41031 and 175056. The authors would like to thank Dr. Milica Apostolović Stojanović for excellent assistance in the preparation of this manuscript.

5. References

[1] Darnell JE Jr. STATs and gene regulation. Science 1997; 277(5332):1630-1635.
[2] Bowman T, Garcia R, Turkson J Jove R. STATs in oncogenesis. Oncogene 2000; 19(21):2474-2488.
[3] Konjević G, Jović V, Jurisić V Radulović S, Jelić S, Spuzić I. IL-2-mediated augmentation of NK-cell activity and activation antigen expression on NK- andT-cell subsets in

patients with metastatic melanoma treated with interferon-alphaand DTIC. Clin Exp Metastasis 2003; 20(7):647-655.

[4] Catlett-Falcone R, Dalton WS, Jove R. STAT proteins as novel targets for cancer therapy. Curr Opin Oncol. 1999; 11(6): 490–496.

[5] Quesnelle KM, Boehm AL, Grandis JR. STAT-mediated EGFR signaling in cancer. J Cell Biochem. 2007; 102(2): 311-319.

[6] Kaplan MH, Grusby MJ. Regulation of T helper cell differentiation by STAT molecules. J Leukoc Biol. 1998; 64(1): 2-5.

[7] Konjević G, Spuzić I. The possibilities of modulation of NK cell activity. Glas Srp Akad Nauka 2002; (47): 89-101.

[8] Konjević G, Mirjačić Martinović K, Vuletić A, Babović N. In-vitro IL-2 or IFN-α-induced NKG2D and CD161 NK cell receptor expression indicates novel aspects of NK cell activation in metastatic melanoma patients. Melanoma Res. 2010; 20(6): 459-467.

[9] Konjević G, Mirjačić Martinović K, Vuletić A, Radenković S. Novel aspects of in vitro IL-2 or IFN-α enhanced NK cytotoxicity of healthy individuals based on NKG2D and CD161 NK cell receptor induction. Biomed Pharmacother. 2010; 64(10): 663-671.

[10] Bromberg JF. Stat proteins and oncogenesis. J Clin Invest. 2002; 109(9): 1139–1142.

[11] Sansone P, Bromberg J. Targeting the interleukin-6/jak/stat pathway in human malignancies. J Clin Oncol. 2012; 30(9): 1005-1014.

[12] Kisseleva T, Bhattacharya S, Braunstein, Schindler CW. Signaling through the JAK/STAT pathway, recent advances and future challenges. Gene 2002; 285(1-2): 1-24.

[13] Benekli M, Baer MR, Baumann H, Wetzler M. Signal transducer and activator of transcription proteins in leukemias. Blood 2003; 101(8): 2940-2954.

[14] Gupta S, Yan H, Wong LH, Ralph S, Krolewski J, Schindler C. The SH2 domain of Stat1 and Stat2 mediate multiple interactions in the transduction of IFN alpha signals. EMBO J. 1996; 15(5): 1075-1084.

[15] Zhang X, Blenis J, Li HC, Schindler C, Chen-Kiang S. Requirement of serine phosphorylation for formation of STAT-promoter complexes. Science 1995; 267(5206): 1990-1994.

[16] Imada K, Leonard WJ. The Jak-STAT pathway. Mol Immunol. 2000; 37(1-2): 1-11.

[17] Ihle JN. The STAT family in cytokine signaling. Curr Opin Cell Biol. 2001; 13(2): 211–217.

[18] Remy I, Wilson IA, Michnick SW. Erythropoietin receptor activation by a ligand-induced conformation change. Science 1999; 283(2): 990-993.

[19] Chatterjee-Kishore M, Wright KL, Ting JP, Stark GR. How Stat1 mediates constitutive gene expression: A complex of unphosphorylated Stat1 and IRF1 supports transcription of LMP2 gene. EMBO J. 2000; 19(15): 4111–4122.

[20] Horvath CM. STAT proteins and transcriptional responses to extracellular signals. TIBS 2000; 25(10): 496–502.

[21] McBride KM, Banninger G, McDonald C, Reich NC. Regulated nuclear import of the STAT1 transcription factor by direct binding of importin-a. EMBO J. 2002; 219(7): 1754–1763.

[22] Decker T, Kovarik P. Serine phosphorylation of STATs. Oncogene 2000; 19(21): 2628–2637.

[23] Goh KC, Haque SJ, Williams BR. p38 MAP kinase is required for STAT1 serine phosphorylation and trascriptional activation induced by interferon. EMBO J. 1999; 18(20): 5601–5608.

[24] Ceresa BP, Pessin JE. Insulin stimulates the serine phosphorylation of the signal transducer and activator of transcription (STAT3) isoform. J Biol Chem. 1996; 271(21): 12121-12124.

[25] Jain N, Zhang T, Kee WH, Li W, Cao X. Protein kinase C delta associates with and phosphorylates Stat3 in an interleukin-6-dependent manner. J Biol Chem. 1999; 274: 24392-24400.

[26] Briscole J, Kohlhuber F, Muller M. JAKs and STATs branch out. Trends Cell Biol. 1996; 6(9): 336–340

[27] Starr R, Willson TA, Viney EM, Murray LJ, Rayner JR, Jenkins BJ, et al. A family of cytokine-inducible inhibitors of signalling. Nature 1997; 387(6636):917-921.

[28] Hagihara K, Nishikawa T, Sugamata Y, Song J, Isobe T, Taga T et al. Essential role of STAT3 in cytokine-driven NF-_B-mediated serum amyloid A gene expression. Genes Cells. 2005; 10(11): 1051–1063.

[29] Yuan ZL. Guan YJ, Chatterjee D, Chin YE. Stat3 dimerization regulated by reversible acetylation of a single lysine residue. Science 2005; 307(5707): 269–273.

[30] Ray S, Sherman CT, Lu M, Brasier AR. Angiotensinogen gene expression is dependent on signal transducer and activator of transcription 3-mediated p300/cAMP response element binding protein-binding protein coactivator recruitment and histone acetyltransferase activity. Mol Endocrinol. 2002; 16(4): 824–836.

[31] Ponti D, Costa A, Zaffaroni N, Pratesi G, Petrangolini G, Coradini D et al. Isolation and in vitro propagation of tumorigenic breast cancer cells with stem/progenitor cellproperties. Cancer Res. 2005; 65(13): 5506–5511.

[32] Yang XJ, Seto E. HATs and HDACs: from structure, function and regulation to novel strategies for therapy and prevention. Oncogene 2007; 26(37): 5310-5318.

[33] Kim KI, Zhang DE. UBP43, an ISG15-specific deconjugating enzyme: expression, purification, and enzymatic assays. Methods Enzymol. 2005; 398 491-499.

[34] Zhao J. Sumoylation regulates diverse biological processes. Cell Mol Life Sci. 2007; 64(24): 3017–3033.

[35] Giandomenico V, Simonsson M, Gronroos E, Ericsson J. Coactivator dependent acetylation stabilizes members of the SREBP family of transcription factors. Mol Cell Biol. 2003; 23(7): 2587–2599.

[36] Lee JL, Wang MJ, Chen JY. Acetylation and activation of STAT3 mediated by nuclear translocation of CD44. J Cell Biol. 2009; 185(6): 949-957.

[37] Ibarra-Sanchez MJ, Simoncic PD, Nestel FR, Duplay P, Lapp WS, Tremblay ML. The T-cell protein tyrosine phosphatase. Semin Immunol. 2000; 12(4): 379–386.

[38] Aoki N, Matsuda TA. A nuclear protein tyrosine phosphatase TC-PTP is a potential negative regulator of the PRL-mediated signaling pathway; dephosphorilation and deactivation of signal trasducer and activator of transcription 5a and 5b by TC-PTP in nucleus. Mol Endocrinol. 2002; 16(1): 58–69.

[39] Simononic PD, Lee-Loy A, Barder DL, Tremblay ML, McGlade CJ. The T cell protein tyrosine phosphatase is a negative regulator of Janus family kinases 1 and 3. Curr Biol. 2002; 12(6): 446–453.

[40] Shuai K. Modulation of STAT signaling by STAT-interacting proteins. Oncogene. 2000; 19(21): 2638–2644.

[41] Krebs DL, Hilton DJ. SOCS proteins: Negative regulators of cytokine signaling. Stem Cells 2001; 19(5): 378–387.

[42] Starr R, Hilton DJ. Negative regulation of the JAK/STAT pathway. Bioessays 1999; 21(1): 47–52.

[43] Cooney RN. Suppressors of cytokine signaling (SOCS): inhibitors of the JAK/STAT pathway. Shock. 2002; 17(2): 83-90.

[44] Nicola NA, Greenhalgh CJ. The suppressors of cytokine signaling (SOCS) proteins: important feedback inhibitors of cytokine action. Exp Hematol. 2000; 28(10): 1105-1112.

[45] Yu CL, Jin YJ, Burakoff SJ. Cytosolic tyrosine dephosphorylation of STAT5.Potential role of SHP-2 in STAT5 regulation. J Biol Chem. 2000; 275(1):599-604.

[46] Calò V, Migliavacca M, Bazan V, Macaluso M, Buscemi M, Gebbia N, et al. STAT proteins: from normal control of cellular events to tumorigenesis. J Cell Physiol. 2003; 197(2):157-168.

[47] Haura EB, Turkson J, Jove R. Mechanisms of disease: Insights into the emerging role of signal transducers and activators of transcription in cancer. Nat Clin Pract Oncol. 2005; 2(6): 315-324.

[48] Gough DJ, Corlett A, Schlessinger K, Wegrzyn J, Larner AC, Levy DE. Mitochondrial STAT3 supports Ras-dependent oncogenic transformation. Science 2009; 324(5935): 1713-1716.

[49] Levy DE, Darnell JE Jr. STATs: Transcriptional control and biological impact. Nat Rev. 2002; 3(9): 651-662.

[50] Dunn GP, Bruce AT, Ikeda H, Old LJ, Schreiber RD. Cancer immunoediting: from immunosurveillance to tumor escape. Nat Immunol. 2002; 3(11): 991-998.

[51] Konjević G, Jović V, Vuletić A, Radulović S, Jelić S, Spuzić I. CD69 on CD56+ NK cells and response to chemoimmunotherapy in metastatic melanoma. Eur J Clin Invest. 2007; 37(11): 887-896.

[52] Jindal S, Borges VF. The emerging role of cytokines in breast cancer: from initiation to survivorship. CML-Breast Cancer 2011; 23(4): 113-126.

[53] Culig Z. Cytokine disbalance in common human cancers. Biochim Biochim Biophys Acta. 2011; 1813(2): 308-314.

[54] Kortylewski M, Xin H, Kujawski M, Lee H, Liu Y, Harris T, et al. Regulation of the IL-23 and IL-12 balance by Stat3 signaling in the tumor microenvironment. Cancer Cell. 2009; 15(2):114-23.

[55] Olkhanud PB, Damdinsuren B, Bodogai M, Gress RE, Sen R, Wejksza K et al. Tumor-evoked regulatory B cells promote breast cancer metastasis by converting resting CD4+ T cells to T-regulatory cells. Cancer Res. 2011; 71(10):3505-15.

[56] Grivennikov S, Karin E, Terzic J, Mucida D, Yu GY, Vallabhapurapu S et al.IL-6 and Stat3 are required for survival of intestinal epithelial cells and development of colitis-associated cancer. Cancer Cell. 2009; 15(2):103-13.

[57] Wang T, Niu G, Kortylewski M, Burdelya L, Shain K, Zhang S et al. Regulation of the innate and adaptive immune responses by Stat-3 signaling in tumor cells. Nat Med. 2004; 10(1): 48-54.

[58] Sano S, Itami S, Takeda K, Tarutani M, Yamaguchi Y, Miura H et al. Keratinocyte-specific ablation of Stat3 exhibits impaired skin remodeling, but does not affect skin morphogenesis. EMBO J. 1999; 18(17):4657-4668.

[59] Turkson J, Bowman T, Garcia R, Caldenhoven E, De Groot RP, Jove R. Stat3 activation by Src induces specific gene regulation and is required for cell transformation. Mol Cell Biol. 1998; 18(5): 2545-2552.

[60] Garcia R, Yu CL, Hudnall A, Catlett R, Nelson KL, Smithgall T et al. Dicer dependent microRNAs regulate gene expression and functions in human endothelial cells. Circ Res. 2007; 100(8):1164-1173.

[61] Suárez Y, Fernández-Hernando C, Pober JS, Sessa WC. Dicer dependent microRNAs regulate gene expression and functions in human endothelial cells. Circ Res. 2007;100(8):1164-73.

[62] Potente M, Ghaeni L, Baldessari D, Mostoslavsky R, Rossig L, Dequiedt F et al. SIRT1 controls endothelial angiogenic functions during vascular growth. Genes Dev. 2007; 21(20): 2644-2658.

[63] Kuehbacher A, Urbich C, Zeiher AM, Dimmeler S. Role of Dicer and Drosha for endothelial microRNA expression and angiogenesis. Circ Res. 2007; 101(1): 59-68.

[64] O. Warburg. Photosynthesis. Science 1958; 128(3315): 68-73.

[65] Reich NC. STAT3 revs up the powerhouse. Sci Signal. 2009;2 (90):pe61

[66] Lin TS, Mahajan S, Frank DA. Stat signaling in the pathogenesis and treatment of leukemias. Oncogene. 2000; 19(21): 2496-2504.

[67] Kaplan DH, Shankaran V, Dighe AS, Stockert E, Aguet M, Old LJ et al. Demonstration of an interferon gamma-dependent tumor surveillance system in immunocompetent mice. Proc Natl Acad Sci U S A. 1998; 95(13):7556-7561.

[68] Kumar A, Commane M, Flickinger TW, Horwath CM, Stark GR. Detective TNF-alpha-induced apoptosis in Stat1-null cells due to low costitutive levels of caspases. Science. 1997; 278(2543): 1630–1632.

[69] Ouchi T, Lee SW, Ouchi M, Aaroson SA, Horvath CM. Collaboration of signal transducer and activator of transcription 1 (STAT1) and BRCA1 in differential regulation of IFN-g target genes. Proc Natl Acad Sci USA. 2000; 97(10): 5208–5213.

[70] Raven JF, Williams V, Wang S, Tremblay ML, Muller WJ, Durbin JE et al. Stat1 is a suppressor of ErbB2/Neu-mediated cellular transformation and mouse mammary gland tumor formation. Cell Cycle. 2011; 10(5): 794-804.

[71] Widschwendter A, Tonko-Geymayer S, Welte T, Daxenbichler G, Marth C, Doppler W. Prognostic significance of signal transducer and activator of transcription 1 activation in breast cancer. Clin Cancer Res. 2002; 8(10): 3065–3074.

[72] Lesinski GB, Valentino D, Hade EM, Jones S, Magro C, Chaudhury AR et al. Expression of STAT1 and STAT2 in malignant melanoma does not correlate with response to interferon-alpha adjuvant therapy. Cancer Immunol Immunother. 2005; 54(9): 815–825.

[73] Khodarev NN, Beckett M, Labay E, Darga T, Roizman B, Weichselbaum RR. STAT1 is overexpressed in tumors selected for radioresistance and confers protection from radiation in transduced sensitive cells. Proc Natl Acad Sci USA. 2004; 101(6): 1714–1719.

[74] Cai D, Cao J, Li Z, Zheng X, Yao Y, Li W, et al. Upregulation of bone marrow stromal protein 2 (BST2) in breast cancer with bone metastasis. BMC Cancer. 2009; 9:102.

[75] Khodarev NN, Roach P, Pitroda SP, Golden DW, Bhayani M, Shao MY et al. STAT1 pathway mediates amplification of metastatic potential and resistance to therapy. PLoS One. 2009; 4: e5821.

[76] Khodarev NN, Minn AJ, Efimova EV, Darga TE, Labay E, Beckett M et al. Signal transducer and activator of transcription 1 regulates both cytotoxic and prosurvival functions in tumor cells. Cancer Res. 2007; 67(19): 9214–9220.

[77] Cheon H, Yang J, Stark GR. The functions of signal transducers and activators of transcriptions 1 and 3 as cytokine-inducible proteins. J Interferon Cytokine Res. 2011; 31(1): 33-40.

[78] Borden EC, Sen GC, Uze G, Silverman RH, Ransohoff RM, Foster GR et al. Interferons at age 50: past, current, and future impact on biomedicine. Nat Rev Drug Discov. 2007; 6(12): 975–990.

[79] Luszczek W, Cheriyath V, Mekhail TM, Borden EC. Combinations of DNA methyltransferase and histone deacetylase inhibitors induce DNA damage in small cell lung cancer cells: correlation of resistance with interferon stimulated gene expression. Mol Cancer Ther 2010;9(8):2309-2321.

[80] Yang J, Stark GR. Roles of unphosphorylated STATs in signaling. Cell Res 2008;18(4):443–451.

[81] Yu H, Jove R. The STATs of cancer-New molecular targets come of age. Nat. Rev Cancer 2004;4(2):97–105

[82] Reich NC, Liu L. Tracking STAT nuclear traffic. Nat Rev Immunol 2006;6(8):602–612.

[83] Liu L, McBride KM, Reich NC. STAT3 nuclear import is independent of tyrosine phosphorylation and mediated by importin-alpha3. Proc Natl Acad Sci. U.S.A 2005;102(23):8150–8155.

[84] Neupert W, Herrmann JM. Translocation of proteinsinto mitochondria. Annu Rev Biochem 2007;76: 723–749.

[85] Fearnley IM, Carroll J, Shannon RJ, Runswick MJ, Walker E, Hirst J. GRIM-19, a cell death regulatory gene product, is a subunit of bovine mitochondrial NADH:ubiquinone oxidoreductase (complex I). J Biol Chem 2001;276(42):38345–38348.

[86] Lufei C, Ma J, Huang G, Zhang T, Novotny- Diermayr V, Ong CT et al. GRIM-19, a deathregulatory gene product, suppresses Stat3 activity via functional interaction. EMBO J 2003;22(6):1325–1335.

[87] Karnoub AE, Weinberg RA. Ras oncogenes: Split personalities. Nat Rev Mol Cell Biol 2008;9(7):517–531.

[88] Faruqi TR, Gomez D, Bustelo XR, Bar-Sagi D, Reich NC. Rac1 mediates STAT3 activation by autocrine IL-6. Proc Natl Acad Sci. U.S.A 2001;98(16):9014–9019.

[89] Vander Heiden MG, Cantley LC, Thompson CB. Understanding the Warburg effect: The metabolic requirements of cell proliferation. Science 2009;324(5930): 1029–1033.

[90] Wegrzyn J, Potla R, Chwae YJ, Sepuri NB, Zhang Q, Koeck T et al. Function of mitochondrial Stat3 incellular respiration. Science 2009;323(5915):793–797.

[91] Wakao H, Gouilleux F, Groner B. Mammary gland factor (MGF) is a novel member of the cytokine regulated transcription factor gene family and confers the prolactin response. EMBO J 1994;13(9):2182–2191.

[92] Schindler CW. Series Introduction: Jak-STAT signaling in human disease. J Clin Invest 2002;109(9):1133–1137.

[93] Kirken RA, Rui H, Malabarba MG, Howard OM, Kawamura M, O'Shea JJ et al. Activation of JAK3, but not JAK1, is critical for IL-2-induced proliferation and STAT5 recruitment by a COOH-terminal region of the IL-2 receptor beta-chain. Cytokine 1995;7(7):689-700.

[94] Mitra A, Ross JA, Rodriguez G, Nagy ZS, Wilson HL, Kirken RA. Signal transducer and activator of transcription 5b (Stat5b) serine 193 is a novel cytokine induced phospho-regulatory site that is constitutively activated in primary hematopoietic malignancies. J Biol Chem 2012;287(20):16596-16608.

[95] Leonard WJ. Role of Jak kinases and STATs in cytokine signal transduction. Int J Hematol 2001;73(3):271-277.

[96] Yamashita H, Nevalainen MT, Xu J, LeBaron MJ, Wagner KU, Erwin RA et al. Role of serine phosphorylation of Stat5a in prolactin-stimulated beta-casein gene expression. Mol Cell Endocrinol 2001;183(1-2):151–163.

[97] Bunting KD. STAT5 signaling in normal and pathologic hematopoiesis. Front Biosci 2007;12:2807-2820.

[98] Chai SK, Nichols GL, Rothman P. Constitutive activation of JAKs and STATs in BCR-Abl-expressing cell lines and peripheral blood cells derived from leukemic patients. J Immunol 1997;159(10):4720-4728.

[99] Ho JM, Beattie BK, Squire JA, Frank DA, Barber DL. Fusion of the ets transcription factor TEL to Jak2 results in constitutive Jak-Stat signaling. Blood (1999);93(12):4354-4364.

[100] Ilaria RL Jr, Van Etten RA. P210 and P190 (BCR/ABL) induce the tyrosine phosphorylation and DNA binding activity of multiple specific STAT family members. J Biol Chem 1996;271(49): 31704-31710.

[101] Van Etten RA. Aberrant cytokine signaling in leukemia. Oncogene 2007;26(47):6738-6749.

[102] Carron C, Cormier F, Janin A, Lacronique V, Giovannini M, Daniel M et al. TEL-JAK2 transgenic mice develop T-cell leukemia. Blood 2000;95(12):3891-3899.

[103] Nieborowska-Skorska M, Wasik MA, Slupianek A, Salomoni P, Kitamura T, Calabretta B et al. Signal transducer and activator of transcription (STAT)5 activation by BCR/ABL is dependent on intact Src homology (SH)3 and SH2 domains of BCR/ABL and is required for leukemogenesis. J Exp Med 1999;189(8):1229-1242.

[104] Mizuki M, Fenski R, Halfter H, Matsumura I, Schmid, R, Muller C et al. Flt3 mutations from patients with acute myeloid leukemia induce transformation of 32D cells mediated by the Ras and STAT5 pathways. Blood 2000;96(12):3907-3914.

[105] Maurer AB, Wichmann C, Gross A Kunkel H, Heinzel T, Ruthardt M et al. The Stat5-RARα fusion protein represses transcription and differentiation through interaction with a corepressor complex. Blood 2002;99(8):2647-2652.

[106] Buettner R, Mora LB, Jove R. Activated Stat signaling in human tumors provides novel molecular targets for therapeutic intervention. Clin Cancer Res 200;8(4):945–954.

[107] Nikitakis NG, Siavash H, Sauk JJ. Targeting the STAT pathway in head and neck cancer: recent advances and future prospects. Curr Cancer Drug Targets 2004;4(8):637-651.

[108] Tan SH, Dagvadorj A, Shen F, Gu L, Liao Z, Abdulghani J et al. Transcription factor Stat5 synergizes with androgen receptor in prostate cancer cells. Cancer Res 2008;68(1):236-248.

[109] Li H, Ahonen TJ, Alanen K, Xie J, LeBaron MJ, Pretlow TG et al. Activation of signal transducer and activator of transcription 5 in human prostate cancer is associated with high histological grade. Cancer Research 2004;64(14):4774–4782.

[110] Ren S, Cai HR, Li M, Furth PA. Loss of Stat5a delays mammary cancer progression in a mouse model. Oncogene 2002;21(27):4335–4339.

[111] Cotarla I, Ren S, Zhang Y, Gehan E, Singh B, Furth PA. Stat5a is tyrosine phosphorylatedand nuclear localized in a high proportion of human breast cancers. Int J Cancer 2004;108(5):665–671.

[112] Nevalainen MT, Xie J, Torhorst J, Bubendorf L, Haas P, Kononen J et al. Signal transducer and activator of transcription-5 activation and breast cancer prognosis. J Clin Oncol 2004;22(11):2053–2060.

[113] Creamer BA, Sakamoto K, Schmidt JW, Triplett AA, Moriggl R, Wagner KU. Stat5 promotes survival of mammary epithelial cells through transcriptional activation of a distinct promoter in Akt1. Mol Cell Biol 2010;30(12): 2957–2970.

[114] Koppikar P, Lui VW, Man D, Xi S, Chai RL, Nelson E et al. Constitutive activation of signal transducer and activator of transcription 5 contributes to tumor growth, epithelial-mesenchymal transition, and resistance to epidermal growth factor receptor targeting. Clin Cancer Res 2008;14(23):7682-7690.

[115] Garcia R, Yu CL, Hudnall A, Catlett R, Nelson KL, Smithgall T et al. Constitutive activation of Stat3 in fibroblasts transformed by diverse oncoproteins and in breast carcinoma cells. Cell Growth Differ 1997;8(12):1267-1276.

[116] Marotta LL, Almendro V, Marusyk A Shipitsin M, Schemme J, Walker SR et al. The JAK2/STAT3 signaling pathway is required for growth of CD44+CD24- stem cell-like breast cancer cells in human tumors. J Clin Invest 2011;121(7):2723-2735.

[117] Grandis JR, Grenning SD, Chakraborty A, Zhou MY, Zeng Q, Pitt AS et al. Requirement of Stat3 but not Stat1 activation for epidermel growth factor receptor-mediated cell growth in vitro. J Clin Invest 1998;102(7):1385-1392.

[118] Dolled-Filhart M, Camp RL, Kowalski DP, Smith BL, Rimm DL. Tissue microarray analysis of signal transducers and activators of transcription 3 (Stat3) and phospho-Stat3 (Tyr705) in node-negative breast cancer shows nuclear localization is associated with a better prognosis. Clin Cancer Res 2003;9(2):594-600.

[119] Shankaran V, Ikeda H, Bruce AT White JM, Swanson PE, Old LJ et al. IFNgamma and lymphocytes prevent primary tumor development and shape tumor immunogenicity. Nature 2001;410(6832):1107-1111.

[120] Konjević G, Jurisić V, Spuzić I. Association of NK cell dysfunction with changes in LDH characteristics of peripheral blood lymphocytes (PBL) in breast cancer patients. Breast Cancer Res Treat 2001;66(3):255-263.

[121] Konjevic G, Radenkovic S, Srdic T, Jurisic V, Stamatovic Lj, Milovic M. Association of decreased NK cell activity and IFNγ expression with pSTAT dysregulation in breast cancer patients. J BUON 2011;16(2):219-226.

[122] Konjevic G, Jurisic V, Jovic V, Vuletic A, Mirjacic Martinovic K, Radenkovic S et al. Investigation of NK cell function and their modulation in different malignancies. Immunol Res 2012;52(1-2):139-156.

[123] Jarnicki AG, Lysaght J, Todryk S, Mills KH. Suppression of antitumor immunity by IL-10 and TGF-beta-producing T cells infi ltrating the growing tumor: infl uence of tumor environment on the induction of CD4+ and CD8+ regulatory T cells. J Immunol 2006;177(2):896-904.

[124] Zwirner NW, Fuertes MB, Girart MV, Domaica CI, Rossi LE. Cytokine-driven regulation of NK cell functions in tumor immunity: role of the MICA-NKG2D system. Cytokine Growth Factor Rev 2007;18(1-2):159-170.

[125] Critchley-Thorne RJ, Simons DL, Yan N, Miyahira AK, Dirbas FM, Johnson DL et al. Impaired interferon signaling is a common immune defect in human cancer. Proc Natl Acad Sci USA 2009;106(22):9010-9015.

[126] Lesinski GB, Kondadasula SV, Crespin T, Shen L, Kendra K, Walker M et al. Multiparametric flowcytometric analysis of inter-patient variation in STAT1 phosphorylation following interferon alfa immunotherapy. J Natl Cancer Inst 2004;96(17):1331-1342.

[127] Varker KA, Kondadasula SV, Go MR Lesinski GB, Ghosh-Berkebile R, Lehman A et al. Multiparametric flow cytometric analysis of signal transducer and activator of transcription 5 phosphorylation in immune cell subsets in vitro and following interleukin-2 immunotherapy. Clin Cancer Res 2006;12(19):5850-5858.

[128] Konjević G, Spuzić I. Stage dependence of NK cell activity and its modulation by interleukin 2 in patients with breast cancer. Neoplasma 1993;40(2):81-85.

[129] Konjević G, Spuzić I. Evaluation of different effects of sera of breast cancer patients on the activity of natural killer cells. J Clin Lab Immunol 1992;38(2):83-93.

[130] Wang T, Niu G, Kortylewski M Burdelya L, Shain K, Zhang S et al. Regulation of the innate and adaptive immune responses by Stat-3 signaling in tumor cells. Nat Med 2004;10(1): 48–54.

[131] Grandis JR, Drenning SD, Chakraborty A, Zhou MY, Zeng Q, Pitt AS et al. Requirement of Stat3 but not Stat1 activation for epidermal growth factor receptor-mediated cell growth in vitro. J Clin Invest 1998;102(7):1385-1392.

[132] Fernandes A, Hamburger AW, Gerwin BI. ErbB-2 kinase is required for constitutive stat 3 activation in malignant human lung epithelial cells. Int J Cancer 1999;83(4):564-570.

[133] Reddy MVR, Chaturvedi P, Reddy EP. Src kinase mediated activation of STAT3 plays an essential role in the proliferation and oncogenicity of human breast, prostate and ovarian carcinomas. Proceeding in Abstract book: Proc Am Assoc Cancer Res 1999; 40: Abstract No.376.

[134] Gao B, Shen X, Kunos G Meng Q, Goldberg ID, Rosen EM et al. Constitutive activation of JAK-STAT3 signaling by BRCA1 in human prostate cancer cells. FEBS Lett 2001;488(3): 179-184.

[135] Niu G, Bowman T, Huang M Shivers S, Reintgen D, Daud A et al. Roles of activated Src and Stat3 signaling in melanoma tumor cell growth. Oncogene 2002;21(46):7001-7010.

[136] Lowenberg B, Touw IP. Hematopoietic growth factors and their receptors in acute leukemia. Blood 1993;81(2):281-292.

[137] Xia Z, Sait SN, Baer MR Barcos M, Donohue KA, Lawrence D et al. Truncated STAT proteins are prevalent at relapse of acute myeloid leukemia. Leuk Res 2001;25(6):473-482.

[138] Niu G, Wright KL, Huang M, Song L, Haura E, Turkson J et al. Constitutive STAT3 activity upregulates VEGF expression and tumor angiogenesis. Oncogene 2002;21(13): 2000-2008.

[139] Skorski T, Nieborowska-Skorska M, Wlodarski P, Wasik M, Trotta R, Kanakaraj P et al. The SH3 domain contributes to BCR/ABL-dependent leukemogenesis in vivo: role in adhesion, invasion, and homing. Blood 1998;91(2):406-418.

[140] Mitchell TJ, John S. Signal transducer and activator of transcription (STAT) signalling and T-cell lymphomas. Immunology 2005;114(3):301-312.

[141] Maurer AB, Wichmann C, Gross A, Kunkel H, Heinzel T, Ruthardt M et al. The Stat5-RARα fusion protein represses transcription and differentiation through interaction with a corepressor complex. Blood 2002;99(8):2647-2652.

[142] Yue P, Turkson J. Targeting STAT3 in cancer: how successful are we? Expert Opin Investig Drugs 2009;18(1):45-56.

[143] Walker SR, Frank DA. STAT Signaling in the Pathogenesis and Treatment of Cancer. In: Frank DA. (ed.) Signaling Pathways in Cancer Pathogenesis and Therapy. New York Dordrecht Heidelberg London: Springer; 2012. p95-108.

[144] Shodeinde AL, Barton BE. Potential use of STAT3 inhibitors in targeted prostate cancer therapy. Onco Targets and Therapy 2012;5:119-125.

[145] Nelson EA, Walker SR, Weisberg E, Bar-Natan M, Barrett R, Gashin LB et al. The STAT5 inhibitor pimozide decreases survival of chronic myelogenous leukemia cells resistant to kinase inhibitors. Blood 2011;117(12):3421–3429.

[146] Hendry L, John S. Regulation of STAT signalling by proteolytic processing. Eur J Biochem 2004;271(23-24):4613-4620.

[147] Chan KK, Oza AM, Siu LL. The statins as anticancer agents. Clin Cancer Res 2003;9(1):10-19.

Permissions

The contributors of this book come from diverse backgrounds, making this book a truly international effort. This book will bring forth new frontiers with its revolutionizing research information and detailed analysis of the nascent developments around the world.

We would like to thank Yahwardiah Siregar, for lending her expertise to make the book truly unique. She has played a crucial role in the development of this book. Without her invaluable contribution this book wouldn't have been possible. She has made vital efforts to compile up to date information on the varied aspects of this subject to make this book a valuable addition to the collection of many professionals and students.

This book was conceptualized with the vision of imparting up-to-date information and advanced data in this field. To ensure the same, a matchless editorial board was set up. Every individual on the board went through rigorous rounds of assessment to prove their worth. After which they invested a large part of their time researching and compiling the most relevant data for our readers. Conferences and sessions were held from time to time between the editorial board and the contributing authors to present the data in the most comprehensible form. The editorial team has worked tirelessly to provide valuable and valid information to help people across the globe.

Every chapter published in this book has been scrutinized by our experts. Their significance has been extensively debated. The topics covered herein carry significant findings which will fuel the growth of the discipline. They may even be implemented as practical applications or may be referred to as a beginning point for another development. Chapters in this book were first published by InTech; hereby published with permission under the Creative Commons Attribution License or equivalent.

The editorial board has been involved in producing this book since its inception. They have spent rigorous hours researching and exploring the diverse topics which have resulted in the successful publishing of this book. They have passed on their knowledge of decades through this book. To expedite this challenging task, the publisher supported the team at every step. A small team of assistant editors was also appointed to further simplify the editing procedure and attain best results for the readers.

Our editorial team has been hand-picked from every corner of the world. Their multi-ethnicity adds dynamic inputs to the discussions which result in innovative outcomes. These outcomes are then further discussed with the researchers and contributors who give their valuable feedback and opinion regarding the same. The feedback is then collaborated with the researches and they are edited in a comprehensive manner to aid the understanding of the subject.

Apart from the editorial board, the designing team has also invested a significant amount of their time in understanding the subject and creating the most relevant covers. They scrutinized every image to scout for the most suitable representation of the subject and create an appropriate cover for the book.

The publishing team has been involved in this book since its early stages. They were actively engaged in every process, be it collecting the data, connecting with the contributors or procuring relevant information. The team has been an ardent support to the editorial, designing and production team. Their endless efforts to recruit the best for this project, has resulted in the accomplishment of this book. They are a veteran in the field of academics and their pool of knowledge is as vast as their experience in printing. Their expertise and guidance has proved useful at every step. Their uncompromising quality standards have made this book an exceptional effort. Their encouragement from time to time has been an inspiration for everyone.

The publisher and the editorial board hope that this book will prove to be a valuable piece of knowledge for researchers, students, practitioners and scholars across the globe.

List of Contributors

Gianpiero Di Leva and Michela Garofalo
The Ohio State University, Department of Molecular Immunology, Virology and Medical Genetics. Columbus, OH, USA

Wei Liu and James M. Phang
Metabolism and Cancer Susceptibility Section, Basic Research Laboratory, Frederick National Laboratory for Cancer Research, NIH. Frederick, MD

Ho-Hyung Woo and Setsuko K. Chambers
Arizona Cancer Center, University of Arizona, Tucson, AZ, USA

Tiziana Triulzi, Elda Tagliabue and Patrizia Casalini
Molecular Targeting Unit, Department of Experimental Oncology and Molecular Medicine,
Fondazione IRCCS, Istituto Nazionale dei Tumori, Milan; Italy

Marilena V. Iorio
Start-Up Unit, Department of Experimental Oncology and Molecular Medicine, Fondazione IRCCS
Istituto Nazionale dei Tumori, Milan; Italy

Tetsuo Hirano
Life Science Group, Graduate School of Integrated Arts and Sciences, Hiroshima University, Kagamiyama, Higashihiroshima, Hiroshima, Japan

Leanna Cheung, Jayne E. Murray, Michelle Haber and Murray D. Norris
Children's Cancer Institute Australia for Medical Research, Lowy Cancer Research Centre, UNSW, Sydney, Australia

Gordana Konjević
Institute of Oncology and Radiology of Serbia, Laboratory for Immunology Medical Faculty, University of Belgrade, Serbia

Sandra Radenković, Ana Vuletić, Katarina Mirjačić Martinović and Tatjana Srdić
Institute of Oncology and Radiology of Serbia, Laboratory for Immunology

Vladimir Jurišić
Medical Faculty, University of Kragujevac, Serbia